Pharmacology
DeMYSTIFIED

Pharmacology
DeMYSTIFIED

Mary Kamienski, PhD, RN, FAEN, FAAN, FNP, ENP, CEN

Jim Keogh, DNP, RN-BC

Second Edition

Mc
Graw
Hill
Education

New York   Chicago   San Francisco   Athens   London   Madrid
Mexico City   Milan   New Delhi   Singapore   Sydney   Toronto

Pharmacology Demystifed, Second Edition

Copyright © 2018 by McGraw-Hill Education. All rights reserved. Except as permit-ted under the United States Copyright Act of 1976, no part of this publication may be reproduced or distributed in any form or by any means, or stored in a data base or retrieval system, without the prior written permission of the publisher.

Previous edition's copyright © 2006 by The McGraw-Hill Companies, Inc.

1 2 3 4 5 6 7 8 9 LCR 22 21 20 19 18 17

ISBN 978-1-259-86259-5
MHID 1-259-86259-3

This book was set in Minion Pro by Cenveo® Publisher Services.
The editors were Susan Barnes and Cindy Yoo.
The production supervisor was Rick Ruzycka.
Project management was provided by Kritika Kaushik, Cenveo Publisher Services.

Library of Congress Cataloging-in-Publication Data

Names: Kamienski, Mary, editor. | Keogh, James Edward, 1948- editor. |
    Preceded by (work): Kamienski, Mary. Pharmacology demystified.
Title: Pharmacology demystified / editors, Mary C. Kamienski and Jim Keogh.
Description: Second edition. | New York : McGraw-Hill, 2017. | Series:
    Demystified | Preceded by Pharmacology demystified / Mary Kamienski,
    Jim Keogh. c2006. | Includes index.
Identifiers: LCCN 2017043912 (print) | LCCN 2017044754 (ebook) | ISBN
    9781259862601 (E-book) | ISBN 1259862607 | ISBN 9781259862595
    (paperback) | ISBN 1259862593 (paperback)
Subjects: | MESH: Pharmaceutical Preparations | Drug Therapy | Examination
    Questions
Classification: LCC RM301.12 (ebook) | LCC RM301.12 (print) | NLM QV 18.2 |
    DDC 615/.1—dc23
LC record available at https://lccn.loc.gov/2017043912

McGraw-Hill Education books are available at special quantity discounts to use as premiums and sales promotions or for use in corporate training programs. To contact a representative, please visit the Contact Us pages at www.mhprofessional.com.

This book is dedicated in memory of my sister Joan.

—Mary Kamienski

This book is dedicated to Anne, Sandy, Joanne, Amber-Leigh Christine, Shawn, Eric, and Amy, without whose help and support this book could not have been written.

—Jim Keogh

About the Authors

Mary Kamienski, PhD, RN, FAEN, FAAN, FNP, ENP, CEN, is a professor at the Rutgers School of Nursing. She is the Specialty Director of the Family Nurse Practitioner in Emergency Care track and teaches the curriculum as well as leadership in the Doctor of Nursing Practice.

Jim Keogh, DNP, RN-BC, is an assistant professor at New York University and is on the faculty of St. Peter's University in Jersey City, New Jersey. He is board-certified in Psychiatric-Mental Health Nursing and is the author of more than 87 books, 20 of them on nursing published by McGraw-Hill.

Contents

Introduction

One of the most important roles of the nurse is to administer medications. Understanding how a drug interacts with the human body will help a nurse administer drugs safely to patients.

Pharmacology Demystified shows you:

- How drugs work
- How to calculate the proper dose
- How to administer drugs
- How to evaluate the drug's effectiveness
- How to avoid common errors when administering drugs
- And much more

You might be a little apprehensive learning pharmacology, especially if you have little, if any, experience with drugs. Pharmacology can be mystifying. However, it becomes demystified as you read *Pharmacology Demystified* because your knowledge of basic science is used as the foundation for learning pharmacology.

As you'll see in Chapter 1, each element of pharmacology is introduced by combining just the pharmacology element with facts you already know from your study of basic science.

Pharmacology is different than other basic science that you've learned—but not so different that you won't be able to quickly build upon your present knowledge base. All you need is a working knowledge of basic science—and *Pharmacology Demystified*—to become knowledgeable in pharmacology.

By the end of this book, you'll have an understanding of drugs that are used to cure common disorders. You'll know how they work, their side effects, adverse effects, and when they are not to be administered to patients. Furthermore, you'll learn how long it takes the drug to take effect and how long the therapeutic effect lasts.

A Look Inside

Pharmacology can be challenging to learn unless you follow the step-by-step approach that is used in *Pharmacology Demystified*. Topics are presented in a systematic order—starting with basic components and then gradually moving on to those features found on classy web sites.

Each chapter follows a time-tested formula that first explains the topic in an easy-to-read style and then shows how it is used in a working web page that you can copy and load yourself. You can then compare your web page with the image of the web page shown in the chapter to be sure that you've coded the web page correctly. There is little room for you to go wrong.

Chapter 1   An Inside Look at Pharmacology

The mere mention of drugs brings all sorts of images to mind. However, these impressions are based on our experience as patients. Healthcare providers have a different view because they see drugs as an arsenal to combat disease. A drug is more than a pill. It is a compound of chemical elements that interacts with the body's chemistry causing a chain reaction of events. Healthcare providers need a thorough understanding of a drug's action in order to effectively prescribe and administer the drug to the patient. Therefore, you begin in Chapter 1 learning the basic concepts of pharmacology.

Chapter 2   Drug Action and Drug Interactions

Drugs are not magical. They follow proven scientific principles to interact with cells in your body to bring about a pharmaceutical response—cure your ills. In this chapter you'll learn about the scientific principles that seem to miraculously make you better when you feel rotten all over. You will learn how drugs stimulate your body's own defense mechanism to stamp out pathogens that give you the sniffles or cause serious diseases.

Chapter 3   Pharmacology and the Nursing Process

Remember from your last hospital stay being awakened from a deep sleep by a nurse saying, "time to take your medicine." The nurse didn't enjoy disturbing you. It was part of standard nursing procedures used to administer medication. You'll learn about those procedures in this chapter so you too can wake up your patients to give them medication.

Chapter 4   Substance Abuse

Drugs can wipe out microorganisms that attack our body. However, some drugs can be abused resulting in an individual becoming dependent on the medication. Substance abuse is the most publicized aspect of pharmacology—and the one least understood by patients and healthcare professionals. This chapter explores drugs that are commonly abused and discusses how to detect substance abuse.

Chapter 5   Principles of Medication Administration

Administering medication can be downright dangerous unless you follow time-tested procedures that assure that the patient receives the right drug in the right dose at the right time using the right route. In this chapter, you'll learn how this is done and how to avoid common errors that could harm your patient.

Chapter 6   Route of Administration

The way a drug is administered to a patient is called a route. Your job is to administer medication using the best route to achieve the desired therapeutic effect. This depends on a number of factors that include the type of medication and the patient's condition. In this chapter, you'll learn how to administer drugs.

Chapter 7   Dose Calculations

Although a prescriber specifies a dose of a medication for a patient, a different dose may be on hand requiring you to calculate the actual dose. With intravenous medication, the prescriber usually orders a dose to be infused over a specific period of time. You must calculate the drip rate to properly set the IV. This chapter shows you how to calculate doses of medication.

Chapter 8   Herbal Therapy

Herbal therapy is used to treat the common cold, infections, diseases of the GI tract, and about anything else that ails you. Herbs are naturally grown and don't have the quality standards found in prescription and over-the-counter medications. You'll learn about the therapeutic effect of herbal therapies in this chapter and the adverse reactions patients can experience when herbal therapy is combined with conventional therapy.

Chapter 9 Vitamins and Minerals

Vitamins and minerals build a strong, healthy body, so you've been told when you were growing up. It is true. A balanced diet provides the vitamins and minerals you need to stay healthy. However, many patients don't have a balanced diet and therefore experience vitamin and mineral deficiencies. In this chapter, you'll learn about vitamins and minerals and how to provide vitamin therapy and mineral therapy for your patients.

Chapter 10 Fluid and Electrolyte Therapy

Some diseases and treatment of disease can cause an imbalance in the body's fluids and electrolytes needed for muscle contraction and other functions. Administering electrolyte therapy to the patient restores balance. You'll learn how this is done.

Chapter 11 Nutritional Support Therapies

Nutrients are given to patients who are at risk for malnutrition caused by disease and by treatment given to cure the disease. Nutrients are also given to strengthen the patient following a trauma such as surgery. In this chapter, you'll learn about nutritional support therapies, how to prepare them, how to administer them, and how to avoid any complications that might arise.

Chapter 12 Inflammation

Fortunately, most times the pain goes away and the inflammation subsides relatively quickly and doesn't interfere with daily activities. In this chapter, you'll learn about the process of inflammation and the medications that are prescribed to reduce the redness, swelling, warmth, and pain that is associated with inflammation.

Chapter 13 Antimicrobials—Fighting Infection

The immune system produces antibodies that seek out, attack, and kill microbials. However, this natural defense isn't sufficient for some patients leaving them with a runny nose, headache, and fever. They need to call in the cavalry. The cavalry is a medication that kills the invading microbial. You'll learn about antimicrobial medication in this chapter.

Chapter 14 Respiratory Diseases

The common cold can be annoying. However, some respiratory diseases—such as emphysema—are debilitating and can slowly choke the life out of a person. In this chapter, we'll explore common respiratory diseases and learn about the medications that are used to manage the symptoms of the disease.

Chapter 15 Nervous System Drugs

The nervous system is our Internet over which sensory impulses travel the neural pathways to the brain where they are interpreted and analyzed for an appropriate response. Sometimes disease or other disorders cause the impulse to go astray or be misinterpreted. Drugs can be prescribed that restore the function of the nervous system. You'll learn about those drugs in this chapter.

Chapter 16 Narcotic Agonists

Make the pain go away. That's what most of us want when we hurt. However, pain is subjective and can be difficult for healthcare providers to manage with the appropriate medication. This chapter explores pain and how healthcare providers assess and manage pain. You'll also learn about narcotic and nonnarcotic analgesics and how they are used to treat pain.

Chapter 17 Immunologic Agents

When the immune system is compromised through diseases including HIV, the body loses its ability to fight off microorganisms and destroys its own abnormal cells, leaving the patient to experience more episodes of infection that can ultimately lead to death. In this chapter, you'll learn about the therapies used to assist the immune system combat preventable diseases and you'll also learn about medications that inhibit the growth of HIV.

Chapter 18 Gastrointestinal System

Problems with the gastrointestinal system can be vomiting, ingesting toxins, diarrhea, constipation, peptic ulcers, and gastroesophageal reflux disease. Each is treatable with the proper medication. In this chapter, you'll learn about common gastrointestinal disorders and the medications that are frequently prescribed to treat these conditions.

Chapter 19 Cardiac Circulatory Medications

When blood vessels become clogged and the heart is unable to pump blood sufficiently, the body loses its ability to distribute oxygen, nutrients, and hormones and remove waste products placing the patient in grave danger. Fortunately, there are medications that can be taken to treat and prevent cardiovascular disorders. In this chapter, you'll learn about drugs that affect the heart and keep the cardiovascular system humming.

Chapter 20 Skin Disorders

Acne, dry skin, a rash, and injuries such as cuts, scrapes, puncture wounds, and burns are some disorders that affect your skin. Some of these are more annoying than endangering to your existence. This chapter discusses using medications to relieve most of the disorders.

Chapter 21 Endocrine Medications

Hormones are messengers that influence how tissues, organs, and other parts of your body function. An overproduction or underproduction of hormones can cause the body to function improperly. Hormones are brought back into balance by using endocrine medications, which are discussed in this chapter.

Chapter 22 Disorders of the Eye and Ear

Common eye and ear disorders rarely result in loss of sight and hearing once the disorder is diagnosed and treated with the proper medication. This chapter takes a look at common disorders that affect the eyes and the ears and discusses drugs that are used to treat those disorders.

Chapter 23 Geriatric Considerations

The elderly are at increased risk for negative health consequence due to increased or excessive number of medications that they are simultaneously taking. In this chapter, you learn about the most commonly prescribed medications for the elderly population and the impact multiple medications has on the physiological response of a geriatric patient.

chapter 1

An Inside Look at Pharmacology

The mere mention of drugs causes all sorts of images to run through our minds: the magic pill that made you feel better when you were under the weather, the stinging injection that left your arm sore for days, the handful of capsules that cost a month's pay, and even the vision of furtive street-corner exchanges.

These impressions are from our experiences as patients or consumers. Healthcare providers, however, view drugs differently because drugs are integral components of the arsenal used to combat the diseases and the physiological changes that disrupt the activities of daily living.

A drug is more than a pill. It is a compound of chemical elements that interact with the body's chemistry, causing a chain reaction of events. Drugs are administered to achieve intended therapeutic effects. However, most drugs also have side effects. Some side effects are desirable, and some are not. Healthcare providers must have a thorough understanding of each drug's action in order to effectively prescribe and administer the drug and to evaluate each patient's response to the medication.

Throughout this book you will learn about drugs: how they work, their intended therapeutic effects, their adverse effects, their interactions with other drugs, how they are prescribed, and how they are administered. However, before learning these details, let us begin in this chapter by discussing the basic concepts of pharmacology.

1. Pharmacology Defined

Pharmacology is the study of chemicals—drugs—on living tissues and how those chemicals help diagnose, treat, cure, and prevent disease or correct the pathophysiology of living tissues. The term pharmacology is derived from two Greek words: *pharmakon*, the Greek word for drugs, and *logos*, the Greek word for science.

Pharmacology is rooted in folklore and tradition that dates back to ancient times when knowledge of the medicinal effects of plants was passed down through generations. By 1240 A.D., pharmacology moved from the realm of home remedies to a science where drug standards were established and a measuring system was developed—called the apothecary system—that was used to measure quantities of drugs. Because drugs can vary in strength and purity, pharmacological standards have been developed that govern the manufacture and control of drugs. The *United States Pharmacopeia and the National Formulary* (USP-NF) is the only official book of drug standards in the United States. Each drug that is included in the USP-NF has met the standards of quality, purity, and strength, and the letters USP following its official name indicate that it is listed in the USP-NF. Accurate dosage and the reliability of the effect that the drug will have on a patient will depend on the purity and strength of the drug. Purity is the dilution or mixture of a drug with other materials to render it in a form that can be administered. The action strength of drugs may vary. The strength of drugs from plants can depend on where the plant is grown, the age at which the plant is harvested, and how the harvest is preserved. Drug packaging standards determine what information needs to be displayed on packages of drugs. You will learn more about these standards later in this book.

In addition to these standards, a number of important laws have been enacted to control the sale and distribution of drugs.

1938 Food, Drug, and Cosmetic Act

Before 1938 there was no control over the manufacture of pharmaceuticals. This changed when a drug company distributed a sulfa drug to treat pediatric patients. The drugs turned out to be a chemical similar to antifreeze. It was highly toxic and killed more than 100 people, including children.

In response to public demands and requests, the United States Congress passed the 1938 Food, Drug, and Cosmetic Act. This act required the following measures:

- Drugs must be proven safe for use before they can be sold.
- All drug manufacturing facilities must be inspected.
- Safe tolerance levels must be identified to prevent the risk of accidental patient poisoning.
- Cosmetics and therapeutic devices be controlled.

1952 Durham-Humphrey Amendment to the Food, Drug, and Cosmetic Act

Until 1952, anyone could distribute drugs. With the passage of the Durham-Humphrey amendment to the Food, Drug, and Cosmetic Act of 1938, a group of drugs was defined that could be purchased only if the patient had a prescription from a licensed practitioner.

1962 Kefauver-Harris Amendment to the Food, Drug, and Cosmetic Act

The Food, Drug, and Cosmetic Act of 1938 was amended once more in 1962 with the passage of the Kefauver-Harris Amendment. This amendment tightened controls on drug safety by requiring drug manufacturers to use standard labeling of drug contain-ers. The drug label lists adverse reactions and contraindications or reasons why the drug should not be used.

1970 Comprehensive Drug Abuse Prevention and Control Act

By 1970, there was widespread abuse of prescription drugs. In an effort to contain this problem, Congress passed the Comprehensive Drug Abuse Prevention and Control Act. This act categorized controlled substances according to a schedule that was based on the potential for drug abuse.

- Schedule I is reserved for the most dangerous substances that have no recognized medicinal use.
- Schedule II drugs have high abuse potential with accepted medicinal uses.
- Schedule III drugs have high abuse potential with accepted medicinal uses.
- Schedule IV and V drugs have lower abuse potential with accepted medicinal uses.

2. The Source of Drugs

Ask a child where milk comes from, and you might be surprised by her or his answer that it comes from the grocery store. The same might be true if you ask an adult where drugs come from and you receive the response "the drugstore." Both are correct answers, but neither identifies the true source.

Drugs can be purchased from a drugstore, but the origins are from one of four sources, described in the following paragraphs.

Plants

A number of plants have medicinal qualities and have been used for centuries as natural remedies for injuries and illnesses. Pharmaceutical firms harvest these plants and transform them into drugs that have a specific purity and strength sufficient to treat diseases and disorders.

An example of a drug that comes from a plant is digitalis. Digitalis is produced from leaves of the foxglove plant and is used to treat congestive heart failure and cardiac arrhythmias. Digitalis also strengthens the force of the contractions of the heart.

Animals

By-products of animals, including humans, are a source for drugs because they contain hormones that can be reclaimed and given to patients who need increased hormonal levels to maintain homeostasis.

For example, Premarin (conjugated estrogen) is a drug that contains estrogen that is recovered from mare urine. This is used as hormonal therapy to manage menopausal symptoms. Insulin is another hormonal drug that is used to regulate blood sugar levels in patients with diabetes mellitus. Insulin can be recovered from humans using DNA technology.

Minerals

Our body requires trace elements of minerals in order to maintain homeostasis. Minerals are inorganic crystal substances that are found naturally on Earth. Patients lacking an adequate level of these materials may take specific mineral-based drugs to raise the level of minerals.

For example, an iron supplement is a common mineral-based drug that is given to patients who suffer from iron deficiency anemia, a condition that can lead to fatigue and shortness of breath. Iron is a natural metal that is an integral part of body proteins such as hemoglobin, which carries oxygen throughout the body. Minerals are obtained from animal and plant sources.

Synthetic/Chemical Derivatives

Great strides in molecular biology and biochemistry enable scientists to create synthetic drugs referred to as synthetic drugs. A synthetic drug is produced using chemical synthesis, a process in which chemical derivatives are rearranged to form a new compound.

Sulfonamides are a common group of synthesized drugs that are used to treat many infections, including bronchitis, pneumonia, and meningitis. Sulfonamides are designed to prevent the growth of bacteria. They are also used to treat allergic reactions and coughing, as well as antifungal and antimalarial conditions. Sulfonamides are present in diuretic agents, antidiabetic medications, and some COX-2 inhibitors, which will be discussed later.

Herbals

Herbals are nonwoody plants. Some have medicinal qualities classified as a dietary supplement—not a drug. Unlike drugs that are governed by the US Food and Drug Administration (FDA), dietary supplements are not tested or regulated and can be sold over the counter without a prescription. This lack of monitoring means that there are no standards for purity and strength for herbals. Two packages of the same herbal distributed by the same company might have different purity and strength levels, which would render the effect of the herb unreliable. There is no control over the manufacturing process, and this can lead to contamination. The law prohibits distributors of herbals from claiming that an herbal can cure a disease. They can only state the effect of the herbal on the body. For example, the manufacturer can say that an herbal increases blood flow to the heart, but cannot claim that the herb prevents heart disease.

Herbals can lead to unwanted side effects and undesirable interactions with prescription drugs. For example, ginkgo biloba inhibits platelet aggregation (grouping to form clots) if taken with Coumadin (warfarin), which is an anticoagulant. The result can be increased bleeding and stroke. Garlic interacts with protease inhibitors used to treat human immunodeficiency virus (HIV) and decreases the effectiveness of the prescribed medication. The interaction of herbals with other drugs can be unpredictable and even dangerous. Healthcare providers should encourage patients to reveal any herbal preparations they are taking.

3. Drug Names

One of the most confusing aspects of pharmacology is naming drugs. A drug is given three names. Each is used in a different area of the drug industry. These names are the drug's chemical name or formula, generic name, and brand name.

Chemical Name

The chemical name identifies chemical elements and compounds that are found in the drug. The chemical name is important to chemists, pharmacists, and researchers who work with drugs at the chemical level.

A chemical name may seem unfamiliar to anyone who is not a chemist and is difficult for most people to pronounce. For this reason, names other than the chemical name are assigned to a drug. Here is the chemical name for a commonly used drug: N-acetyl-p-aminophenol.

Generic Name

The generic name of a drug is the universally accepted name and is considered the official proprietary name for the drug. The generic name appears on all drug labels and is the official name listed in official sources such as the *Physician's Desk Reference* (PDR). The pharmaceutical company that patents a drug has exclusive rights to sell it until the patent expires. When the patent expires, other drug manufacturers may distribute the drug under the drug's generic name or create a brand name. The generic version of a drug may be less expensive than the original drug, and the cost is usually reimbursed by insurance companies. An example of a generic name for a commonly used drug is acetaminophen. The generic name is easier to read and pronounce than the drug's chemical name, N-acetyl-p-aminophenol.

Brand/Trade Name

Drug companies often select and copyright a trade or brand name for their drug. This restricts the use of this name to that particular company. Many brand names may exist for the same chemical compound.

Brand-name drugs may be more costly than generic drugs and are only partially reimbursed or not covered at all by insurance companies.

A brand name for acetaminophen is Tylenol (acetaminophen; patented by Johnson & Johnson Pharmaceuticals).

An example of the correct documentation of the generic and brand name of a drug is: furosemide (Lasix). This drug is a diuretic agent used for many patients with hypertension (high blood pressure) or cardiac (heart) disease.

4. Prescription Versus Over-the-Counter Drugs

The 1952 Durham-Humphrey Amendment to the Food, Drug, and Cosmetic Act requires that certain classifications of drugs be accessible only by prescription from a licensed healthcare practitioner. These are commonly referred to as prescription drugs or "legend drugs" because the drug label must display the legend "Caution: Federal law prohibits dispensing without prescription." on the label of the drug.

The following drugs fall under this classification:

- Those given by injection
- Hypnotic drugs (drugs that depress the central nervous system)
- Narcotics (drugs that relieve pain, dull the senses, and induce sleep)
- Habit-forming drugs
- Drugs that are unsafe unless administered under the supervision of a licensed practitioner
- New drugs that are still being investigated and not considered safe for indiscriminate use by the public

Nonprescription drugs are called over-the-counter (OTC) drugs and are available to the public without prescription. Some OTC drugs were at one time available by prescription, but later were considered safe for use by the public or reformulated for OTC use. Some drugs can be sold in lower doses OTC, while higher doses of the same drug require a prescription as per FDA requirements.

5. Drug Effects

Drugs have multiple effects on the body. Some effects are desirable, and some are not. The therapeutic effect is the intended physiological effect or the reason why the drug is being given. A therapeutic effect can be the drug's action against a disease such as an antibiotic that destroys bacteria. Another physiological effect can be side effects that occur in the body such as nausea and vomiting or a skin rash. A side effect is a physiological effect that is not the intended action such as the drowsiness that occurs when a patient takes an antihistamine. Some side effects are beneficial, while other effects can be adverse and harmful to a patient.

Healthcare providers must identify all known side effects of a drug and weigh any adverse effects with the therapeutic effect before administering a drug. Patients must also be informed about expected side effects and must be provided instructions about how to manage adverse side effects if at all possible.

For example, female patients may be instructed to drink buttermilk and eat yogurt when taking a broad-spectrum antibiotic in order to prevent a possible vaginal yeast infection, which is a common adverse effect of broad-spectrum antibiotics. Additionally, a female patient should be instructed to use other forms of birth control when taking this medication because antibiotics lower the effectiveness of birth control pills.

Often patients will discontinue the use of a medication because the side effects are so unpleasant. Antihypertensive medications (blood pressure medicine) can cause side effects such as drowsiness or the inability to achieve an erection in a male. Patients may decide that this effect is undesirable and may discontinue the use of the pre-scribed drug. Patients should be encouraged to discuss any and all side effects with the healthcare provider. Frequently, there are alternative medications that can be pre-scribed. Abruptly discontinuing the use of a drug may not be in the best interest of a particular patient. Some drugs may be gradually decreased in dosage and frequency. Sometimes patients might discontinue taking a drug because they feel better; however, the conditions being treated are still present. Some examples of these types of medica-tion are antibiotics and antidepressants.

6. Drug Safety

Drugs must undergo rigorous testing before being approved by the FDA for use in humans. The initial testing is done with animals to determine the toxicity of the drug. Acute toxicity is the dose that is lethal or kills 50% of the laboratory animals tested. The testing is also done to determine what symptoms are experienced by the animals and the time when the symptoms appear.

Subchronic toxicity studies, conducted in at least two animal species, usually con-sist of daily administration of the drug for up to 90 days. Physical examinations and laboratory tests are performed during and at the end of the study to see what organs may have been adversely affected by the drug.

Chronic toxicity studies, which also conducted in at least two species, usually last the lifetime of the animal, but the length of the study may depend on the intended duration of drug administration to humans. Three dose levels are used, varying from a nontoxic low-level dose to a dose that is higher than the expected therapeutic dose and is toxic when given over a long period of time. Physical examinations and labora-tory tests are performed to determine which organs are affected and whether the drug has the potential to cause cancer (whether it is carcinogenic).

Animal studies enable scientists to develop a therapeutic index (TI) for the drug. The TI is the ratio between the median lethal dose and the median effective dose. The healthcare practitioner uses the TI to determine the safe dose that should be admin-istered to achieve the intended effect.

Some drugs have a narrow margin of safety and require that the blood plasma levels be monitored frequently to ensure that the drug stays within the therapeutic range. Drugs that have a wide margin of safety do not require that the plasma levels be moni-tored. Digitalis (digoxin) is an example of a drug that has a narrow margin of safety and requires frequent monitoring of plasma levels.

Pharmaceutical scientists also learn how the drug is absorbed, distributed, metabolized, and excreted once it is administered to animal subjects. This knowledge helps the scientists predict how the drug will react when administered to humans.

Tests are also conducted in laboratory test tubes that can determine the metabolism of the drug in humans, which may be different from that in animals. These are called in vitro studies. Once animal studies are successfully completed, the drug is ready for human trials, during which human subjects are administered the drug. There are three phases of human trial.

Phase I: Initial Pharmacological Evaluation

In Phase I drug trials, the drug is given to a small number of healthy volunteers to determine safe dosage levels. The purpose is to document the dose level at which signs of toxicity first appear in humans, determine a safe tolerated dose, and determine the pharmacokinetics of the drug. Pharmacokinetics will be discussed in Chapter 2. Volunteers who give consent to participate are monitored closely during this phase. Permission must be obtained from the FDA to conduct Phase I clinical trials.

Phase II: Limited Controlled Evaluation

The purpose of Phase II evaluation is to monitor drug effectiveness and any possible side effects. Individuals with the targeted disease participate in this phase of drug trials. For example, antihypertensive (blood pressure–lowering) drugs will be administered to patients who have hypertension (high blood pressure) to determine the drug's effectiveness or optimal dose response range and for side effects. The number of participants is larger than that in Phase I trials but rarely exceeds 100 persons, and every effort is made to include only those human subjects who have no other disorders or diseases.

Phase III: Extended Clinical Evaluation

Phase III drug trials include many physicians and large groups of participants. When enough information has been collected to justify continued use of the drug, a New Drug Application (NDA) is submitted to the FDA. Usually, more than 4 years has passed between the drug's selection and the filing of the NDA.

Phase IV studies are also called postmarketing follow-up. Phase IV studies are voluntarily conducted by pharmaceutical companies. These studies continue after the FDA has approved the drug and often include subjects such as pregnant women, children, and the elderly. Manufacturers can find low-level side effects or can find that a drug is toxic and must be removed from market. The FDA continues to monitor new drugs even after they are marketed.

Drugs also undergo tests to determine the possible effects on a fetus. As a result of these tests, drugs are classified using the following pregnancy categories.

Category A
Adequate and well-controlled studies indicate no risk to the fetus in the first trimester of pregnancy or later.

Category B
Animal reproduction studies indicate no risk to the fetus; however, there are no well-controlled studies in pregnant women.

Category C
Animal reproduction studies have reported adverse effects on the fetus; however, there are no well-controlled studies in humans, but potential benefits may indicate use of the drug in pregnant women despite potential risks.

Category D
Positive human fetal risk has been reported from investigational or marketing experience, or human studies. Considering potential benefit versus risk may, in selected cases, warrant the use of these drugs in pregnant women.

Category X
Data on any reported fetal abnormalities and positive evidence of fetal risk in humans are available from animal and/or human studies. The risks involved clearly outweigh the potential benefits. These drugs should not be used in pregnant women.

7. Locating Drug Information

Before administering a drug to a patient (see Chapter 4), healthcare providers need to know the following information about the drug:

- **Generic and Trade Names**: The generic name is the official name of the drug; the trade name is the drug's brand or proprietary name.
- **Clinical Uses and Indications for Use:** This information describes the purpose of the drug and when the drug is to be given to a patient.
- **Mechanism of Action:** This information describes how the drug works.
- **Adverse and Side Effects and Toxicity:** This information identifies any nontherapeutic effects of the drug, that is, effects other than the intended therapeutic effect.
- **Signs and Symptoms to Monitor:** This information identifies the patient's physiological response that must be evaluated after the drug is administered.

- **What to Teach the Patient:** This information specifies the instructions that must be given to the patient before and after the drug is administered.

This information is available in product inserts, various drug handbooks for nurses, and computerized pharmacology databases and in the following publications:

- *American Hospital Formulary Service (AHFS) Drug Information:* This reference source is published by the American Society of Hospital Pharmacists, Inc. and contains an overview of every drug.
- *United States Pharmacopeia Dispensing Information:* This reference source is published by the US Pharmacopeial Convention and highlights clinical information, which is the same as that provided in the drug inserts found in packages of drugs.
- *Physician's Desk Reference (PDR):* This reference source is published by Medical Economics, with the financial support of the pharmaceutical industry, and contains the same information as found in the package drug inserts.
- *Physician's GenRx:* This reference source is published by the C.V. Mosby Company and includes comprehensive drug information, product identification charts, and product ratings by the FDA. It also contains cost comparisons between drugs.
- *Handbook of Nonprescription Drugs:* This handbook is published by the American Pharmaceutical Association and contains comprehensive information on OTC drugs, including the primary minor illnesses that the drug is used to treat.
- *Medline Plus* (**http://www.nlm.nih.gov/medlineplus/druginformation.html**): This is an online database produced by the US National Library of Medicine and the National Institutes of Health (in Bethesda, MD) and contains information about prescription and OTC drugs and devices as well as warnings and drug recall information.

8. Drug Orders

A drug order, also called a medical prescription, is an instruction from a healthcare provider to administer a medication to a specific patient. A healthcare provider such as a physician, a dentist, a podiatrist, an advanced practice nurse (APN), and any other authorized licensed healthcare provider can write a drug order. Physician assistants can also write a drug order but require the cosignature of a physician.

All drug orders are written on a prescription pad or on an order sheet if they are written in a healthcare institution. Sometimes orders are written into a computerized drug order system. A verbal drug order is sometimes given but must be followed up with a written drug order within 24 hours.

Drug orders are written using the abbreviations shown in Table 1–1 and must contain the following information:

TABLE 1–1	Commonly Used Abbreviations for Drug Orders	
Direction	L (in circle)	Left
	R (in a circle)	Right
Dose	aa	Of each
	c̄	With
	DS	Double strength
	elix.	Elixir
	fl or fld.	Fluid
	gtt	Drop
	NS or N/S	Normal saline
	q.s.	A sufficient amount/as much as needed/quantity sufficient
	s̄	Without
	s̄s̄ or ss	One half
	SR	Sustained release
	XL	Long acting
	XR	Extended release
Form	amp	ampule
	aq	water
	c	Cup
	cap or caps	Capsule
	EC	Enteric coated
	mix	Mixture
	sol or soln	Solution
	supp	Suppository
	susp	Suspension
	syp or syr	Syrup
	tab	Tablet
	Tr or tinct	Tincture
	ung. or oint	Ointment
Method	gt or GT	Gastrostomy tube
	I.D.	Intradermal
	I.M.	Intramuscular
	I.V.	Intravenous
	IVPB	Intravenous piggyback
	IVSS	Intravenous soluset

(Continued)

TABLE 1–1	Commonly Used Abbreviations for Drug Orders (Continued)	
Method (Cont.)	KVO	Keep vein open (a very slow infusion rate)
	NGT	Nasogastric tube
	n.p.o.	Nothing by mouth
	Per	Through or by
	Per os or p.o.	By or through mouth
	p.r.	By rectum
	s.c. or S.C. or s.q.*	Subcutaneous
	sl or SL	Sublingual
	S&S	Swish and swallow
	vag	Vaginally
Part	A.D. or AD*	Right ear
	A.S. or AS*	Left ear
	A.U. or AU*	Both ears
	OD*	Right eye
	os*	Mouth
	OS*	Left eye
	OU*	Both eyes
	Rect*	Rectum
Time	$\bar{a}$	Before
	ad.lib	As desired
	b.i.d. or bid	Twice a day
	d.c. or D/C	Discontinue
	h or hr	Hour
	h.s.	At bed time
	min	Minute
	o.d. or OD	Once a day
	$\bar{p}$	After
	p.c.	After meals
	p.r.n.	When necessary
	q.	Every, each
	q.a.m.	Every morning
	q.d. or qd*	Every day or once a day
	q.h. or qh	Every hour

(Continued)

TABLE 1–1 Commonly Used Abbreviations for Drug Orders (Continued)		
Time (Cont.)	q2h, q4h	Every two hours, every four hours
	qhs or q.h.s.*	Every night at bedtime
	q.i.d. or qid	Four times a day
	q.o.d. or qod*	Every other day
	s.o.s.	Once if necessary
	stat or STAT	Immediately or at once
	t.i.d. or tid	Three times a day
	t.i.w.*	Three times a week

*The Joint Commission for Accreditation of Hospitals Organization (JCAHO) has recommended that these abbreviations not be used to decrease the chance of errors. However, some hospitals and providers continue to use them when writing medications orders.

- Date on which the order (prescription) was issued; the time when the order is written is required for inpatient orders
- Name of the drug and whether a generic form of the drug can be substituted for a brand-name drug
- Drug dose
- Route of administration
- Frequency and duration of administration
- Special instructions such as withholding or adjusting dosage on the basis of nursing assessment, laboratory results, or drug effectiveness
- Signature of the prescriber

Types of Drug Orders

There are four types of drug orders: routine, one-time, PRN, and STAT:

Routine Order: This is an ongoing order given for a specific number of doses or number of days. An example would be as follows: 1/31/05 7:30 P.M. Lasix (furosemide) 40 mg, PO (orally; per os), qd (every day; signature). (Inpatient orders.) This is an order to give 40 milligrams of Lasix by mouth once a day. Once-a-day medications are generally given around 9 A.M. or 10 A.M. according to the healthcare institution or patient choice if at home. Lasix is a diuretic agent. Another variation would be as follows: 1/31/05—furosemide 40 mg—take one (1) tablet by mouth once a day in the morning. The order number #30 indicates how many tablets the pharmacy will dispense (signature). The routine order should also indicate whether the drug can be substituted with another generic form and how many refills can be issued. (Outpatient prescriptions.)

One-Time Order: This is a single dose given at a particular time. An example would be as follows: Demerol 50 mg with Vistaril 25 mg IM (intramuscularly) at 10 A.M. or 2 h (hours) before call to the OR (operating room). This is an order to give Demerol (meperidine) 50 milligrams with Vistaril (hydroxyzine) 25 milligrams intramuscularly at 10 A.M. or two hours before call to the operating room.

PRN Order: The PRN (pro re nata; as necessary) order is an order to give a medication if specific criteria exist, such as a headache, a fever, or pain, and at the patient's request. An example would be as follows: Advil 600 mg PO q6h PRN for mild to moderate knee pain. This is an order to give Advil (ibuprofen) 600 milligrams by mouth every 6 hours as needed for mild to moderate knee pain.

STAT: This is a single-dose order to give at once or immediately (statim). An example would be as follows: Give Benadryl 50 mg PO Stat. This is an order to give Benadryl (dyphenhydramine) 50 milligrams by mouth immediately.

There are also protocols for administering medications. This is a set of criteria that indicates under what conditions a drug may be given. There are two types of protocols: standing orders and flow diagrams (algorithms). Standing orders are an officially accepted set of orders to be applied by nurses, physician assistants, and paramedics in the care of patients with certain conditions or under certain circumstances. For example, for patients who are not breathing and have no heartbeat, an algorithm (flow diagram) has been developed to administer different medications such as epinephrine and other cardiac stimulants to resuscitate the individual. Other standing orders include orders for Tylenol (acetaminophen) 600 mg q4h by mouth or per rectum for a temperature >101.4°F (>38.56°C).

9. The "Five Rights" of Drug Administration

There are five traditional "right" or recommended actions that should be followed when giving medication. These are to determine the right patient, right drug, right dose, right time, and right route. Five additional rights include the right assessment, documentation, education, evaluation, and the right to refuse.

Right Patient

The "right patient" means that the healthcare provider gives the drug to the right (correct; appropriate) patient. Each time a drug is administered, the healthcare provider must verify who the patient is by the person's identification bracelet. This is the preferred method as opposed to identifying a patient by asking his or her name. Some patients will answer "yes" to any name, and two patients can have similar-sounding names or the same name. Some patients are not mentally alert and do not remember their names. Again, check the patient's identification every time medication is administered.

Right Drug

Healthcare providers must be sure that the drug is the correct medication for the patient. This, too, leads to errors. Healthcare providers may ask any of the following questions:

"Was this the drug prescribed on the medication order?"

"Is the medication order legible and complete?"

"Why is the patient receiving this medication?"

"Is the medication consistent with the patient's condition?"

"Does the patient have any food or drug allergies?"

Healthcare providers check the expiration date and return the medication to the pharmacy if it has expired. If the medication is used past its expiration date, the effect on the patient can be unpredictable.

Healthcare providers check the medication label 3 times before administering the drug: first, when taking the medication from the shelf or drawer; next, before pouring the drug, and finally, after pouring the drug before disposing of the drug packaging.

Right Dose

The dose on the medication order must be within recommended guidelines. The healthcare provider should have a general idea of the correct dose before performing any drug calculations, and should check with a pharmacist or another appropriate provider if the calculated dose varies too much from this estimated dose. Some drug calculations should always be checked by two or more individuals if the calculation is complicated, if the drug has potentially harmful side effects, or if the dose is either too large or too small. Medications that are wrapped and labeled or prefilled for the exact dose are preferred and can reduce the risk of error.

Healthcare providers should also ensure that they are using the proper system of measurement when calculating a dose (see Chapter 4).

Right Time

The healthcare provider will also ask "Is it the correct time to administer the drug?" The time is specified in the drug order and may be given a half hour before or after the stated time depending on the policy of the hospital or healthcare facility.

How often a drug is given depends on the half-life of the drug. A drug's half-life is the amount of time for one-half of the drug to be eliminated from the body. A drug with a short half-life must be administered more frequently than a drug with a long half-life in order to maintain a therapeutic level of the drug in plasma.

The use of military time can avoid A.M. and P.M. errors.

Healthcare providers should check whether their patients are scheduled for diagnostic test or other procedures that might interfere with the administration of medications. They should determine whether their patients should receive the medication even if they are scheduled to be on an NPO (nothing by mouth) regimen.

Healthcare providers should also make sure that medication is given in coordination with meals. Some drugs must be given with meals, while other drugs are given for a specific period before or after a meal.

Where possible, the medication schedule is adjusted to conform to the patient's lifestyle, which may differ from the normal schedule. For example, Digoxin might be scheduled for 10 A.M. to conform to hospital policy, but the patient can take Digoxin any time in the morning. This becomes important once the patient is discharged and takes medication at home.

Right Route

The healthcare provider must also determine the proper routine to administer the drug to ensure that the patient's body properly absorbs it. Here are the common routes:

- **Oral (by Mouth):** liquid, elixir, suspension, pill, tablet, and capsule
- **Sublingual (under the Tongue):** pill, tablet, and capsule
- **Buccal (between the Gum and the Cheek):** pill, tablet, and capsule
- **Topical (Applied to the Skin):** cream, ointment, and patch
- **Inhalation (Nose, Eye, Ear):** liquid, cream, and ointment
- **Insertion (Rectal, Vaginal):** suppository
- **Intradermal (beneath the Skin):** injection
- **Subcutaneous (beneath the Skin):** injection
- **Intramuscular (in Muscle):** injection
- **Intravenous (in the Vein):** injection
- **Nasogastric and Gastronomy Tubes:** liquid
- **Transdermal:** patches

The healthcare provider should make sure that the patient can swallow if the route of the medication is by mouth and should stay with the patient until the medication is swallowed. Enteric-coated or timed-release drugs should not be crushed or mixed.

Caution should be used when administering intravenous medications because the body quickly absorbs these drugs. Therefore, healthcare providers need to know expected side effects, effects that occur when the drug is first given, effects that the drug has during its therapeutic peak, and duration of the drug's action. Caution should be used when administering any medication via this route.

Self-administration of medication (SAM) is the normal practice for patients in the home and workplace. This method is also used in some acute and long-term care institutional settings. In these settings the nurse gives the patient a packet of medications with instructions that are kept at the bedside. The patient takes the medication according to the instructions and advises the nurse when she or he has done so. This practice helps patients learn how to manage their medications and prepares them for discharge and use of these medications at home. This method is often used with oncology (cancer) patients and maternity patients.

Patient-controlled analgesia (PCA) is a common method of administering intravenous pain medication for many patients. This will be discussed further in a Chapter 15.

Right to Refuse Medication

A mentally competent patient has the right to refuse medication. Refusal is documented on the patient record. Patients should be advised of the consequences of the refusal to take the medication such as worsening of the condition. As a general rule, every effort is made to encourage the patient to take the medication. However, no one should physically force a patient to take medication.

Right to Education

The patient has the right to be told about the medication that is about to be administered. The patient is given the following information:

- The name of the medication
- Why the medication is given
- What the medication looks like
- How much of the medication to take
- When to take the medication
- When not to take the medication
- What side effects, adverse effects, and toxic effects to expect

This information is discussed in the best way that the patient can most easily understand. The healthcare provider should avoid speaking in medical terminology and, instead, use common words and expressions that are familiar to the patient—and always in the language that the patient speaks. Interpreters should be used with patients who do not speak English.

Patients should be asked to provide feedback that they understand everything about the medication. It is common for healthcare providers to ask patients to describe in their own words what was told to them about the medication.

Patients are also shown how to keep track of multiple medications. Typically, patients are encouraged to keep lists of medications. These lists should include the medication names dosages, times the medications are to be taken, and the name and phone numbers of the prescribers who ordered the medications.

Summary

Pharmacology is the study of drug effects on living tissue and how drugs cure, prevent, or manage diseases. Drugs are derived from plants, animals, and minerals, and are synthesized in the laboratory. Each drug has three names: the chemical name, the generic name that is considered the official name for the drug, and the brand name, which is used by the manufacturer who marketed the drug.

There are two general classifications of drugs: prescription and OTC drugs. Prescription drugs are also known as "legend drugs" and must be prescribed by an authorized healthcare provider. Over-the-counter drugs can be purchased with or without a prescription.

Drugs have three effects: (1) the intended therapeutic effect to fight or prevent a disease or disorder, (2) a side effect that is not harmful, and (3) an adverse effect that is harmful to a varying degree. Some drugs can also cause an allergic response in some patients. Healthcare providers must know about these effects before administering medications to their patients. Furthermore, the patients must be informed of these effects.

Before a drug is manufactured and released for public use, it must undergo a series of tests that begin with animal studies and follow through to clinical studies on humans. Animal studies determine the TI for the drug. Clinical studies determine the intended therapeutic effect, adverse effects, and side effects that the drug has on humans.

A drug is prescribed to a patient by writing a drug order or medical prescription. A drug order specifies, among other things, the name of the drug, the dose, the administration route, and the frequency. Only an authorized healthcare provider can order drugs. There are four types of drug orders: routine, one-time, PRNs, and STAT orders. There are also standing orders or protocols.

There are five right actions to take when giving medications. These are to give the right patient the right drug, in the right dose, at the right time, by the right route.

Patients also have the right to refuse medication and the right to education about the medication.

With this overview of pharmacology under your belt, let's take a closer look at how drugs work by exploring the principles of drug action and drug interactions in the next chapter.

QUIZ

1. **A brand name of a drug is**
   - (a) the non-trademarked name given by the original drug manufacturer.
   - (b) the trademarked name given by the drug manufacturer.
   - (c) the official nonproprietary name for the drug.
   - (d) the universally accepted name.

2. **Schedule I controlled substances**
   - (a) cannot be prescribed.
   - (b) can be prescribed only by a physician.
   - (c) can be purchased over the counter.
   - (d) are approved for medical use.

3. **The 1938 Food, Drug, and Cosmetic Act**
   - (a) established categories of drugs.
   - (b) standardized labeling for drugs.
   - (c) established who could prescribe drugs.
   - (d) requires drug manufacturers to prove that their drugs are safe.

4. **Herbals are tested and regulated by the Food and Drug Administration.**
   - (a) True
   - (b) False

5. **All drug side effects are harmful.**
   - (a) True
   - (b) False

6. **Drugs come from**
   - (a) animals.
   - (b) humans.
   - (c) plants.
   - (d) all of the above.

7. **PO in a drug order means by rectum.**

   (a) True
   (b) False

8. **A drug order that requires the drug to be given immediately is called a**

   (a) one-time order.
   (b) PRN order.
   (c) STAT order.
   (d) standing order.

9. **A patient does not have the right to refuse medication.**

   (a) True
   (b) False

10. **The number of times that a drug is given to a patient can be determined by the half-life of the drug.**

    (a) True
    (b) False

chapter 2

Drug Action and Drug Interactions

"Just give me the magic pill to make me normal again." You probably said something like that the last time you felt under the weather and your home remedies didn't make you feel better. You might have even reached the point when you'd welcome an injection of a miracle drug if it would get you back on your feet quickly.

Drugs aren't miracles and have nothing to do with magic, although you might think differently when your nose is running, your eyes are watering, and you feel rotten all over. A drug is a chemical compound specifically designed to combat disease.

In this chapter, you will be introduced to the scientific principles that describe how drugs interact with cells in your body to bring about a pharmaceutical response that either directly attacks the pathogen that is causing your sniffles or stimulates your body's own defense mechanism to stamp them out.

1. Drug Actions

Drug action is the physiochemical interaction between the drug molecule and molecules in the body that alters a physiological process in the body in one of three ways:

- **Replacement:** The drug replaces an existing physiological process such as insulin secretion.
- **Interruption:** The drug interferes with a physiological process. This occurs, for example, when an antihypertensive (blood pressure–reducing) drug interferes with the process that constricts blood vessels, and may cause blood pressure to rise. The blood vessels remain dilated, and pressures remain normal or drop.
- **Potentiation:** The drug stimulates a physiological process, as in the case of furosemide (Lasix), a diuretic agent that stimulates the kidneys to excrete urine.

A drug action begins when the drug enters the body and is absorbed into the bloodstream, where it is transported to receptor sites throughout the body (see "Pharmacokinetics," in this chapter). Once the drug hooks onto a receptor site, its pharmacological response begins. The *pharmacological response* is the intended therapeutic effect that reduces or eliminates the disease or other pathological processes and makes the patient well.

Drugs exert multiple actions. These include the primary effect and other secondary effects as well. The *desired effect* is what makes the patient well or prevents the disease or disorder. Any secondary effect—that is, any effect other than the desired one—is known as a *side effect*. Some side effects are desirable and others are undesirable (see "Side Effects," in this chapter).

The strength of a drug action is determined by the quantity of the drug that is administered (the dose) and how often the drug is given (the frequency). For example, a patient with a sore throat can be administered a large dose of an antibiotic—a *loading dose*—on the first day of treatment and a normal or maintenance dose for the next 5 days.

Drug activity is divided into three phases:

- **Pharmaceutic Phase:** This phase occurs after the drug is given and involves disintegration and dissolution of the dosage form.
- **Pharmacokinetic Phase:** This is the way the drug is absorbed, distributed, and eliminated.
- **Pharmacodynamic Phase:** This is the effect the drug has on the body.

Pharmaceutic

The *pharmaceutic phase* is the form of the drug such as a tablet, a capsule, a liquid, an elixir, or a syrup. The drug in solid form must disintegrate prior to *dissolution*, a process by which a drug goes into solution before it becomes available for absorption. Drugs contain one active ingredient and multiple added inactive ingredients. The *active ingredient* is the substance that causes the pharmaceutical response. *Inactive ingredients*, also called *excipients*, are substances that have no

TABLE 2–1 Rate-Limiting Time Rating for Drug Forms

Preparation	Absorption Rate (Fastest to Slowest)
Lipid-soluble nonionized liquids, elixirs, syrups	1
Water-soluble ionized liquids, elixirs, syrups	2
Suspension solutions	3
Powders	4
Capsules	5
Tablets	6
Coated tablets	7
Enteric-coated tablets	8

pharmaceutical response but facilitate delivery of the drug. These are inert substances, also referred to as "fillers," that give the drug its shape and size. The coating around tiny particles of a capsule that causes a timed-release action of the drug is an inactive ingredient.

Nearly 80% of all drugs are administered orally (PO) and are carried to the small intestine by the gastrointestinal (GI) tract, where the drug is absorbed into the bloodstream. The time necessary for the drug to disintegrate and dissolve so that it can be absorbed is called the *rate-limiting time*.

A drug has a higher rate-limiting time (Table 2–1) if it is absorbed in acidic fluids rather than alkaline fluids. Children and the elderly have a lower pH in their GI tracts, and therefore drugs are absorbed more slowly than in a healthy adult.

Some drugs are more effective if absorbed in the small intestine rather than the stomach. However, the stomach is more acidic than the small intestine. Therefore, pharmaceutical manufacturers place an enteric coating around the drug that resists disintegration in the stomach. The coating disintegrates in the alkaline environment of the small intestine. Enteric coating is also used to delay the onset of the pharmaceutical response and to prevent food that has entered the stomach from interfering with the dissolution and absorption of the drug.

TIP

Never crush a capsule that contains enteric release beads or is coated for timed release. The form of a drug influences the drug's pharmacokinetics and pharmacodynamics.

Pharmacokinetics

Pharmacokinetics is the study of the drug concentration during absorption, distribution, and elimination of a drug in the patient. About 80% of all drugs are administered orally and flow through the GI tract into the small intestine. The membrane of the small intestine absorbs drug particles, passing them into the bloodstream, where plasma circulates the particles throughout the body. Drug molecules move to the intended site of action in the plasma, but sometimes this journey can be limited because the molecules have to enter the interior of a cell or body compartment through cell membranes. These membranes could be in the skin, the intestinal tract, or any other intended site of action. Drug particles then become attached to receptor sites, resulting in their therapeutic effect.

Drug particles are absorbed in one of three ways: by passive diffusion, active diffusion, or pinocytosis.

Passive Diffusion

Passive diffusion is the flow of drug particles from a high concentration to a low concentration—similar to the flow of water downstream. There is a higher concentration of water upstream than there is downstream. There is no energy expended in passive diffusion because drug particles are moving along the natural flow.

Active Diffusion

In *active diffusion*, drug particles swim upstream against the natural flow when there is a higher concentration of plasma than there is of drug particles. Drug particles do not have sufficient energy to effectively oppose the natural flow without help. Assistance comes from an enzyme or protein carrier that transports drug particles upstream across the membrane and into the plasma. The enzyme or protein carrier expends energy to move drug particles.

Pinocytosis

Pinocytosis is the process of engulfing the drug particle and pulling it across the membrane. This process is similar to placing an item in a box and shipping the box to a friend. The friend opens and removes the item from the box when it arrives.

Absorption Rate

Absorption begins where the drug is administered. This can be by mouth, by injection, through the skin, and through many other sites. How quickly the drug becomes therapeutic will depend on how rapidly it is absorbed. How long the drug will be effective and how much drug is needed will depend on the route of administration, the dose of the drug, and the dosage form (tablet, capsule, or liquid).

The absorption rate of a drug is influenced by a number of factors that might increase or decrease the rate. This is similar to determining the additional amount of gasoline that is used to drive a motor vehicle at higher speeds. Absorption is affected by many factors, including pain, stress, hunger, fasting, food consumption, and pH. Hot, solid, fatty foods can slow absorption, such as, for example, when someone eats a large hamburger before taking medication. Even exercise—which is usually beneficial for the body—affects absorption of a drug. During exercise, circulation to the stomach is diverted to other areas of the body, and drug absorption is decreased.

Circulation

Blood flow to the site of administration of the drug will help increase the rate of absorption. An area that contains many blood vessels and has good circulation will help absorb the drug quickly and circulate it to the intended site(s). When a patient is in shock and has a low blood pressure due to decreased circulation (blood flow), drugs may not be absorbed very quickly.

Route of Administration

The rate at which drug particles are absorbed is determined by the number of blood vessels that are present in the area where the drug is administered. Drug particles are absorbed nearly instantaneously if the drug is injected intravenously (IV). A slower absorption rate occurs if the drug is administered intramuscularly (IM). The IM rate is dependent on the number of blood vessels that are present at the injection site. For example, a drug is absorbed more rapidly in the deltoid (arm) muscle than in the gluteal (buttock) muscle because there are more blood vessels in the deltoid muscle. Drugs injected in subcutaneous (SC) tissue are absorbed more slowly than those injected IM because there are fewer blood vessels in SC tissues than in muscles.

Solubility

Drug particles dissolve in either lipid (fat) or water. Lipid-soluble drugs are absorbed more quickly than water-soluble drugs because membranes in the GI tract are composed of lipids, making those membranes a perfect highway for lipid-soluble drugs to move from the GI tract and into the bloodstream. However, membranes of the GI tract do not directly absorb large water-soluble molecules, so a carrier must be used to transport the water-soluble drugs across the GI membrane and into the bloodstream.

This additional step causes water-soluble drugs to be absorbed more slowly than fat-soluble drugs.

pH Level

The *pH level* of a drug determines how easily drug particles will be absorbed in the GI tract. Those drugs that are a weak acid—such as aspirin—can pass rapidly across the GI tract membrane, whereas weak-base drugs—such as an antacid—are absorbed more slowly than a weak acidic drug. Strong acids and bases destroy cells and are not absorbed.

The *drug concentration* will also affect the rate of absorption. If a high concentration of the drug is given, it will tend to be absorbed more rapidly. Sometimes larger (loading or priming) doses of a drug may be given that will exceed the amount that the body can excrete. When this is the case, the drug becomes therapeutic much sooner. After the first large dose, small maintenance doses will help maintain the therapeutic effect.

The *form* (solid, powder, or liquid) in which the drug is given can affect the absorption rate. Drugs can be processed during manufacture to add other ingredients that will help or hinder absorption.

Bioavailability

Not all drug particles reach the circulatory system. Some particles are misdirected or destroyed during the absorption process. For example, hydrochloric acid in the stomach destroys some drug particles before they can pass through the membrane and into the bloodstream.

The percentage of a dose that reaches the bloodstream is called the *bioavailability* of a drug. Typically, between 20% and 40% of drugs that are administered orally reach the bloodstream. This is called the *first-pass effect* and indicates the beginning of the metabolism of a drug that is given orally. After a drug is absorbed in the GI tract, it is carried to the liver, and metabolism occurs. Sometimes very little of the drug remains available for a therapeutic effect after the first pass. Only drugs administered IV have a 100% bioavailability because they are directly injected into the vein.

Pharmaceutical manufacturers must consider bioavailability when determining the correct dose for a drug. For example, the dose for a drug administered PO (orally) might be several times higher than if the same drug is administered IV.

Several factors alter bioavailability:

- **Form:** Tablet, capsule, slow-release, liquid, transdermal patch, suppository, and inhalation.
- **Route:** PO (by mouth), topical, parenteral, and rectal.

- **Gastrointestinal Tract:** The ability of the mucosa (lining) in the GI tract impacts the ability to absorb drug particles and the ability to move food through the digestive tract.
- **Food:** Drug particles for some drugs are absorbed more effectively if they are ingested with certain foods, while other foods may slow down or block absorption.
- **Drugs:** Some drugs increase or decrease another drug's absorption when both drugs are ingested simultaneously.
- **Liver Metabolism:** Liver dysfunction can prevent or delay the metabolism of a drug.
- **Concentration:** A higher portion of active ingredient in a dose increases the number of drug particles that are absorbed.
- **Cell Membrane:** Single-layer cell membranes, such as those found in the intestine, increase absorption, whereas some drugs are absorbed more slowly in multiple layers, such as skin.
- **Surface Area:** A larger surface area, such as that of the small intestine, absorbs drugs more rapidly than does a smaller area such as in the stomach.

Drug Concentration

A drug contains an active ingredient, which produces the therapeutic effect, and other materials that impart the drug form and provide protection. The percentage of active ingredient in a given dose is referred to as the *drug concentration.*

There are generally two levels of concentration: *primary loading*, where a large concentration is used to achieve a rapid therapeutic effect such as the first dose of an antibiotic, and the *maintenance dose*, where a typical concentration of the drug is used to provide an ongoing therapeutic effect such as subsequent doses of an antibiotic.

Distribution

Once absorbed, drug particles are transported in blood plasma. These are referred to as "free" drugs because they are not bound to any receptor sites. Only free drugs can cause a pharmacological response. Drugs bind to proteins in plasma, usually albumin or globulins. These drug-protein complexes decrease the concentration of free drug in the circulation. This protein-drug molecule is too large to pass through the membrane of a blood vessel and is not available for therapeutic use. This process can be reversed when a free drug is excreted from the body. When the drug molecule is released from the protein, the drug becomes free and can be absorbed for use. Drugs affect those areas of the body that have more abundant blood supplies first, such as the heart, liver, kidney, and brain, and then flow to areas with less blood supply, such as muscles and fat.

Drugs accumulate in an area of the body and form a reservoir by binding to tissues. This is referred to as *drug pooling*. There are two types of pooling: (1) *protein binding*, in which a drug binds to plasma proteins, and (2) *tissue binding*, in which fat-soluble drugs are stored in adipose (fatty) tissue. Inderal (propranolol) is a heart medication that is highly bound to the receptor site, and only about 7% of free drug is available for use at a given time. Thiopental (pentothal) is an anesthetic agent that is stored in fat tissue. In addition, some drugs, such as the antibiotic tetracycline, tend to be stored in bones, and this process can interfere with growth of fetal skeletal tissues, which, in turn, can result in discolored teeth if such drugs are administered to children under 8 years of age.

Distribution of drugs is affected by three factors, described below.

Level of Plasma Protein

A low level of plasma protein and albumin might not provide a sufficient number of binding sites for drug particles. This may result in a buildup of drugs that can reach a toxic level. This can occur in the presence of liver or kidney disease or if the patient is malnourished, resulting in low albumin levels (hypoalbuminemia). The elderly are susceptible to hypoalbuminemia. Healthcare professionals should monitor patients' plasma protein and albumin levels and the protein-binding percentages of all drugs before administering any drugs to their patients.

Blood Flow

There must be adequate blood flow to target areas of the body; otherwise, insufficient drug particles will reach affected parts of the body. Drugs can also be stored in fat, bones, muscle, and the eyes. Drugs that accumulate in fat are called *lipid-soluble* and remain in the circulatory system for about 3 hours because there is low blood flow in fat tissue.

The body also has a *blood-brain barrier* that enables passage of only lipid-soluble drugs—such as general anesthetics and barbiturates—into the brain and cerebral spinal fluid (CSF). The only way for nonlipid soluble drugs to enter the brain is if they are instilled intrathecally, that is, injected directly into the CSF, bypassing the blood-brain barrier.

Competing Drugs

Two drugs administered simultaneously might compete for the same binding sites, preventing some drug particles from finding a binding site. The result is an accumulation of free drug that could reach toxic levels. Two drugs that are highly protein-bound—such as Coumadin (warfarin) and Inderal (propranolol)—will compete for the protein sites. This can cause serious problems and can result in toxic levels of one or both of the drugs when increased amounts of free drug become available.

Other Factors

Abscesses, exudates, body glands, cysts, and tumors hinder the distribution of drugs in the body. In addition, antibodies do not distribute well at abscess and exudate sites. The placenta metabolizes some drugs, rendering them inactive and thereby protecting the fetus from drugs given to the mother. However, steroids, narcotics, anesthetics, and some antibiotics can penetrate the placental barrier and result in adverse effects to the fetus.

Elimination

Drugs accumulate in a reservoir *and are gradually absorbed and eventually eliminated by the body. This metabolism—called biotransformation* occurs in the liver, where enzymes inactivate a drug by transforming it into a more water-soluble compound that can be excreted from the body. Elimination occurs mainly through the kidneys, although some drugs are also eliminated in bile, feces, lungs, sweat, and breast milk.

Patients suffering from liver diseases are susceptible to drug toxicity because the diseased liver no longer metabolizes the drug sufficiently to allow elimination through the kidneys. The result is a buildup of the drug, which can eventually lead to a toxic effect on the body.

The amount of time for half of the drug concentration to be eliminated from the body is called the drug's *half-life* and is a crucial measurement used to determine how often to administer the drug. Some drugs have a short half-life ($t_{1/2} < 8$ hours), while other drugs have a longer half-life ($t_{1/2} > 24$ hours).

For example, digoxin has a half-life of 36 hours. This means that there will be a steady state of digoxin in the serum after 5–7 days. This is referred to as the *steady-state serum concentration*; the drug will not have a therapeutic effect before this concentration level is obtained.

Children and the elderly might be unable to absorb or eliminate drugs. This can result in toxicity if additional doses are given before the previous dose is eliminated from the body. Free drugs, water-soluble drugs, and unchanged drugs are filtered by the kidneys and eliminated through urine. Protein-bound drugs do not filter through the kidneys until the drug is released from the protein.

The quantity of drugs that can be excreted by the kidneys is influenced by the pH of the urine, which normally is between 4.5 and 8.0. Acidic urine (pH 4.5) eliminates weak-base drugs; alkaline urine (pH 8.0) eliminates weak-acid drugs. The pH of urine can be altered to increase the elimination of certain drugs. For example, urine can be rendered more alkaline by giving the patient sodium bicarbonate or made more acidic by giving the patient high doses of vitamin C or ammonium chloride.

Kidney disease decreases the *glomerular filtration rate* (GFR) and thereby reduces the quantity of drugs that can be eliminated by the kidneys. This can result in drug toxicity. A similar effect can be caused by a decrease in blood flow to the kidneys.

Kidney function is tested by the creatinine clearance test. A decrease in GFR causes an increase in creatinine in serum and a decrease in creatinine in urine. The results of the creatinine clearance test vary with age and whenever there is decreased muscle mass.

In some situations, it is important to reduce the excretion of a drug to prolong the drug's therapeutic effect, such as with penicillin. Giving the patient another drug, such as probenecid, blocks excretion of penicillin.

Drugs can be excreted artificially through the use of dialysis, which is a common treatment for certain types of drug overdose. Drugs that are excreted by the kidneys can be eliminated using hemodialysis. These drugs include stimulants, depressants, and some nonnarcotic analgesics.

Drugs that are metabolized by the liver are secreted into bile and then passed through the intestines and eliminated in feces. During this process, the bloodstream might reabsorb fat-soluble drugs and return them to the liver, where they will be metabolized, and they will then be eliminated by the kidneys. This process is called the *enterohepatic cycle*.

The lungs eliminate drugs that are intact, and not metabolites such as gases and anesthetic drugs. The rate at which these drugs are eliminated corresponds to the respiratory rate. Some drugs, such as ethyl alcohol and paraldehyde, are excreted at multiple sites. Small amounts are excreted by the lungs, and the remainder are excreted by the liver and the kidneys. Volatile drugs, such as anesthetics and drugs that are metabolized to CO_2 and H_2O, are excreted through the lungs.

Sweat and salivary glands do not serve as major routes of drug elimination because elimination depends on the diffusion of lipid-soluble drugs through the epithelial cells of the glands. However, side effects of drugs, such as rashes and skin reactions, can be seen at these sites. Some intravenously administered drugs are excreted into saliva and cause the patient to taste the drug. Eventually, drugs that are excreted into saliva are swallowed, reabsorbed, and eliminated in urine.

Many drugs or their metabolites are excreted in mammary glands. These include narcotics such as morphine and codeine. Diuretics and barbiturates, which are weak acids, are less concentrated in breast milk. However, even small amounts of drugs can accumulate, causing an undesirable effect on an infant receiving breast milk.

2. The First-Pass Effect

The most common route of drug administration is orally (PO), when the patient swallows a pill. The drug is then absorbed into the GI tract and enters the portal circulation system, where drug particles are transported through the portal vein into the liver, where the drug is metabolized. This is referred to as the *first-pass effect*.

Not all drugs are metabolized in the liver. Some drugs bypass the first-pass effect by sublingual administration (under the tongue) or buccal administration (between the gums and the cheek), where they are absorbed directly into the bloodstream from the mouth. These drugs do not enter the stomach, where the hydrochloric acid might destroy drug particles. Other drugs go directly to the liver through the portal vein and also bypass the stomach. These drugs are then metabolized in the liver, and much of the drug may be eliminated and not available to ensure a therapeutic effect. Sometimes these adverse effects are so great that none of the drug will be available for use if it is administered by mouth. The drug must then be given in very high doses or parenterally (intramuscularly or intravenously) to bypass the liver.

3. Pharmacodynamics

Pharmacodynamics is a drug's effect on the physiology of the cell and the mechanism that causes the pharmaceutical response. A drug delivers two types of effects: the primary effect and the secondary effect. The *primary effect* is the reason for which the drug is administered. The *secondary effect* is a side effect that may or may not be desirable.

For example, diphenhydramine (Benadryl) is an antihistamine. Its primary effect is to treat symptoms of allergies. Its secondary effect is to depress the central nervous system (CNS), causing drowsiness. The secondary effect is desirable if the patient needs bedrest, but undesirable if the patient is driving a car.

A period of time passes after a drug is administered until the pharmaceutical response is realized. This is referred to as the drug's *response time*. There are three types of response time: onset, peak, and duration.

The *onset response time* is the time for the minimum concentration of drug to cause the initial pharmaceutical response. Some drugs reach the onset time in minutes, and other drugs take days. The *peak response time* is that time during which the drug reaches its highest blood or plasma concentration. The *duration* is the length of time during which the drug maintains the pharmaceutical response.

The response time is plotted on a *time–response curve* that shows the onset response time, the peak response time, and the duration. All three parameters are used when administering the drug in order to determine the therapeutic range—when the drug will become effective, when it will be most effective, and when it will no longer be effective. The time–response curve is also used to determine when a drug is expected to reach a toxic level.

For example, data obtained from the time–response curve of an analgesic are used for pain management. Once the peak response time is reached, the effectiveness of the drug to block pain diminishes. The time–response curve indicates when the pharmaceutical response is no longer present, indicating that an additional dose should be administered to the patient.

Receptor Theory

The pharmaceutical response is realized when a drug binds to a receptor on the cell membrane. These receptors are referred to as *reactive cellular sites*. The activity of the drug is determined by that drug's ability to bind to a specific receptor. The better the fit, the more biologically active the drug. Receptors are proteins, glycoproteins, proteolipids, or enzymes. Depending on the drug, binding either initiates a physiological response by the cell or blocks a cell's physiological response.

Receptors are classified into four families:

1. **Rapid Cell Membrane–Embedded Enzymes:** Drugs in this category bind to the surface of the cell, causing an enzyme inside the cell to initiate a physiological response.

2. **Rapid Ligand-Gated Ion Channels:** Drug in this category span the cell membrane, causing ion channels within the membrane to open, resulting in the flow of primarily sodium and calcium ions into and out of the cell.

3. **Rapid G-Protein-Coupled Receptor Systems:** Drugs in this category bind with the receptor, causing the G protein to bind with guanosine triphosphate (GTP). This, in turn, causes an enzyme inside the cell to initiate a physiological response or causes the ion channel to open.

4. **Prolonged Transcription Factor Systems:** Drugs in this category bind to the transcription factors on the DNA within the nucleus of the cell and cause these transcript factors to undergo physiological changes.

A drug that causes a physiological response is called an *agonist*, and a drug that blocks a physiological response is referred to as an *antagonist*. The effect of an antagonist is determined by the inhibitory (I) action of the drug concentration on the receptor site. An inhibitory action of 50 (I_{50}) indicates that the drug effectively inhibits the receptor response in 50% of the population.

Agonists and antagonists lack specific and selective effects. They are called *nonspecific* and have nonspecificity properties. Each receptor can produce various physiologic responses. Cholinergic receptors are located in the bladder, heart, blood vessels, lungs, and eyes. A cholinergic stimulator or blocker will affect all of these sites. These drugs are also called *nonspecific* or are assumed to have nonspecificity properties. A drug that is given to stimulate the cholinergic receptors will decrease the heart rate and blood pressure, increase gastric acid secretion, constrict bronchioles, increase urinary bladder contraction, and constrict the pupils. The effects may be either beneficial or harmful.

4. Categories of Drug Action

Drugs are categorized by the type of action they cause in the body. There are four types of response:

- **Stimulation or Depression:** Drugs in this category either increase or depress cellular activity.
- **Replacement:** Drugs in this category replace an essential body compound such as insulin or estrogen.
- **Inhibition:** Drugs in this category, such as penicillin, interfere with the processes occurring within bacterial cells by limiting bacterial growth or eliminating the bacteria.
- **Irritation:** Drugs in this category stimulate cells to cause a natural response that has a therapeutic effect such as a laxative that stimulates the colon wall to increase movement of the colon resulting in defecation.

5. Therapeutic Index and Therapeutic Range

Drugs have a pharmaceutical response as long as the dose remains within the drug's margin of safety. Some drugs have a broad margin of safety. This means that a patient can be given a wide range of dose levels without experiencing a toxic effect. Other drugs have a narrow margin of safety, where the slightest change in dosage can result in an undesirable adverse side effect.

The drug's *therapeutic index* (TI) identifies the margin of safety of the drug and is defined as a ratio between the therapeutic dose in 50% of people or animals and the lethal dose in 50% of animals. The *therapeutic dose* is denoted as ED_{50}, and the *lethal dose* in animals is denoted as LD_{50}. The closer the ratio is to 1, the greater the danger of toxicity:

$$TI = LD_{50}/ED_{50}$$

Drugs that have a low TI are considered to have a narrow margin of safety. These drugs require that the plasma levels be monitored and that the dosages be adjusted in order to prevent the occurrence of toxic effects.

The plasma drug levels must be within the therapeutic range, which is also known as the *therapeutic window*. The therapeutic window ranges between the *minimum effective concentration* (MEC) for obtaining the desired pharmaceutical response and the *minimum toxic concentration* (MTC). The MEC is achieved by administering a *loading dose*, which is a large initial dose given to achieve a rapid plasma MEC.

Peak and Trough Levels

The plasma concentration of a drug must be monitored for drugs that have a narrow margin of safety or low TI. The concentration is measured at two points. These are the peak drug level and the trough level.

The *peak drug level* is the highest plasma concentration at a specific time. The peak drug level indicates the rate at which a drug is absorbed in the body and is affected by the route of drug administration. Drugs administered intravenously have high (or rapidly rising) peak drug levels, whereas drugs taken orally have low (or slowly rising) peak drug level because these drugs need time to be absorbed and distributed. Blood samples are drawn at peak times according to the route used to administer the drug. This is usually 30–90 minutes after drug administration.

The *trough drug level* is the lowest plasma concentration of the drug and measures the rate at which the drug is eliminated. Blood should be drawn immediately before the next dose is given regardless of the route of drug administration.

Side Effects

A drug can have a side effect in addition to its pharmaceutical response. A *side effect* is a physiologic effect other than the desired effect. Sometimes side effects are predictable, and at other times they are not and may be unrelated to the dosage. Some side effects are desirable, and others are undesirable.

A severely undesirable side effect is referred to as an *adverse reaction* that occurs unintentionally when a normal dose of the drug is given to a patient. For example, an adverse reaction might be anaphylaxis (cardiovascular collapse).

Some adverse reactions are predictable according to age and weight of the patient. Young children and the elderly are highly responsive to medications because of an immature or declining hepatorenal function. Body mass also influences the distribution and concentration of a drug. The dosage must be adjusted for elderly patients in proportion to body weight or body surface area.

Drug effects can also be related to other factors. These include the following:

1. **Gender:** Women typically are smaller than men and have a different proportion of fat and water, which affects absorption and distribution of the drug. Pharmacokinetics in women is affected by lower body weight, slower GI emptying, and slower filtration through the kidneys. Women also have a greater sensitivity to certain drugs and are 50–75% more likely to have an adverse drug reaction.

2. **Environment:** Cold, heat, sensory deprivation or overload, and oxygen deprivation at high altitudes create environmental factors that might interact with a drug.

3. **Time of Administration:** A drug might be influenced by the presence or absence of food in the patient's gastrointestinal tract or by the patient's cortiocosteroid secretion rhythm. In addition, circadian cycle, urinary excretion pattern, fluid intake, and drug-metabolizing enzyme rhythms all might influence a drug's effect.

4. **Pathologic State:** A drug can react differently if the patient is experiencing pain, anxiety, circulatory distress, or hepatic and/or renal dysfunction.

5. **Idiosyncracy:** This is an unpredictable and inexplicable abnormal response that could result if the patient over- or under-responds to the drug or if the effect of the drug differs from the effect that was expected.

6. **Tolerance:** The patient has a decreased physiologic response after repeated administration of the drug. This is common following inhalation or ingestion of tobacco, opium alkaloids, nitrites, and ethyl alcohol. The dosage must be increased to achieve the desired pharmaceutical response.

7. **Drug Dependence:** This can be either a physical or a psychological dependence. With a physical dependence, the patient experiences an intense physical disturbance when the drug is withdrawn. With psychological dependence, the patient develops an emotional reliance on the drug.

8. **Drug Interaction:** The administration of one drug increases or decreases the pharmaceutical response of a previously administered drug.

9. **Synergism:** A more desirable pharmaceutical response is achieved through the interaction of two drugs that are administered.

10. **Potentiation:** Concurrent administration of two drugs increases the pharmaceutical response of one of those drugs.

11. **Toxic Effect:** This occurs when the administered drug exceeds the therapeutic range through an overdose or by the drug accumulating in the patient.

12. **Tachyphylaxis:** This occurs when the patient builds a tolerance to the drug due to the frequency in which the drug is administered. This occurs with administration or ingestion of narcotics, barbiturates, laxatives, and psychotropic agents. The patient may eventually need more of the drug to reach the desired effect.

13. **Placebo Effect:** The patient receives a psychological benefit from receiving a compound that has no pharmaceutical response. A third of patients taking a placebo experience the placebo effect.

14. **Pharmacogenetic Effect:** A drug effect varies from a predicted response because of the influence of a patient's genetic factors. Genetic factors can alter the metabolism of the drug and may result in an enhanced or diminished pharmaceutical response.

15. **Allergic Reactions:** If a patient was previously sensitized to a specific drug, administration of that drug might trigger that patient's immunologic mechanism, which could result in allergic symptoms. Antibodies are produced the first time that the drug is introduced to the patient, creating a sensitivity to that drug. The next time the drug is given to the patient, it reacts with the antibodies and results in the production of histamine. Histamine causes allergic symptoms to occur. The patient should not take any drug that causes an allergic reaction.

There are four types of allergic reactions:

- **Anaphylactic Reaction:** This is an immediate allergic response that is potentially fatal.

- **Cytotoxic Reaction:** This is an autoimmune response that results in hemolytic anemia, thrombocytopenia, or lupus erythematosus (blood disorders). In some cases, it takes months for the reaction to dissipate.

- **Immune Complex Reaction:** This response is also referred to as *serum sickness* and usually results in angioedema (a type of swelling that affects deeper layers in the skin often around the face and lips), arthralgia (sore joints), fever, swollen lymph nodes, and splenomegaly (large spleen). The immune complex reaction can appear within 3 weeks after the drug is administered.

- **Cell-Mediated Response:** This is an inflammatory skin reaction that is also known as *delayed hypersensitivity*.

Summary

A drug exerts a physiochemical action with the physiological process of the body, resulting in a pharmaceutical response. A drug might replace a missing element such as a hormone, interrupt a physiological process, or stimulate the occurrence of a physiological process. In addition to a therapeutic effect, drugs may have side effects that can be desirable or undesirable.

The strength of a drug action is determined by the dose administered to a patient and how frequently it is administered. The first dose is called a *loading dose* or *priming dose* and consists of a large concentration of the drug. Subsequent doses are called *maintenance doses* and consist of a normal concentration of the drug.

Drug activity is divided into the pharmaceutic phase, the pharmacokinetic phase, and the pharmacodynamic phase. The *pharmaceutic phase* is the disintegration and dissolution of a drug taken orally. The *pharmacokinetic phase* is the mechanism used to absorb, distribute, and eliminate a drug. The *pharmacodynamic phase* is a drug's effect on the physiology of the cell and the mechanism that causes the pharmaceutical response.

Drugs bind to receptors on the cell membrane at locations called *reactive cellular sites*. Receptors are proteins, glycoproteins, proteolipids, or enzymes. Depending on the drug, binding either initiates a physiological response by the cell or blocks a cell's physiological response. A drug that causes a physiological response is called an *agonist*. A drug that blocks a physiological response is called an *antagonist*.

The safety of a drug is identified by the drug's *therapeutic index* (TI). A low TI indicates that a drug has a narrow margin of safety, requiring that the drug's peak level and trough levels be closely monitored. A high TI indicates that a drug has a broad margin of safety and does not require frequent monitoring of the patient and the serum drug level.

Now that you have a good understanding of the theory of how drugs work, in the next chapter we will consider the practical aspects of pharmacology and see how pharmacology is used in the nursing process.

QUIZ

1. The pharmacokinetic phase is
   (a) the form of the drug.
   (b) the way the drug is absorbed, distributed, and eliminated.
   (c) the effect the drug has on the body.
   (d) none of the above.

2. The ingredient in a drug that causes a physiological response is called
   (a) D-fill.
   (b) excipient.
   (c) D-active.
   (d) particle.

3. The method in which a drug is absorbed by flowing from a high concentration to a low concentration is called
   (a) active diffusion.
   (b) pinocytosis.
   (c) passive diffusion.
   (d) absorption rate.

4. All drugs are absorbed immediately when they are administered.
   (a) True
   (b) False

5. Lipid-soluble drugs are absorbed more quickly than water-soluble drugs.
   (a) True
   (b) False

6. Bioavailability is
   (a) the quantity of drug in a vial.
   (b) the quantity of drug injected into the body.
   (c) the number of drug particles in a dose.
   (d) the percentage of a dose that reaches the bloodstream.

7. Primary loading is the first measured quantity of drug that is eliminated from the body.
   (a) True
   (b) False

8. A drug that causes a nonspecific physiological response is called a(n)
   (a) agonist.
   (b) metabolite.
   (c) protein.
   (d) molecule.

9. Insulin is a type of inhibition drug.

    (a) True

    (b) False

10. The therapeutic index identifies the margin of safety of the drug.

    (a) True

    (b) False

chapter 3

Pharmacology and the Nursing Process

Anyone who has spent a few nights in a hospital bed remembers being awakened from a sound sleep by a nurse saying, "Time to take your medication." Try as you might to ignore the request, you can't win. The voice simply becomes more insistent until you have no choice but to open your eyes.

Patients are also awakened sometimes so that the nurse can check their vital signs. The purpose of this is to determine whether the medication is having an effect or whether the patient is experiencing an undesirable side effect. In cases where the patient is being treated with a narrow-spectrum antibiotic, blood may be drawn to determine whether the antibiotic is working on the infection.

Administering medication, evaluating the patient's response, and determining whether the drug is working as planned are pharmacology-specific activities that are part of the nursing process. You were introduced to pharmacology in Chapters 1 and 2. This chapter takes a look at the nursing process as it relates to giving medications.

1. The Nursing Process

The *nursing process* is a systematic way for a nurse to decide how to treat the patient's responses to health and illness. There are five steps in the nursing process:

1. Assessment

2. Diagnosis

3. Planning

4. Intervention or implementation

5. Evaluation

Assessment is data collection. During the assessment step, the nurse is gathering subjective and objective data from the patient that will later be used to arrive at a nursing diagnosis. Subjective data are information that is reported by the patient, such as "I'm feeling warm." Objective data are information that can be measured or observed, such as the patient's temperature or the color of the patient's skin. Assessment data may include results of laboratory or X-rays.

Diagnosis is the patient's condition, which is determined by analyzing data collected during the patient's assessment. The data could lead the nurse to determine that the patient has more than one problem. This diagnosis is referred to as a *nursing diagnosis*. A nursing diagnosis is different from a medical diagnosis. For example, a nurse might diagnose an alteration in mobility in a patient who has had a stroke. A physician or an advanced nurse practitioner might determine the medical diagnosis, which is cerebral vascular accident (CVA). The nurse might also determine that this patient has a potential for alteration in nutrition because she/he is having difficulty swallowing because of the stroke.

The *plan* is how the nurse proposes to care for the patient. The plan takes the form of a care plan that itemizes the patient's nursing diagnosis. Each nursing diagnosis will have an expected outcome or goal. The care plan contains at least one nursing intervention for each nursing diagnosis, the expected outcome for each intervention, and how the nurse will evaluate the outcome. For example, the final outcome goal for an alteration in mobility might be to have the patient get out of bed and ambulate without assistance. However, the interventions will begin with getting the patient out of bed and to the chair or assisting the patient to walk short distances each day. The plan also includes carrying out the physician/provider orders.

The *intervention* consists in executing the plan. For example, the nurse will assist the patient to the chair the first time and might delegate the task to a nursing assistant thereafter if the patient does not experience any problems.

The *evaluation* step of the nursing process determines whether the intervention worked. For example, the nurse evaluates the patient's response to getting out of bed and also determines whether the patient continues to get out of bed on a daily basis. If the patient's progress in getting out of bed continues to be unproblematic, the nurse may change the interventions to include walking short distances in addition to getting out of bed and may increase those distances each day. When the patient is able to get out of bed and walk without assistance, the final goal will have been achieved. Evaluation should also include a patient's response to medications. For example, if the patient received acetaminophen for a fever, the evaluation should include the patient's temperature.

The nursing process is circular. If the nurse determines during the evaluation step that the intervention did not work or that the expected outcome has not been achieved, the nurse begins the nursing process again, starting with the assessment step, and then revises the care plan as the patient's problem changes. The nursing process is repeated until the patient's problem(s) is resolved.

Assessment Related to Drugs

During the assessment phase, the nurse systematically collects, verifies, and analyzes patient-related data. A portion of the assessment process directly relates to administering medication to the patient.

Before administering medication to a patient, the nurse must make the assessments described in the following paragraphs.

Validity of the Drug Order

A drug order must be written by a physician, a dentist, a physician assistant, or an advanced practice nurse and contain the following information:

- The date and time when the order is written
- The name of the drug
- The dosage
- The route of administration
- The frequency of administration
- The duration (how long the patient is to receive the drug)
- The signature of the prescriber

Identifying the Brand and Generic Names of the Drug

Drugs are known under several names:

- The chemical name used by pharmacists and researchers
- The generic name, which is the official (proprietary) nonproprietary name that is universally accepted
- The brand name, which is the name chosen by the drug manufacturer
- The official name that appears in the USP-NF

Reasons for Using a Specific Drug

The nurse is required to know why the drug is given to the patient and what symptoms a patient exhibits to indicate that that specific drug should be administered. The nurse needs to understand what outcomes should be expected when giving the medication. For example, if the patient is given a medication to prevent or control nausea, the outcome should be that the patient will no longer be nauseous. The nurse cannot rely solely on the prescriber because the patient's condition might have changed since the assessment. Furthermore, there is always a potential for error in the order. An order can be erroneous for various reasons. These include, but are not limited to, writing an order or a prescription for the wrong patient, for a drug to which the patient is allergic, for a drug that will interact adversely with another drug that the patient is taking, at a dose that is too small or too large relative to the patient's weight, or simply for the wrong drug. Medication errors can be reduced or eliminated if everyone involved in the process uses critical thinking skills and checks and double-checks the orders, the patient, and the medication.

How the Drug Works

It is critical that the nurse understand how the drug is absorbed, distributed, metabolized, and eliminated before administering it to the patient. One of these mechanisms might be malfunctioning. For example, the patient might have lower-than-expected urinary output and might thus be unable to excrete the drug in normal volume, which could result in a potential toxic buildup in the body.

The nurse must also know the drug's onset of action, peak action, and duration of action. As you'll recall from Chapter 2, *onset* is the time period when the drug reaches the minimally effective concentration in the plasma. The *peak action* is when the drug reaches the maximum concentration in the plasma. The *duration* is the length of time the therapeutic action will last.

Agents That Might Interact With the Drug

The effectiveness of a drug can be influenced by interactions with food, herbal remedies, and other drugs that alter or modify the drug's action. Such interactions might increase, decrease, or neutralize the drug's effectiveness. The nurse must be aware of known or potential interactions in order to avoid them.

Potential Side Effects and Toxicity of the Drug

A *side effect* is a physiological response in the patient's body that is not related to the drug's primary action. Some side effects are beneficial, whereas other side effects—such as nausea and vomiting—are undesirable. By knowing a drug's possible side effects, the nurse can prepare to manage them before the patient is given the drug.

The nurse must also know the toxicity of a drug. A drug's *toxicity* is the drug concentration in plasma and accumulation in tissues that exceeds the drug's therapeutic range.

Signs and Symptoms to Be Monitored

The nurse must note the signs and symptoms that indicate whether the patient is having an adverse reaction to a drug or whether the drug has reached toxic levels. These indications may not be present for minutes, hours, and even days after the drug is administered.

What the Patient Should Know About the Drug

Many drugs are self-administered by patients after they leave the healthcare facility. Therefore, it is important that the nurse identify any information about the drug that the patient needs to know in order to administer it properly.

Availability, Expiration Date, and Cost of the Drug

The drug that is ordered may not be available in the healthcare facility. The nurse must ensure that the drug is available and that the drug on hand has not yet expired if it is available. For example, a healthcare facility might have a very low requirement for a particular drug, and the drug in stock might be old and have passed the expiration date.

The cost of the drug is important to know for a number of reasons. Some drugs are not covered by the patient's health insurance because they are expensive. The insurance company may cover the cost of a similar, less expensive, medication. In addition, many patients do not have sufficient insurance to cover medications and cannot afford to fill an expensive prescription. Nurses should ask patients about their insurance coverage and whether they can afford to purchase the medication if their insurance will not cover the cost. Many patients might stop taking an important medication simply because they lack sufficient funds to pay for it.

Patient Information

Before administering a drug, the nurse must review information about the patient to ensure that the patient will not have an adverse reaction to the drug. The nurse must determine the following:

- Does the patient have any allergies to the drug or to food that might be given along with the drug?
- Has the patient's condition changed since the drug was ordered?
- What is the patient's age?
- What is the appropriate dose of the drug according to the patient's weight?

- What is the patient's gender?
- Is the patient pregnant?
- What is the patient's primary language?
- Are there any religious or cultural influences that would cause the patient to resist taking the medication?
- Does the patient know and understand the purpose of the medication?
- Does the patient's history include taking vitamins, birth control pills, and herbal remedies?
- Does the patient use illegal drugs or alcohol?
- Does the patient have a tolerance for the drug that is being administered?
- Are there any genetic factors that might cause an adverse reaction by taking the medication?
- Are there any emotional factors that could affect the patient's ability to take the drug?
- Are there any contraindications for the medication that are indicated by taking the patient's vital signs and reviewing her or his current laboratory and diagnostic tests?
- Is the patient's mental status sufficient to understand why the particular medication is being administered? Will someone be available to monitor the patient?
- Can the patient afford the medication?
- Will family members or friends be with the patient to monitor for side effects and toxicity?
- Is the patient scheduled to undergo tests, procedures, or other activities and to receive medication at the same time?
- Is the patient scheduled to receive medication during visiting hours?
- Is the patient required to have a procedure performed, such as insertion of an IV or feeding tube, before medication is administered?

Obtaining this information may sound overwhelming to the new nurse. However, much of this information will have already been obtained when the patient was admitted in the hospital or arrived at the office or clinic for care.

2. Nursing Diagnosis

The nurse develops a nursing diagnosis after analyzing information gained from assessing the patient. A *nursing diagnosis* is a statement that describes the patient's actual or potential response to a health problem that the nurse is licensed and competent to treat. The North American Nursing Diagnosis Association (NANDA) developed a guide used by many nurses to arrive at a nursing diagnosis.

A physician or an advanced practitioner uses the medical diagnosis to prescribe a treatment for combating the disease. This might involve medication and/or a change in the patient's lifestyle. A nurse uses the nursing diagnosis to develop a comprehensive quality care plan to restore the patient to a state where she/he can return to activities of normal living.

For example, a physician might diagnose a patient as having diabetes and might prescribe glucose monitoring and insulin injections to control the disease. The nursing diagnosis might be a knowledge deficit about the disease and the medications employed to treat it. The nurse teaches the patient how to monitor glucose and give injections as well as how to identify adverse side effects of the medication and of the disease. Furthermore, the nurse determines whether the patient has the financial, social, and mental capacity to self-medicate. The nurse then develops a plan to enlist the healthcare team to assist the patient if the patient lacks the capacity.

The nursing diagnosis consists of a problem statement that identifies the potential or actual health problem that the nurse is licensed and expected to treat. A nursing diagnosis may also include the cause of the problem—such as alteration in mobility related to right-sided paralysis—which are factors related to or associated with the patient's problem and the symptoms that manifested the problem.

A common nursing diagnosis related to drug therapy might be as follows:

- **Knowledge Deficit of Disease and Medication Related to Inability to Understand English:** This occurs when the patient doesn't understand the language used by healthcare professionals, such as when healthcare is provided in English, and English is the patient's second language.

- **Risk for Injury Related to Side Effect(s) of the Drug:** The patient may be given medication such as narcotic analgesics for pain that impairs the patient's activities of normal daily life such as driving an automobile.

- **Alteration in Thought Processes Related to Drug Action:** Some drugs such as barbiturates, sedatives, and mood-altering medication may interrupt the patient's normal thought process, which could confuse the patient and the patient's family and friends if they are unaware of the potential side effect(s) of the drug.

- **Constipation Related to Drug Action or Side Effect(s):** Morphine sulfate and other opioids cause a reduction in intestinal movement resulting in constipation that might make the patient uncomfortable. Knowing this, the nurse might instruct the patient about foods and fluids that might increase intestinal motility, such as bran, and increased water intake.

- **Fluid Volume Deficit Related to Drug Action:** Diuretic medication such as furosemide (Lasix) causes the patient to lose more than the normal volume of fluid in an effort to counteract a disease that results in fluid retention. The nurse alerts the patient to the likely increase in urination and also monitors the patient's fluid intake and output to ensure that the patient maintains an adequate fluid level.

- **Breathing Pattern Ineffective Related to Drug Side Effect(s):** Opioids, such as morphine sulfate, can reduce the patient's breathing to a level where the patient's respiration is no longer effective. This might mean not moving enough air or blowing off too much CO_2. The nurse should monitor the patient's respiratory rate on a regular basis.

3. Patient Care Plan

Once a nursing diagnosis is reached, a care plan is developed that describes how the healthcare team will address the patient's problems. The care plan should contain the following information:

- Nursing diagnosis
- Expected outcomes—goal statement
- Interventions based on a scientific and medical rationale needed to achieve the goal
- How to measure each outcome

Goal Statement

At the heart of the care plan is a *goal statement* that specifies an expected outcome of the healthcare team's intervention with the patient. Think of a goal statement as what you want to happen to the patient. For example, a typical goal is that a patient will report a reduction in pain level from 8 to 4 on a scale of 0 to 10 in 3 hours.

A goal statement is a *nursing order* that must be patient-centered and specify a desired behavior to occur at a specified time. The behavior must be observable and measurable, and the goal statement must specify criteria for measuring the behavior.

Ideally, both the nurse and the patient develop and accept the goal. If the patient's decision-making ability is impaired, then the patient's family or another support person becomes the patient's advocate in the planning process. It is critical that the patient adopt the goal statement; otherwise, the goal might not be achieved. For example, if the patient does not believe in taking pain medication, then a goal of reducing pain by taking analgesics will not be met. The nurse will then have to explore alternatives to pain medication such as a massage or imagery. The care plan should be shared with the patient's family, the healthcare team, and others who are caring for the patient to ensure that everyone will be working toward the same goals.

Deadlines and Measurement

It is important that the care plan establish realistic deadlines for reaching the goal; otherwise the patient and the patient's caregivers will become frustrated if the goal is not met. For example, it is not realistic to assume that the patient will no longer cough after taking dextromethorphan (Robitussin DM) simply because the medication does not provide an instant cure for coughing. A more realistic goal is for the frequency of the patient's coughing to decrease after each dose. The deadline might be for the patient to take dextromethorphan for 48 hours and report a decrease in frequency of coughing and experience uninterrupted rest. This goal is both observable and measurable because the nurse can observe whether the patient is coughing and can measure the frequency of the cough to determine whether the goal is reached.

Interventions

The care plan must also specify the intervention for each goal statement. An *intervention* is a clear statement that specifies the action that must be taken to achieve the goal statement. An intervention must complement the goal statement, use available resources, follow protocols established by the healthcare facility, and always keep the patient's safety in mind.

There are three types of intervention.

Nurse-Initiated Intervention

A *nurse-initiated intervention* is a nursing order performed independently by the nurse on the basis of a scientific rationale that benefits the patient in a predicted way, such as removing a blanket to lower the patient's temperature.

Physician or Advanced Practice Intervention

This type of intervention is a dependent function issued by a physician or an advanced practitioner that is carried out by a nurse, such as administering prescribed medication to the patient.

Collaborative Intervention

A *collaborative intervention* is an activity performed among multiple healthcare professionals, such as physical therapy for the patient.

Evaluation

Each outcome on the care plan must be evaluated to determine whether the goal is achieved. Once all goals on the care plan are reached, the care plan no longer exists.

The patient no longer exhibits symptoms of the nursing diagnosis. However, if at least one goal is not realized, reassessment or data collection should occur. This would include reassessing the patient and other factors, such as schedules, availability of resources, and developing new goals, interventions, and evaluations.

4. Teaching the Patient About Drugs

A critical nursing responsibility is to educate the patient and the patient's family about the medication that is administered to the patient or that is self-administered by the patient. Teaching should be conducted in a comfortable environment in a language that both the patient and the patient's family understand. Use appropriate charts, graphs, audio, and videotapes as necessary. Always provide enough time for questions and answers. Avoid rushing. If the information cannot be presented in one session, plan several sessions. It is always a good idea to give the patient and family members material that they can take home and review at their leisure. It is very important that written information be at a reading level that can be understood by the patient and family.

Demonstrate how the patient or family members are to administer medication. For example, show the proper injection techniques if the patient requires insulin injections or the correct use of bronchodilator inhalers for asthma. Do not assume that they can administer the medication after seeing you do it. Make sure to have the patient and family members show you how they plan to give the medication. This is especially critical when medication is given using a syringe, topical drugs, and inhalers. The patient and the caregiver must have the necessary visual acuity, manual dexterity, and mental capacity to prepare and administer medication.

Prompt the patient and family members to give you feedback from your lesson and demonstration by asking the following questions:

- What things help you take your medicine?
- What things prevent you from taking your medication?
- What would you do if you forget to take your medication?
- What would you feel if you are taking too much of the medication?
- What would you feel if you experience side effects from taking the medication?
- Is there anything you could do to reduce side effects of the medication?

It is very important that the patient and family members be informed about the signs and symptoms of an allergic response to the medication such as urticaria (hives), swollen lips, hoarse voice, difficulty breathing, and shortness of breath—an indication of life-threatening anaphylaxis.

In addition to the signs and symptoms of an allergic response, you must also discuss side effects and toxic effects of the medication and any dietary considerations the patient must follow while on the medication.

Some patients require several medications. Therefore, the nurse needs to develop a medication plan to help the patient manage the medication schedule. Common techniques include the following:

- A multicompartment dispenser to hold a daily or weekly supply of medication
- A timer to remind the patient when to take the medication
- Color-coded envelopes where each color represents an hour or a day
- A written record of when medication should be administered and when it was administered

5. Impact of Cultural Influences in Drug Administration

The cultural background of the patient and the patient's family can impact the administration of medication. Cultural influences are learned values, beliefs, customs, and behavior. These influences include the patient's belief about health, such as the following:

- What healthcare can do for the patient
- The patient's susceptibility to disease
- The benefits of taking steps to prevent disease
- What makes a patient seek healthcare
- What makes a patient follow healthcare guidelines

For example, a patient who is a coal miner may believe that all coal miners will eventually develop lung cancer. In that case, the patient may feel that there is no benefit in smoking cessation. Another patient may avoid taking pain medication for fear of becoming addicted to it.

Some cultures have their own beliefs about how to prevent and cure disease. For example, although garlic does lower blood pressure, taking garlic as an herbal cure might be dangerous if the patient is also taking antihypertensive medication, because the patient's blood pressure could be lowered to a dangerous level. Herbal remedies are preferred by some cultures over traditional Western medicine, and some patients continue herbal treatment even when a mild illness progresses to a critical level.

The beliefs of healthcare providers can differ from those of their patients. A patient may refuse any treatment because of the sole belief in the healing power of prayer. Healthcare providers must be nonjudgmental and must tolerate alternative beliefs in healthcare, even if those beliefs are potentially harmful to the patient. When confronted with cultural differences that can result in an adverse effect to the patient, healthcare providers can educate the patient about the benefits of medications and treatment and the risk that the patient is exposed to by not following the recommended treatment. This information is sometimes best given while the healthcare provider is assessing the patient. The nurse should be careful to remain nonjudgmental about the patient's decisions.

Cultural beliefs can also influence who makes healthcare decisions for the family. In most cultures, women are typically responsible for managing the family's health. However, in some cultures, although the female is responsible for providing and obtaining care, the oldest male is seen as the head of the family and the authority figure for making overall decisions such as when to access healthcare.

The way in which the patient communicates with healthcare providers is greatly influenced by individual culture. Here are factors to consider when communicating with a patient:

- Try to avoid direct eye contact, as this might not be appropriate.
- Ask the patient how she/he should be addressed. Always address the patient formally until the patient gives permission to be addressed informally.
- Know how the patient perceives time (eg, day/night, sunrise/sunset). Otherwise, the patient may be unable to comply with the appropriate medication schedule.
- Maintain the patient's personal space. Always ask permission to invade the personal space to perform a procedure. In some cultures, patients do not want anyone standing or sitting too close, and they feel uncomfortable if someone touches them.
- Consider food beliefs and rituals as related to illnesses. Some patients believe that the more you eat, the healthier you will become. Other people restrict certain foods for religious reasons.
- Evaluate the family's attitude toward the elderly. The elderly are revered in some cultures, and the family may go to great lengths to care for them. In other cultures, the family leaves the elderly to die peacefully without interference.

Ethnic Considerations

Besides cultural differences, there are also ethnic and racial differences in the physiological response to drugs. As you'll recall from Chapter 2, *pharmacogenetics* is the study of the influence of genetics on drug responses. For example, children with Reye's syndrome, which affects primarily the liver, cannot metabolize aspirin because of a genetic defect.

Similarly, a genetic factor in African-Americans renders them less responsive to β-blocking agents used in cardiac and antihypertensive medications. Asians have a genetic factor that causes undesirable side effects when they are given the typical dose of benzodiazepines [diazepam (Valium)] alprazolam (Xanax), tricyclic antidepressants, atropine, and propranolol (Inderal). Therefore, a lower dose must be given.

6. Mother and the Fetus

Many drugs cross the placenta, but only some of them can adversely affect the fetus because of the immature fetal metabolism and slower excretion rates. Waste products are excreted into the amniotic fluid and then absorbed by the mother or swallowed by the fetus.

Alcohol, barbiturates, and narcotics—such as diphenhydramine (Benadryl), amobarbital (Amytal), diazepam (Valium), codeine, heroin, methadone, morphine, and propoxyphene (Darvon)—that are used during pregnancy can lead to harmful effects on the newborn. Use of these drugs during pregnancy can create an addiction in the newborn. The baby will go into withdrawal from the drug after birth. This can result in hyperactivity, crying, irritability, seizures, and even sudden death.

When taken by the mother during the first trimester, some drugs have a teratogenic effect on the fetus, which can result in fetal defects. This includes mutagenic (causing genetic mutation) or carcinogenic (causing cancer) effects. These drugs include thalidomide (Thalomid), which causes abnormal limb development, and cocaine, which can cause miscarriages, fetal hypoxia (lack of oxygen), low-birth-weight infants, tremors, strokes, increase in stillbirth rates, congenital heart disease, skull defects, and other malformations.

Adverse side effects of the drug on the fetus can be avoided by carefully checking the Pregnancy Category of the medication before the medication is administered to a pregnant woman. Regardless of the Pregnancy Category of the drug, always carefully observe the pregnant patient after administering medication to ensure that the patient does not manifest any observable adverse response.

7. Pediatrics

Special care must be given when administering medication to pediatric patients because their organs are immature and they might have difficulty absorbing, distributing, and excreting the medication. This is especially true with neonatal patients. Neonatal patients can receive some medication through breast milk. However, because the mother has already metabolized and excreted the medication, less than the original dose is passed into breast milk.

Other medications cannot be given to a mother who is breastfeeding because of the toxic effect of the medication on the baby (unless breastfeeding is interrupted for

24–72 hours). These medications include amphetamines, bromocriptine, cocaine, cyclophosphamide, cyclosporine, doxorubicin, ergotamine, gold salts, lithium, methotrexate, nicotine, and phenindione.

Organs in the neonate might be unable to tolerate the normal doses of some medications. For example, the stomach lacks acid, gastric emptying time is prolonged, the liver and kidneys are immature, and there is a decrease in protein binding.

Administering Medication to Pediatric Patients

There is no standard dose for pediatric patients. The dose is calculated using the patient's weight or body surface area. Some OTC medications specify a dose that is based on the child's age, but these are really based on the average weight of a child within that age range. The dose can become problematic if the child's weight is lower or higher than the average weight of that age group. If a child with a very low weight receives an age-related dose, this might result in an undesirable adverse effect from the medication. When a child who is heavier than average receives an age-related dose, the drug may not have a therapeutic effect.

Before administering medication to a pediatric patient, the healthcare team should consult with the parents to ascertain whether the patient has allergies to food, medications, and the environment; has a family history of allergies; has had any experience with medications and illnesses; or is taking any other medication or herbal remedies.

8. The Elderly

More than 30% of all prescriptions and more than 50% of all OTC medications in the United States are consumed by patients who are over 60 years of age. It is this group of patients who are 3 times more likely to be admitted to a healthcare facility for an adverse reaction to medication; 51% die from these reactions, and 70–80% of the adverse reactions are dose-related.

There are several important reasons for such a high occurrence of adverse response to medication, including the following:

- Multiple medications may be prescribed without discontinuing current medication (polypharmacy), causing an interaction between drugs; see Chapter 2.
- Medication can impair mental and physical capacity, leading to accidental injury.
- Age can increase the sensitivity to drugs and drug-induced disease.
- Absorption of medication is altered because of an increase in gastric pH.

- Distribution of the medication is affected because of a decrease in lean body mass, increased fat stores, a decrease in total body water, decreased serum albumin, and a decrease in blood flow and cardiac output.
- Metabolism changes as enzymatic activity decreases with age and with decreased liver function (as in Reye's syndrome).
- Excretion is impaired because of decreased kidney function.

Assessing the Elderly

Begin assessing an elderly patient by obtaining a complete history of medications used by the patient. This includes all prescription drugs, OTC drugs, home remedies, vitamins, and herbal treatments. Make sure that you determine the medications that have been prescribed and medications that the patient actually takes. Include those that are taken at the patient's discretion. Some patients do not take all of the medications that are prescribed to them because of the cost of the medication or some unpleasant or undesirable side effects. Also note how often the medications are taken.

List all practitioners who prescribed medications for a particular patient, including the patient's primary physician, orthopedist, cardiologist, or other specialist. Create a list of all pharmacies providing medication to that patient. Review the expiration dates for all medications. Ask your patients how they self-medicate, whether they maintain a medication schedule, and if they ever forget to take their medication. If they do, ask what medications they've skipped and what they do when they forget or skip a dose.

Determine whether a particular patient has any barriers to taking medication safely such as allergies, physical handicaps, memory loss, cultural beliefs, and financial constraints. Also, ascertain whether the patient has support from family, friends, and neighbors. Most importantly, be aware of the cost of medication prescribed to the patient. Many elderly patients live on fixed incomes and may be unable to purchase expensive medications—even if the benefit outweighs the cost. Always keep medication for the elderly simple and to a minimum.

Summary

There are five steps in the nursing process: assessment, diagnosis, planning, intervention, and evaluation. The assessment step collects data about the patient that are analyzed and applied to arrive at a nursing diagnosis. A care plan is then developed that describes what must be done to address the symptoms of the nursing diagnosis. The care plan is then enacted during the intervention step, and the results are then evaluated. The care plan terminates if the goals of the plan are achieved or revised if the goals are not achieved. Before any medication is given to a patient, the nurse must assess a number of factors that include the drug order, drug actions, interactions, and contraindications.

Educating the patient about medication is an important responsibility for the nurse. The nurse must explain why the medication is given and how the patient can self-medicate. The nurse must also make sure that the patient and the family know the signs and symptoms of adverse side effects from the medication as well as any toxic effects and dietary considerations to follow while taking the medication.

Cultural factors typically influence patients' beliefs about health and can impact medication prescribed to treat their illnesses. Nurses must put aside their own opinions about those beliefs and work within those limitations when caring for their patients.

Genetic, ethnic, and racial differences play a role in the physiological response to drugs. Some groups of patients are less responsive to certain medications because of genetic factors; other groups of patients can experience a toxic effect because of hereditary traits.

Drugs can have different effects on the very young and the elderly because of physiological changes in their bodies. The very young have immature organs that are not yet able to metabolize, absorb, distribute, and excrete certain drugs.

Likewise, the elderly have mature organs that might have lost the capability to properly process medication. Furthermore, the elderly may require multiple medications simultaneously, which can result in drug interactions that produce adverse side effects.

QUIZ

1. **A medical diagnosis**
   - (a) is the same as a nursing diagnosis.
   - (b) identifies the disease that affects the patient.
   - (c) is a problem statement that identifies the potential or actual health problem.
   - (d) is none of the above.

2. **An expected outcome is**
   - (a) the patient's condition after a care plan is executed.
   - (b) the goal of a care plan.
   - (c) an adverse reaction to a medication.
   - (d) a side effect to a medication.

3. After the patient is shown how to self-medicate, the nurse should
   (a) show a film to the patient on self-medication.
   (b) make sure that the patient's family is shown how to medicate the patient.
   (c) make sure that the patient has the prescription for the medication.
   (d) ask the patient to demonstrate how she/he will self-medicate.

4. A healthcare provider should administer medication to a patient even if the patient's cultural beliefs disagree with receiving the medication.
   (a) True
   (b) False

5. An infant receives a full dose of the drug given to its mother during breastfeeding.
   (a) True
   (b) False

6. A dose for a pediatric patient is determined by
   (a) the patient's weight.
   (b) the patient's height.
   (c) the patient's age.
   (d) the patient's sex.

7. Adverse reaction to medication is a leading cause of death in elderly patients.
   (a) True
   (b) False

8. Which of the following is a standard type of intervention?
   (a) Nurse-initiated intervention
   (b) Physician- or advanced-practitioner-initiated intervention
   (c) Collaborative intervention
   (d) All of the above

9. Knowledge deficit related to language difficulties is a common nursing diagnoses related to drug therapy.
   (a) True
   (b) False

10. NANDA is a guide to nursing diagnosis.
    (a) True
    (b) False

chapter 5

Principles of Medication Administration

Administering medication to a patient can be tricky and downright dangerous unless special precautions are followed to ensure that the patient receives the right drug, the right dose, given at the right time, and using the right route, and that it is given to the right (intended) patient. These criteria are called the "five rights" of medication administration. In this chapter you'll learn the proper way to administer medication and how to avoid common errors that frequently result in improper medication administration that can potentially harm the patient. You'll also learn how to assess the patient to determine whether she/he experiences the intended therapeutic effect of the medication.

1. The Nursing Process and Medication Administration

Assessing the patient is the first step in administering medication. This might seem unusual because the prescriber—prior to writing the prescription for the medication—will have already assessed the patient. However, the patient's condition can change between the prescriber's assessment and the time when the medication is administered. Assessing the patient also provides a baseline for comparison of the patient's reaction to the medication after administering the medication.

The assessment is divided into two areas. First is a general assessment that is necessary for every medication. Then there is an assessment that is required for specific drugs. The general assessment must determine the following criteria:

- **Whether the Therapeutic Action of the Drug Is Appropriate for the Patient:** This, too, appears to be unusual because the prescriber will already have made this determination. However, the nurse is responsible for independently verifying that the drug is appropriate for the patient. This is done by reading the diagnosis in the patient's chart and looking up the medication in the drug manual, which will state the approved use of the drug. If use of that particular drug is not recommended for the patient's condition, then the nurse should contact the prescriber. Nurses may not administer drugs that are being used for purposes other than those approved by the US Federal Drug Administration (FDA). It is important to realize that in some situations, the prescriber will be using the drug for a secondary therapeutic effect that addresses the patient's condition, which is acceptable if that purpose is FDA-approved.

- **Whether the Route Is Appropriate for the Patient:** Some drugs can be administered through more than one route. Although the prescriber specifies a route in the medication order, the patient's current condition might indicate that a different route is appropriate. For example, the prescriber might order antibiotics PO. However, the patient might have a very high fever that requires immediate relief by administration of antibiotics IV. In another situation, the patient might experience stomach pains and vomiting, which is a clear indication that PO is not the desired route. If the route is no longer appropriate, then the nurse should contact the prescriber and obtain an order to use an alternate route that is appropriate for the patient's condition.

- **Determining the Proper Dose for the Patient:** The prescriber will specify the dose in the medication order. Sometimes the dose does not match the prepared dose that the nurse has on hand, thus necessitating that the nurse calculate the dose. For example, the prescriber might write a medication order for 800 mg of ibuprofen. The nurse might have on hand 200-mg tablets and thus will calculate that the patient must be administered 4 of these tablets. With some drugs, the prescriber will order a dose according to the weight of the patient. It is the nurse's responsibility to calculate the actual dose after weighing the patient. For example, the prescriber may order Depakote (divalproex sodium) 10 mg/kg. The patient weights 176 lb. The nurse has 200 mg/5 mL on hand and calculates that the correct dose for the patient is 20 mL. (You'll learn how to perform this calculation in Chapter 7.)

- **Assessment for Contraindications:** The patient might have developed a condition since being assessed by the prescriber that renders administration of the medication inappropriate. The nurse must review the drug's profile in the drug manual to determine the drug's contraindications and then determine whether they apply to the patient. If so, then the nurse must contact the prescriber to advise of the patient's condition. This is particularly important as different healthcare professionals might prescribe the patient drugs. For example, the patient might be scheduled for an angiogram in 24 hours and the prescriber might have a standing medication order for Glucophage. Glucophage reacts with contrast dyes and therefore cannot be administered to the patient within 24 hours of any dye procedures such as an angiogram. However, withholding medications should be done only after the healthcare provider has been notified.

- **Assessment for Side Effects and Adverse Reactions to the Drug:** Drugs can have known side effects, one of which the patient can tolerate and others that result in an adverse reaction. The nurse must review the profile of the drug in the drug manual to determine any side effects and adverse reactions that it might cause and must monitor the patient for such signs and symptoms. The nurse should alert the patient to the possible side effects before administering the medication. In addition, the nurse should prepare to handle a possible adverse reaction that the patient might have to a medication. For example, some opioids such as morphine sulfate can cause respiratory depression. Narcan (naxalone) can reverse the effects of opioids. Keeping Narcan available when administering morphine sulfate in high doses or to a patient who has never received morphine is a safety precaution that is imposed to avoid adverse outcomes.

2. Assessment Required for Specific Drugs

Besides contraindications, the drug's profile in the drug manual also provides the nurse with the pharmacologic response of the drug (see Chapter 2)—how the drug works in the body. Knowing this, the nurse can assess the patient to determine whether the patient's body will be able to metabolize and eliminate the medication.

Here are the areas that the nurse needs to consider:

- **Absorption:** The patient must be able to absorb the medication. For example, medication administered PO is absorbed in the GI tract (stomach and small intestine). A patient with GI disturbances such as vomiting or diarrhea will not be able to absorb the medication.

- **Distribution:** Once absorbed, the medication must be distributed throughout the body. In order for this to occur, some drugs must bind to protein, which carries drug particles through the veins and arteries. If the patient has low protein levels, some drug particles are unable to bind to the protein and the unbound drug particles are free drug, which can possibly produce a toxic effect. For example, Dilantin (phenytoin) binds to albumin. If the patient has a low albumin level, there will be less Dilantin bound to protein. The patient will be receiving the proper therapeutic dose, but because much of it is not bound to protein, the serum levels of free drug will be too high, causing toxicity.

- **Metabolism:** The liver breaks down drugs so that they can be excreted from the body. If the patient's liver is not functioning properly, then the drug particles are not metabolized and cannot be excreted from the body. This results in a buildup of the drug and can possibly cause toxicity in the patient. It is important to remember that inadequate liver function is not always caused by liver disease. Age influences liver function. For example, newborns have an immature liver, while an elderly person may have decreased liver function.

- **Excretion:** The kidney is the main organ that excretes medication, although some medication is excreted in bile, feces, respiration, saliva, and sweat. The patient is unable to excrete drugs if these routes are not functioning properly. The nurse should be aware of the route in which the drug is excreted from the body and then determine whether that route is fully functional before administering the medication to the patient.

In addition to the pharmacologic response of the drug, the nurse must also assess other aspects of the patient and the medication:

- **Age:** The very young and the elderly are more sensitive to drugs than is the average adult because there is a decrease in gastric secretion, resulting in poor absorption through the GI tract. The elderly are particularly sensitive to barbiturates and CNS depressants. Therefore, it is critical that the nurse assess the patient's age before administering medication and carefully monitor very young and elderly patients afterward for adverse side effects.

- **Body Weight:** The prescriber might order medication given at the recommended dose. However, the recommended dose is typically for a patient whose body weight is within the average range (70 kg for an adult). The medication might have a different effect if the patient's body weight falls outside this range. For example, the recommended dose might be too strong for a very thin patient, resulting in a toxic effect. Similarly, the recommended dose might be too low for an obese patient and never reach the therapeutic level. This is particularly important to assess when administering medications such as antineoplastics (anticancer drugs), where a low therapeutic level can have a nontherapeutic effect for the patient, resulting in an undesirable outcome. Using body weight to determine drug dose will avoid this problem.

- **Pharmacogenetic:** Genetic factors might seriously influence the response to a drug. Depending on the medication, a patient might have a genetically based adverse reaction to the drug. Therefore, in assessing the patient, the nurse must ascertain whether the patient's parents, siblings, or other close relatives have had an adverse reaction to the medication.

- **Time:** Medication must be given to the patient at the most opportune time during the day to ensure that the therapeutic effect is attained. Some drugs are effective only if taken with meals, while other medications cannot be taken with meals. Similarly, certain drugs are more effective if taken at bedtime. Every agency will have a policy regarding the time when the medication should be given and the range of time allowed. For example, a medication scheduled for 10 A.M. may be given between 9:30 and 10:30 A.M.

- **Food-Drug Interaction:** Certain types of foods can adversely affect the drug's therapeutic effect by increasing, delaying, and even preventing absorption of the medication. Furthermore, food may cause the patient to experience an adverse reaction, as in the case with phenelzine sulfate (Nardil), which is a monoamine oxidase (MAO) inhibitor antidepressant. Nardil cannot be given with foods that were prepared with bacteria or molds or foods containing a tyramine preservative, such as cheese, sour cream, beer, wine, figs, raisins, bananas, and avocados. The nurse must assess whether the drug has a contraindication with food and must educate the patient about this food-drug interaction.

- **Drug-Drug Interaction:** The nurse should be aware that the combination of drugs administered to the patient may have a negative effect. Some drugs when administered together might increase or decrease the therapeutic effectiveness of either or both medications by competing for the same receptor sites in the body. Furthermore, a combination of some medications may produce toxicity or a fatal condition such as anaphylaxis. Sometimes there is more than one provider prescribing medications. The prescribers should be notified before medications are administered if there is a possibility of a drug-drug interaction.

- **Drug History, Tolerance, and the Cumulative Effect:** Continued use of a medication might lessen the therapeutic effect of the drug because the patient's body becomes tolerant to the medication. The nurse must assess the patient's drug history and monitor the patient for signs and symptoms indicating that the drug is having a therapeutic effect. One such example would be the absence of seizures if the patient is taking phenytoin (Dilantin), an antiseizure medication. Another concern is the drug buildup in the patient's body. The patient may be unable to metabolize and excrete the medication as rapidly as new doses are administered. The result is a cumulative effect that can cause toxicity. The patient should be monitored for signs of drug buildup. For example, ataxia (muscular incoordination), nystagmus (rhythmic oscillation of eyes), and double vision are signs of toxic levels of Dilantin.

3. Administering Medication

Medication can be administered once the nurse assesses the patient and determines that the medication can be administered safely. The nurse follows implementation procedures for administering medication.

- **Checking the Prescriber's Medication Order:** The initial step in administering medication is to read the medication order that is written by the prescriber to ensure that the proper medication, in the correct dose, is administered to the patient. The prescriber's medication order is found in the patient's chart.

- **Checking the Medication Administration Record (MAR) or Electronic Medical Record (EMR):** *The medication administration record* is a transcription of the prescriber's medication order. Often the MAR is a computer-generated document, but sometimes there will be handwritten entries in the MAR. Compare the MAR with the prescriber's medication order to ensure that the proper medication, dose, and other aspects of the medication order have been properly transcribed. Many medications are entered directly into the EMR by the prescriber. This avoids the possibility of an error in transcription. However, the nurse is still responsible for checking all of the above before administering the drug.

- **Checking All Medications Prescribed to the Patient:** The nurse should check all medications prescribed to the patient even if she/he will not be administering all of these medications while taking care of the patient. The MAR/EMR lists all medications that the patient receives, including those already given to the patient and medication that has been discontinued. It is critical for the nurse to review all medications and not only those that will be given on the nurse's shift because previous medications may still be active in the patient's body. Remember that some drugs have a long half-life, which may result in a potential conflict with another medication days after it was administered to the patient.

- **Checking the Patient's Allergies:** Although the patient's chart might indicate the absence of any allergies to medication or food, the nurse must review whether the patient has any allergies before administering medication. Sometimes the patient might not have recalled any allergies during the history taking, but will recall an allergy after being questioned again by the nurse later.

- **Creating Your Own Medication Administration Worksheet:** Although the MAR/EMR lists medications and the times when they are to be administered, the patient may be scheduled for tests and procedures that conflict with the medication schedule. It is best to create a medication administration worksheet that schedules the medication and the patient's other activities, so that there will be only one schedule for that patient.

- **Checking PRN Medications:** It is common for some medications to be administered to the patient by the nurse on an as-needed basis (PRN) such as analgesics (pain medication). The nurse must determine the type(s) and time of PRN medication administration before giving any further medication. This avoids any potential interaction between medications.

Preparing the Medication

After ensuring that the medication can be administered properly to the patient, you (the nurse) can administer it by following these steps:

1. Wash your hands. This is the best way to prevent infection.

2. Prepare the medication that you will be giving at this time. Do not prepare all medications at once. It is possible that someone else may have to administer the other medications. You should *never* give medication that someone else has prepared.

3. Prepare medications in a quiet area to ensure that you will not be interrupted.

4. Double-check your math when calculating doses. Have a colleague verify your calculations if necessary.

5. Make sure that all of the patient's medications that will be administered during the shift are available and in the correct dose and quantity.

6. Compare the medication with that listed on the MAR/EMR. Sometimes the pharmacy substitutes a generic drug for a brand-name drug. Always look up the medication in the drug manual if you do not recognize the name of the drug.

7. Check the name of the medication 3 times: (a) when you remove it, (b) when you prepare it, and (c) before returning it to the drawer or disposing of its wrapper or container. If the medication is wrapped, then bring the wrapper with you to the patient's room and check the wrapper again before administering the medication to the patient.

At the Patient's Bedside

After medication is prepared, it is taken to the patient's room, where you (the nurse) will administer it to the patient. In doing so, you must follow precautions to ensure that the medication is administered safely. Here is how it is done:

1. Wash your hands.

2. Introduce yourself to the patient.

3. Ask the patient to state her/his complete name. Do not assist the patient by asking "Are you Mr. Jones?" The patient should state her/his name without your help if possible.

4. Compare the patient's name and number on the patient's identification band against the patient's name and number on the MAR.

5. Question the patient regarding any allergies to food or medication. The patient may be aware of food allergies such as shellfish, but may be unaware of allergies to medication. However, patients who are allergic to shellfish are also allergic to some medications.

6. Examine the patient's identification band to see if there is any history of allergies. Allergies may be noted on the identification band.

7. Assist the patient into a comfortable position to administer the medication.

8. Ascertain whether the patient knows what medication is being administered and the reason why this medication was prescribed. The response provides insight into the patient's knowledge about her/his condition and treatment. This will give you a perfect opportunity to educate the patient about her/his condition, treatment, and medication.

9. Make sure that the patient sees the medication and knows whether it is a tablet or a liquid. Stop immediately if the patient doesn't recognize the medication as the drug that she/he received previously. Recheck the order. The dose may have changed, a different medication may have been substituted, or there may be an error in the medication. Always pay attention to the patient's response and recheck the order.

10. Make sure that you have baseline vital signs, laboratory results (often referred to as "labs"), and other patient data before administering the medication. To determine the patient's reaction to the drug, the baseline can be compared to vital signs, labs, and other patient data taken after the patient receives the medication.

11. Instruct the patient about the possible side effects of the medication, and take precautions to ensure the patient's safety, such as raising the bedside rails and instructing the patient to remain in bed until the side effects subside.

12. Stay with the patient until all the medications have been swallowed. Remember that the patient has the right to refuse medication. Notify the prescriber if this occurs.

13. Properly dispose of the medication and the supplies used to administer it. Do not leave the medication at the patient's bedside unless required to do so by the medication order.

14. Wash your hands before leaving the patient's room.

15. Document in the MAR/EMR that you administered the medication to the patient.

Handy Tips When Administering Medication

Medication can leave a bitter or otherwise unpleasant taste in the patient's mouth. You can minimize this adverse effect by giving the patient ice chips prior to administering the medication. Ice chips numb the taste buds so that the patient will be unable to taste the medication.

Give unpleasant-tasting medications first, followed by more pleasant-tasting liquids. This shortens the time during which the patient experiences the unpleasant taste. The patient is left with the more pleasant-tasting medication in her/his mouth. Use the liquid form of the medication where possible because most patients find it easier to ingest a liquid. Offer water after giving a medication unless water is contraindicated.

Administer medication to a patient who needs extra assistance in swallowing it after you give medication to your other patients. In this way, you can devote the necessary time to assist this patient without being pressured to administer medication to your other patients.

Avoid Medication Errors

Medication errors are the most common cause of patient injuries in a hospital. It is therefore critical that the nurse avoid situations that frequently result in medication errors. If an error occurs, assess the patient and notify the nurse in charge and the physician. Follow your hospital's policy for preparing an incident report. Review the steps that caused the error to occur.

Here are ways to avoid common errors:

- Avoid distractions when preparing medication.
- Avoid conversations while preparing medication.
- Administer only those medications that you prepare.
- Pour or prepare medication only from containers that have complete, easily legible labels.
- Do not transfer drugs from one container to another.
- Do not pour medications directly into your hand.
- Do not give medications that have expired.
- Do not guess about medication and doses. If the medication order is handwritten but not legible, do not guess. Always ask the prescriber.
- Do not administer drugs that are discolored, contain sediment, or are cloudy, unless this is a normal state for the medication.
- Do not leave medications by the bedside or with visitors.
- Keep medications in clear sight. Do not give a particular medication if the patient states that she/he is allergic to it or to that particular drug group or says that it does not look the same as the drug that she/he normally takes.
- Use the patient's name and case number on the identification band to identify the patient.
- Do not administer medication with food or beverages unless the drug manual or prescriber indicates that the medication can be given with food and beverages.

Proper Disposal of Medication

Hospitals have strict policies that govern how unused medications and supplies used to administer medication are handled. Here are steps typically found in hospital policies:

- Do not recap needles.
- Discard needles and syringes in an appropriate container that prevents others from receiving a needle stick.
- Dispose of medication in the sink or toilet and not in the trash.
- Return controlled substances to the pharmacy.
- Dispose of controlled substances in the presence of another licensed healthcare worker who will sign as a witness to the disposal.
- Discard unused solutions from ampules before discarding the ampule.

Administering Medication at Home

The nurse is responsible for educating the patient on how to self-medicate at home by providing the do's and don'ts of administering the medication. The nurse must do or instruct the patient to do the following:

- Store the medication properly. Some medication, such as insulin, should be refrigerated.
- Always label the date and time when the medication was opened.
- Keep the medication in a locked cabinet away from the reach of children and pets.
- Explain the reason why the patient is taking the medication and how often it is given.
- Explain what to do if the patient misses a dose.
- Describe the signs and symptoms of the toxic effect of the medication if the patient takes more than the prescribed dose.
- Describe the signs and symptoms of side effects and adverse reactions that might occur when taking the medication.
- Explain negative interactions that the medication might have with certain foods.
- Develop a system for self-medication for patients who have poor eyesight and decreased mental capacity. For example, a patient can use specially marked containers for each day of the week, and a relative or friend can fill those containers with the appropriate medication. The patient is then taught to open the proper container each day.
- Give the patient a list of medications, doses, and administration frequency, and include the name of the prescriber so that the patient can keep the list in a wallet or pocketbook.
- Suggest that the patient wear a MedicAlert bracelet or other jewelry that identifies the patient as having allergies or chronic illnesses.

4. Evaluating the Patient After Administering Medication

The nurse must assess the patient after administering the medication to determine whether the medication has had the desired therapeutic effect. To do this, the nurse compares the patient's current vital signs, labs, and other pertinent patient data with baseline information. The patient should also be assessed after the medication has reached its onset and peak times. Early or late assessments could be misleading and could provide false information about the effectiveness of the drug.

The nurse must suspend administration of further doses of the medication if the patient shows any signs or symptoms indicating an adverse reaction to the medication. The prescriber must be notified immediately of the patient's condition.

The nurse must also note any side effect of the medication experienced by the patient and how well the patient tolerates the side effect. If the patient has a low tolerance to the side effect, then the nurse needs to notify the prescriber. The prescriber might substitute a different medication or prescribe other medication to alleviate the side effect.

The nurse must determine whether the patient is receiving the intended therapeutic effect from the medication. This is critical when giving pain medication. Doses are often ordered for the average-weight patient. Patients who are very thin or obese may be receiving too much or too little medication. Prescribers are also concerned about patients developing tolerance to or dependence on pain medication and may under-prescribe the dosage or frequency or administration. If the nurse accurately assesses the patient's response to the drug, the dose or frequency may be adjusted to provide appropriate relief from pain.

5. Controlling Narcotics

Special precautions are necessary for storing and handling narcotics because the manufacture, sale, and use of narcotics are controlled by federal legislation. Here are the steps that must be taken to secure narcotics.

- Keep narcotics in a double-locked drawer or a closet.
- One nurse per shift must keep the keys to the narcotic drawer on her/his person.
- A sign-out sheet must be used to control the inventory of narcotics.
- Document on the MAR/EMR or similar records the time(s) when a patient is given a narcotic.

Controlled substances (narcotics) are generally counted at least once per shift. The amount of the drug available is compared with the numbers that have been used for patients and signed for on the narcotics form. Each agency has a policy to govern this activity and to determine what action should be followed if the count is not accurate.

Summary

Assessing the patient is the first step when administering medication. Ensure that the patient is receiving the proper medication at the proper dose because the patient's condition might have changed since the prescriber assessed the patient.

The assessment is divided into two areas. First, a general assessment is required and then assess for specific medications. The general assessment determines several factors that include the right drug, dose, and route for the patient. The assessment also determines the contraindications to and potential side effects and adverse effects of the medication. The specific assessment examines the pharmacologic response of the medication in relation to the patient's capability to absorb, distribute, metabolize, and excrete the medication.

Having determined that the medication is appropriate for the patient, the nurse prepares to administer it by verifying the prescriber's medication order and comparing it to other medications that the patient received to determine potential interactions. The nurse also determines whether the patient has allergies to the medication.

The medication is prepared in a quiet place without any interruptions. At the bedside, the nurse follows safety procedures to ensure that the medication is being administered to the proper patient. The nurse verifies the patient's identity and that the patient knows why the medication is being given. Baseline data (such as vital signs and labs) is obtained by the nurse. They will be compared to similar data collected after the onset of the medication.

The nurse will monitor the patient after the medication is administered and look for signs and symptoms of adverse reactions to the medication.

Now that you have a good understanding of how to administer medication, in the next chapter we'll take a look at the different routes used to administered medication.

QUIZ

1. **The desired action of a medication is called**
   (a) its medication reaction.
   (b) its safety action.
   (c) its therapeutic action.
   (d) none of the above.

2. **What can inadvertently cause a patient to receive an insufficient dose of a medication?**
   (a) Genetic substitution of a brand medication
   (b) Allergies
   (c) Obesity
   (d) Being underweight

3. **Why should Narcan be on hand when administering an opioid?**

   (a) It reverses the narcotic effect.

   (b) It can be substituted for the narcotic.

   (c) It is mixed with a narcotic to extend the peak time of the narcotic.

   (d) It is mixed with a narcotic to shorten the narcotic's onset.

4. **The body weight of a patient can never influence the dose of a medication.**

   (a) True

   (b) False

5. **A patient who is allergic to shellfish may be allergic to some medications.**

   (a) True

   (b) False

6. **The purpose of collecting baseline patient data is**

   (a) to adhere to legal requirements.

   (b) to legally protect the nurse.

   (c) to ensure that they can be compared to data on the patient's condition after the medication is administered, to determine the patient's reaction to the medication.

   (d) to determine the patient's condition before administering the medication.

7. **It is acceptable to administer medication to a patient that is prepared by another licensed practitioner.**

   (a) True

   (b) False

8. **Ice chips are given to the patient prior to administering unpleasant-tasting medication because**

   (a) the ice chips dilute the medication.

   (b) the ice chips numb the taste buds.

   (c) the ice chip moisturizes the oral cavity.

   (d) none of the above.

9. **The prescriber's medication order is compared to the MAR to ensure that the medication has been properly transcribed to the MAR.**

   (a) True

   (b) False

10. **A prescriber's medication order is always accurate and should not be questioned.**

    (a) True

    (b) False

chapter 4

Substance Abuse

Substance abuse is probably one of the most publicized aspects of pharmacology—and the least understood by patients. Substance abuse includes prescribed medications, illicit drugs, and alcohol. Healthcare providers obviously do not prescribe illicit drugs or alcohol to patients. But they do prescribe analgesics (pain relievers), which are controlled medications. They are called *opioid analgesics*, and they work by interacting with nerve cells in the brain and nervous system to produce a euphoric effect as well as to reduce pain. This class of drugs includes oxycodone, hydrocodone, codeine, morphine, fentanyl, and other opioids. Patients—as well as healthcare professionals (see Section 3, "Healthcare Professionals and Substance Abuse," later in this chapter)—can become dependent on these medications. Several studies report that patients who were prescribed opioids when discharged from the emergency department were still using opioid analgesia at 3 months postdischarge. All healthcare providers need to understand the signs of substance abuse and signs and symptoms of withdrawal.

This chapter explores drugs that are commonly abused and discusses how to detect substance abuse.

1. Drug Misuse and Abuse

Substance abuse affects all socioeconomic groups and has become a major medical, social, economic, and interpersonal challenge for society. According to the Centers for Disease Control, 1 in 70 people in the United States is a substance abuser. Of the 20.5 million Americans who had a substance abuse disorder in 2015, 2 million had a disorder involving prescription pain medications.

Medication *misuse* occurs, for example, whenever a person indiscriminately uses a medication that was prescribed for someone else. Medication *abuse* occurs when a person continually self-medicates, resulting in a physical and/or a psychological dependence on the drug.

An *addiction* occurs when a person experiences three or more of the characteristics described in the following four paragraphs over a 6-month period.

Tolerance

Tolerance occurs when an increasingly large dose of the medication is required to achieve the same physiological reaction. It is important to realize that tolerance is not addiction. In some treatments, patients commonly develop a tolerance for a drug, but do not become addicted to it. The prescriber increases the dose to achieve the same therapeutic effect. The medication is discontinued once the treatment is completed.

Withdrawal

Withdrawal is a physiological and/or psychological reaction that a person experiences when a medication is no longer administered. Prescribers properly manage treatment by gradually decreasing the dose and/or frequency of administration of the drug to avoid withdrawal symptoms in a patient.

Increased Dosages

A person who is addicted tends to regularly increase the dosage of the medication in an attempt to increase her/his physiological reaction to the drug, such as reaching a higher state of euphoria for a longer period of time.

Uncontrollable Use

A person addicted to drugs is unable to control the urge to self-medicate. The desire for the drug must be satisfied as quickly as possible.

Taking the Drug—A Scheduled Event

The person spends an inordinate amount of time acquiring the drug, self-medicating, and recovering from the effects of the drug. This scenario is evident with a patient who is addicted to sedatives and whose thoughts are focused on how to obtain the next dose.

A specific time in the day must then be set aside to administer the medication and to avoid contact with other people until the visible effects of the drug have worn off.

Priority Over Activities of Daily Life

Daily activities are scheduled around times when the patient acquires, uses, and recovers from the effects of the drug. Everything else, including family and work, takes a backseat to the addiction.

Addiction Continuing Despite Negative Consequences

Self-medication continues regardless of the repercussions. Individuals who are addicted to drugs will begin to arrive late for work and will then gradually miss entire workdays until they ultimately lose their jobs. However, the self-medication will continue.

2. Behavioral Patterns of Addiction

Besides the clinical signs of addition mentioned in the previous section, certain behavioral patterns are common in a person who abuses medication. These behavioral patterns deviate from what is considered normal behavior.

For example, a substance abuser may fail to adhere to a routine and will be late for work or school or will be absent for the entire day. The person may have poor hygiene and appear disheveled, especially when compared to her/his coworkers or classmates. Family and social relationships become strained, because craving for the drug or being under the influence of the medication makes it nearly impossible for the addicted person to interact normally. The person is also in frequent need of medical attention as a result of self-medication. The medication itself might disrupt normal body functions or place the person in a weakened state and thus vulnerable to harm.

For various reasons, a substance abuser experiences more legal problems than the average person. The police might arrest the person for illegally obtaining or possessing the medication or for driving while under the influence of the drug. A substance abuser is exposed to unsavory characters who are involved in the illicit drug trade. These interactions can create unsafe and violent situations for all people involved.

Denial is the most common behavior exhibited by drug abusers. Because the addiction may be gradual and the abuser is often in an altered mental state as a result of the effects of the drug, the person may be unable to recognize the addiction. As the addiction worsens, the drug abuser is unwilling to admit to the problem and the denial continues.

3. Healthcare Professionals and Substance Abuse

Fans of the television show *ER* may recall how Dr. John Carter became dependent on pain medication that was legally prescribed to treat pain from a nearly deadly attack he experienced in the emergency room. His dependence drove him to steal drugs from the hospital to feed his addiction.

ER is fiction, but its depiction of a healthcare professional becoming a substance abuser is well founded as ≤15% of overall addiction to opioids have been attributed to healthcare professionals for more than 130 years. Many healthcare professionals who become drug abusers feel that they can self-medicate without becoming addicted because they know when to stop taking the medication. Craving for the drug quickly overshadows their critical thinking.

Healthcare professionals self-administer drugs for a number of reasons.

Performance Enhancement

Some healthcare professionals such as interns and residents are on duty for 36 hours at a stretch, during which time they make many critical decisions. Some feel that they need a boost to maintain a high performance level, especially after being on duty for so many hours without sleep.

Self-Treatment

A healthcare provider knows how to recognize symptoms of a disease and knows what medications are used to treat the disease, so it makes sense to self-treat when she/he becomes ill. This is especially true when the healthcare provider is depressed, anxious, or in pain. The information used to diagnose personal illness is subjective, and as the craving for the medication dose increases, it interferes with the objective reasoning that the healthcare provider normally uses when assessing patients.

Easy Accessibility to Drugs

Drugs are available to many healthcare professionals, especially in a healthcare facility where they administer medication. Even under tight controls, drugs can be diverted by healthcare professionals with little chance of being caught. For example, they may give the patient half the prescribed dose and keep the other half for themselves.

Recreational Use

After a long shift, healthcare professionals need to relax. The fastest way to do so may be to take a pill or inject a drug. However, additional doses may be needed to remain in that relaxed mental state. Eventually, the healthcare professional may become addicted to the drug.

4. Detecting Substance Abuse

The term *substance abuser* conjures up images of an unkempt, malnourished person who sleeps on the streets. In reality, the person working alongside you or living in the house across the street from you could be a substance abuser because many substance abusers go to great lengths to hide their addictions.

However, regardless of how well substance abusers try to conceal their addictions, eventually the addictions cause them to change, and it is those changes that become signs of substance abuse. The signs are described in the following paragraphs.

Disorganization

Many of the drugs used to alleviate pain or anxiety can lead to addiction. These drugs alter the thought process. Consequently, individuals are unable to think clearly and logically. Simple tasks can become overwhelming, and eventually an addicted individual will become scattered or disorganized. For example, taking a medication for pain creates a sense of distance from the real world. Trying to add a column of numbers or serve food to customers will become confusing, and an individual may be unable to decide what to do first.

Frequent Absences

Some drugs can create periods of wakefulness that lead to a "crash." The individual may sleep because of fatigue or want to sleep off the effects of a pain or an anxiety-relieving drug that causes drowsiness. Individuals simply don't wake up to go to work, or they may experience periods of withdrawal from reality that result in an inability to remember to go to work or school.

Inability to Get Along With Colleagues

As the addiction worsens, individuals have difficulty with interpersonal relationships for several reasons. One reason is the simple fact that nothing really matters anymore except getting more of the drug. In addition, the disorganization and frequent absences make a drug abuser an unpopular colleague. Coworkers begin to suspect that there is a problem and put pressure on the individual to "clean up her (his) act." This can deteriorate into very unpleasant episodes at work and at home.

Changes in Appearance and Personal Hygiene

The altered mental state experienced by drug abusers also changes their self-perceptions. Addicted individuals may be unaware of how they look or even forget to take a shower and change their clothing regularly. The need to find more of the drug can also be time-consuming and can interfere with regular activities that include personal hygiene.

Slurred Speech During off-Hours

A side effect of the most abused drugs is slurred speech and staggering gait. Responses are slowed, and the individual may appear to be intoxicated. Frequently a drug abuser will make a great effort to appear normal during working or school hours. However, after-hours may become the time to take more of the drug, and the side effects become more pronounced or obvious.

5. Delayed Action

Drug abuse in the healthcare field can go undetected because of the structure of the healthcare industry. Healthcare providers may be less closely supervised than in other industries. For example, physicians work independently and come under scrutiny only in a healthcare facility setting. Furthermore, healthcare professionals are capable of diagnosing and treating themselves, and may not request or want another healthcare provider to perform an objective assessment that might reveal substance abuse. Acknowledging substance abuse may place the individual at risk of suspension or revocation of the license to practice.

There can also be a "white wall of silence" among healthcare professionals to hide their substance abuse tendencies from their colleagues, who might report the abuse. Although the colleagues of a substance abuser might want to help their addicted coworker, no one wants to be responsible for a colleague losing her/his license—or to expose oneself to inadvertently making false accusations.

Silence is not the right course of action. First, there is an ethical obligation to report suspected abuse to protect patients who are being treated by the healthcare provider. Healthcare facilities and regulatory boards are sensitive to the need to maintain confidentiality during the handling of the allegation and subsequent inquiry. Second, the addicted person actually becomes a patient and should be given the best and most appropriate care. That care includes treatment for the addiction. Keeping silent about suspicion of addiction is actually harmful to the substance abuser and violates the ethical responsibilities of the healthcare provider.

Substance abuse is considered a handicap. Therefore, the healthcare provider who is employed by a healthcare facility may be protected by state and federal employment discrimination laws such as the Rehabilitation Act of 1973 (29 USC, § 706). This act requires employers to continue employment of a substance abuser as long as the employee can perform her/his job function and is not a threat to safety or property. This means that the healthcare provider's responsibility might be temporarily reassigned until treatment is completed.

Drug Testing

Drug testing is the most common method used to determine whether a person has taken medication or illicit drugs recently. Many businesses, government agencies, and healthcare facilities require prospective employees to be screened for drugs. In addition, employees might be required to undergo random drug testing or drug testing under special circumstances (such as medication unaccounted for in the work area).

Testing for drug overdose or poisoning is best done with blood. The immediate levels found can determine what treatment would be appropriate. Screening to determine whether someone is using drugs inappropriately is commonly done with urine testing. Urine testing can detect drugs used days or even a week before the test is performed. As false-positive and false-negative results can occur, caution should be exercised when interpreting the results. When asked whether they are taking any kind of medication, individuals should include prescription, OTC, and herbal remedies. For example, traces of diphenhydramine (Benadryl)—a commonly used antihistamine medication—will be found in urine and will cause the person to test positive for methadone.

Whenever the result of a urine test is found to be positive for drugs, the person should undergo another test for that specific medication to confirm the results. Results from the second test are used to identify a false positive that might be generated by the first test. Again, urine testing is done, but the request is to screen only for the specific drug identified in the first test. Blood levels may also be obtained to determine the immediate use of drugs.

Drug testing only gives evidence that the individual has used or been exposed to a drug but does not indicate any particular pattern of drug use or the degree of dependence. Table 4–1 shows the length of time during which traces of popular drugs remain in the body. The most commonly misused and abused drugs are listed in Table 4–2.

6. Substances That Can Be Abused

Nearly all drugs that are abused produce a desirable effect such as altering the state of the mind and filling a void in a person's life. Some professionals believe that a person who has a low threshold for frustration, a fear of failure, and a feeling of

TABLE 4–1 Length of Time That Substances Remain in Urine	
Drug	Time That Substance Is Detectable in Urine
Alcohol	<1 day
Amphetamines	≤1–3 days
Barbiturates	≤1 day short-acting; 2–3 weeks long-acting
Cocaine	≤2–4 days
Methadone	≤3–5 days
Marijuana	
Single use	≤3–5 days
Chronic use	≤29 days
Opioids—short-acting	≤3–4 days
PCP	2–4 days

inadequacy is more likely to abuse drugs. Those who abuse drugs do so because they are bored; feel pressured by their peers; seek relief from conflict, an escape from reality, or pleasure; are affluent and want to experiment; or feel inadequate, ashamed, and depressed.

The following four characteristics describe drugs that are frequently abused:

1. The drug creates an altered state of consciousness.

2. Prolonged use of the drug creates a tolerance to the drug.

3. The desired effect is rapid.

4. Withdrawal symptoms develop if the drug is stopped after prolonged use.

7. Dependence Versus Tolerance

There is an important difference between drug dependence and drug tolerance, although sometimes these terms are used interchangeably. *Drug dependence* occurs when the patient has a psychological and/or physical dependence on the drug that results in withdrawal symptoms that can become unbearable for the patient to endure. Relief comes only when the patient is administered a dose of the drug.

Drug tolerance occurs when the concentration of a drug no longer has a continuing therapeutic effect. This happens because receptor sites in the effective tissues adapt to the prescribed level of drug. The only way to regain the therapeutic effect is to increase the concentration of the drug.

TABLE 4–2 The Most Commonly Misused and Abused Drugs as Reported by the National Surveillance Agency Drug Abuse Warning Network (DAWN)

Drug	Description
Xanthines	This is a class of drugs that includes caffeine. These drugs are used in coffee, tea, chocolate, and colas; affect the CNS; and are the most frequently abused drugs.
Nicotine	This drug is used in tobacco products, affects the CNS, and is one of the most frequently misused and abused drugs.
Ethyl alcohol	This drug is used in distilled spirits and beverages, affects the CNS, and is one of the most frequently misused and abused drugs.
Anticholinergics	This is a class of drugs that includes Robinal, which is referred to as the "date rape" drug and affects the CNS.
Steroids	This is a performance-enhancing drug that affects the CNS.
Amphetamines	This is a class of drugs that includes dextroamphetamine, "dexies," and methamphetamine (commonly referred to as "speed" and "crystal meth"). These drugs affect the CNS.
Pentazocine	This drug creates a morphine-like effect, is also known as Talwin, and affects the CNS.
L-Dopa	This drug is used to alleviate some of the symptoms of Parkinson's disease; it causes an alteration in feelings, thoughts, and perceptions.
Cocaine	This is a leading drug (ie, one of the most frequently abused drugs); its use often results in visits to the emergency department and can cause tachycardia (rapid heart rate), increased blood pressure, chills, fever, agitation, nervousness, confusion, inability to remain still, nausea, vomiting, abdominal pain, increased sweating, rapid breathing, and dilated ocular pupils. Cocaine use can rapidly advance to CNS hemorrhage, congestive failure, convulsions, delirium, and death.
Heroin	This is a leading drug; its use often results in visits to the emergency department. Heroin is a prodrug and is converted in the liver to morphine with the same side effects.
Morphine	This is a leading drug; its use frequently results in visits to the emergency department. Morphine is an opioid narcotic analgesic. Side effects include sedation, decreased blood pressure, increased sweating, flushed face, constipation, dizziness, drowsiness, and nausea and vomiting.
Acetaminophen	This drug is commonly known as Tylenol. It is a leading drug; its use often results in visits to the emergency department. It is commonly used in overdoses and can cause serious kidney problems and death.

(Continued)

TABLE 4–2 The Most Commonly Misused and Abused Drugs as Reported by the National Surveillance Agency Drug Abuse Warning Network (DAWN) (Continued)

Aspirin	This is a leading drug; its use often results in visits to the emergency department. Aspirin abuse can cause gastric (stomach) irritation, which can lead to ulcers and subsequent gastric hemorrhage (bleeding).
Alprazolam	Known as Xanax, this is an antianxiety and antipanic agent. Several of the side effects include episodes of violent and aggressive behavior, seizures, delirium, and other withdrawal reactions.
Marijuana/hashish	These are *Cannabis* drugs that seem to act as CNS depressants. The effects are mental relaxation and euphoria and decreased inhibitions.
Diazepam	This drug, commonly known as Valium, is used for short-term relief of anxiety symptoms. Side effects include drowsiness, fatigue, and ataxia (muscular incoordination). Overdose can result in somnolence (sleepiness), confusion, diminished reflexes, and coma.
Ibuprofen	This is a commonly used nonsteroidal anti-inflammatory drug (NSAID). Side effects and overdose can result in gastrointestinal bleeding or a metabolic acidosis.
PCP/PCP combinations	PCP is a hallucinogenic drug that can cause violent and aggressive behavior.
Lorazepam	This drug is commonly known as Ativan. Its use often causes an alteration in thoughts, feelings, and perceptions.
Benzodiazepines	This medication can cause an alteration in thoughts, feelings, and perceptions.
Amitriptyline	This drug is commonly known as Elavil. It is a mood elevator and can cause an alteration in thoughts, feelings, and perceptions.
Clonazepam	This drug is commonly known as Klonopin. It is used to inhibit seizure activity. Side effects can be mild drowsiness, ataxia, and behavioral disturbances that are manifested as aggression, irritability, and agitation.
d-Propoxyphene	This drug is commonly known as Darvon. It is an opioid analgesic that can cause an alteration in sensory perception, which includes euphoria, dizziness, drowsiness, hypotension, nausea, and vomiting.

Tolerance also has a metabolic effect commonly referred to as *pharmacologic tolerance*. Prolonged exposure to a drug increases its excretion from the body. This means that there is a lower concentration of the drug in the plasma that is distributed throughout the body.

8. Pathophysiologic Changes Occurring in Substance Abuse

Drug abusers frequently exhibit pathophysiologic changes that require treatment concurrently with their drug addiction treatments. These debilitating changes are malnutrition, dehydration, and hypovitaminosis.

In addition, these patients can experience respiratory diseases such as pneumonia, blood clots (pulmonary emboli), and abscesses.

Furthermore, drug abusers rarely use aseptic techniques for administering drugs intravenously, which can lead to localized and systemic infections such as endocarditis (infection of the lining of the heart), HIV, and sepsis (infection of the entire circulatory system). Drug abusers also incur cellulitis (infection in the tissues), sclerosis (scaring of the veins), phlebitis (irritation of veins), and skin abscesses.

Drug abusers are always at risk of overdosing because the active ingredients in illegal drugs are frequently adulterated with dangerous substances such as amphetamines, benzodiazepines, hallucinogens, and alcohol. This renders the potency of the drug unreliable, and the risk of death from an accidental overdose is high. For example, there are medications such as naloxone hydrochloride (Narcan), which is used to reverse an opioid overdose. This medication can be delivered via an intravenous route or intranasally (by nose). There has recently been a move to make this medication available to unlicensed individuals in an attempt to reduce the number of deaths from an opioid overdose.

9. Cultural Aspects of Substance Abuse

The views of drug use differ among cultures around the world. Some drugs considered illegal in one culture are accepted in another culture. Alcohol, caffeine, and nicotine are addictive drugs that are widely accepted in the United States and elsewhere throughout the world.

Cannabis use, on the other hand, is illegal in certain states in the United States and in many other countries. There is much controversy about the use of cannabis, and many states have legalized its use for both medicinal and recreational purposes. Hallucinogens that affect the auditory and visual senses such as peyote are used by Native Americans as part of religious rituals. Coca leaves that contain cocaine are brewed or chewed by people in the mountainous regions of the Andes to decrease hunger, increase work performance, and create a sense of well-being. Methamphetamine is a central nervous system (CNS) stimulant and is used primarily as a recreational drug. It can elevate mood; increase alertness, concentration, and energy; and reduce appetite. At high doses it can cause psychosis, breakdown of skeletal muscle, seizures, and bleeding in the brain. Chronic use can cause rapid mood swings, delusions, and violent behavior. It is highly addictive, and withdrawal symptoms occur quickly when use of the drug is discontinued.

10. Commonly Abused Substances

Commonly abused classes of prescription drugs include opioid painkillers; stimulants; depressants; and Syrup, Purple Drank, Sizzurp, or Lean, which is prescription-strength cough syrup containing codeine and promethazine. Other commonly abused substances include prescription medications and some OTC medications. Also included is alcohol, amphetamines/methamphetamine, anabolic steroids, and bath salts. Bath salts are a new family of drugs that have one or more synthetic chemicals related to an amphetamine-like stimulant found naturally in the khat (*Catha edulis*) plant.

Hallucinogens are drugs that alter perception and feeling. These include lysergic acid diethylamide (LSD), mescaline, psilocybin, and phencyclidine (PCP). *Inhalants* are aerosols and volatile hydrocarbons such as airplane glue and paint thinner that give the drug abuser a "buzz" or feeling of euphoria.

Cannabis Drugs

Cannabis is an extract from the leaves, stems, fruiting tops, and resin of the hemp plant (*Cannabis sativa*). The most common form of cannabis is hashish. Hashish is the resinous material of the cannabis plant. Other forms of this drug include banji, ganga, charas, kif, and dagga. The trade names K2 and Spice refer to a wide variety of herbal mixtures that produce experiences similar to those obtained from marijuana. There active ingredients are synthetic cannabinoid compounds. Use of K2 or Spice can cause a rapid heart rate, vomiting, agitation, confusion, hallucinations, raised blood pressure, and reduced blood supply to the heart. It is highly addictive.

Hashish is classified as a controlled substance, although it is not a narcotic derivative. Hashish also has sedative-hypnotic, anesthetic, or psychedelic properties and is capable of altering perception, thought, and feeling.

Hashish is administered orally by using pipes or cigarettes and can be injected subcutaneously; however, the most potent route is inhalation. Many drug abusers prefer smoking hashish through a water pipe to reduce the irritating effect of the acidic smoke. Some drug abusers grind hashish into a powder and mix it with foods in order to delay absorption of the drug by the body.

Hashish acts to depress the CNS and causes mental relaxation and euphoria, which occur within 15 minutes and lasts for ≤4 hours. The drug abuser experiences a loss of inhibitions. The person's spatiotemporal perception is altered and causes a free flow of ideas to occur. These ideas, however, are disconnected. The person can experience blanks or gaps in memory similar to those experience in an epileptic episode. The user may also have palpitations, loss of concentration, lightheadedness, weakness, tremors, postural hypotension, ataxia (staggering gait), and a sense of floating. As the dosage increases, the effects of the drug progresses from relief to disinhibition, excitement, and anesthesia. Respiratory and vasomotor depression and even collapse can occur with high doses.

Hashish is metabolized in the liver and is eliminated in bile and feces. Only a trace amount of hashish is detectable in urine. Hashish may affect the metabolism of drugs that require protein binding. These include ethyl alcohol, barbiturates, amphetamines, cocaine, opiates, and atropine.

Hashish causes withdrawal symptoms. These include minor discomfort for a few days. Insomnia, anxiety, irritability, and restlessness may persist for a few weeks. The person may have intermittent craving for a few months, which is best treated by exercise. No pharmacological intervention should be given.

Hallucinogens

Hallucinogens are natural and chemically manufactured drugs that alter perception and feeling. These drugs alter the mind and change a person's perception of time, reality, and the environment. Hallucinogens disrupt the normal activity of serotonin, which is a neurotransmitter that sends signals throughout the brain. Hallucinogens cause abnormal activation of serotonin in the part of the brain responsible for coordinating and processing hearing and sight. As a result, people taking hallucinogens hear voices and perceive images that do not exist.

Researchers are uncertain as to whether hallucinogens permanently alter the brain's chemistry; however, some patients who have taken hallucinogens have experienced chronic mental disorders.

The following hallucinogens are commonly used.

LSD

Lysergide, better known as LSD, is a potent hallucinogenic that exerts a psychoactive effect that heightens perception, creates distortions of the body, and causes visual hallucinations. A person taking LSD can experience unpredictable mood swings ranging from euphoria to depression and panic, which is commonly referred to as a "bad trip." LSD also causes hypertension, dilated pupils, hyperthermia, and tachycardia (rapid heart rate).

LSD takes effect within 20 minutes and lasts for ≤2 hours, altering the user's state of consciousness. This can lead to psychosis and trigger flashbacks called *latent psychosis*. The experience is frequently unpleasant.

The combination of acute panic and paranoia is a common side effect that can lead to homicidal thoughts and actions. The toxic effect of LSD causes impaired judgment and toxic delirium. This results in a stage of exhaustion and feeling of emptiness where the person is unable to coordinate thoughts. This fall into depression increases the risk of suicide. Some people who take LSD also enter into a long-term schizophrenic or psychotic reaction. LSD stimulates the uterus and could induce contractions in a pregnant woman.

Healthcare providers treat a person who is under the influence of LSD by using a "talk-down" approach, by talking the patient through the episode in a quiet, relaxed environment. If this approach fails, drug therapy is employed, using a benzodiazepine such as diazepam (Valium). Drugs should be used only along with crisis intervention therapy.

Healthcare providers should avoid administering phenothiazines such as chlorpromazine (Thorazine). These can exacerbate the patient's panic reaction and cause postural hypotension (low blood pressure when standing). Large doses of tranquilizers, use of restraints, and isolating the patient should also be avoided because these strategies are more traumatic than therapeutic.

Mescaline

Mescaline is an alkaloid that is extracted from the flowering heads (mescal buttons) of the peyote cactus. Mescaline causes subjective hallucinogenic effects similar to those of LSD. The extract is a soluble crystalline power that can be dissolved into tea or placed in capsules for ingestion.

This drug takes effect almost immediately and lasts for ~6 hours before it reaches its half-life and is excreted in the urine. People taking mescaline experience anxiety, hyperreflexia, static tremors, and psychic disturbances with vivid visual hallucinations. They also experience abdominal pain, nausea, and diarrhea.

Psilocybin

Psilocybin is extracted from Mexican mushrooms. It produces a subjective hallucinogenic effect that is similar to that from mescaline, but of shorter duration. Psilocybin takes effect within 30–60 minutes after the drug is administered, and its effect can last for ≤6 hours.

People who take this drug experience a pleasant mood, although some users become apprehensive. This results in impaired performance and poor critical judgment. Some people exhibit hyperkinetic (compulsive movements) behavior and inappropriate laughter. The pupils dilate and the person experiences vertigo (dizziness) and ataxia (stagger). They also experience paresthesias (numbness, tingling) and muscle weakness. The drug also induces drowsiness and sleep.

PCP

Phencyclidine (PCP) is a controlled substance that causes hallucinations. Usage can result in assaults, murders, and suicides. PCP was developed in the late 1950s as a dissociative anesthetic that leaves a patient awake but detached from her/his surroundings and unresponsive to pain. Once the drug's hallucinogenic effect was discovered, PCP was withdrawn from use in humans, but its use in veterinary medicine continued. PCP picked up the street name "hog" because of its use with animals.

PCP metabolizes rapidly in the liver and forms a high concentration in urine if consumed in large quantities. A small dose of PCP has a half-life of 30–60 minutes. Larger doses can have a half-life of 1–4 days.

Patients who are under the influence of PCP are flushed and sweat profusely. They experience nystagmus (rapid eye movements), diplopia (double vision), and ptosis (drooping eyelids). These patients also appear sedated and under the influence of an analgesic. They also exhibit the effects of alcohol intoxication with ataxia (staggering gait) and generalized numbness of the extremities.

Patients undergo three stages of psychological effect when using PCP. The first stage is a change in body image and a feeling of depersonalization. This follows with the second stage when the patient's hearing and vision become distorted. The third stage occurs when the patient feels apathy, estrangement, and alienation.

The patient's thoughts become more disorganized. Attention span is impaired, as are motor skills and an overall sense of body boundaries. The drug's hallucinatory effects can occur long after the patient's acute symptoms disappear. These are unpredictable and can occur months after the drug was taken.

The patient can experience psychotic disturbances that are exhibited by paranoid behavior, self-destructive actions, random eye movement, and excitation. These are combined with physiological changes such as tachycardia, hypertension, respiratory depression, muscle rigidity, increased reflexes, seizures, and an unconscious state with open eyes.

There is no known chemical antidote to PCP ingestion. The only treatment is to keep the patient quiet, in a dark room, away from sensory stimuli, and protected from self-inflicted injury. The healthcare provider should not attempt to talk the patient down as the patient can perceive any interaction as a personal attack and may become very violent. The patient is commonly given diazepam (Valium) or haloperidol (Haldol) to counteract antianxiety and antipsychotic effects.

PCP is very toxic, and nurses should be aware of the potential severity of the drug's effects. These effects include hypertensive crisis, intracerebral hemorrhage (bleeding into the brain), convulsions, coma, and death. Patients who have used PCP should be closely monitored.

Inhalants

Inhalants are not drugs. They are volatile hydrocarbons and aerosols that are used to dispense various of chemical products that create a euphoric effect when inhaled. These products include airplane glue, paint thinner, typewriter correction fluid, lighter fluid, nitrous oxide, xylene, toluene, and more than 1000 household and commercial products. Treatment of inhalant abuse employs a symptomatic rather than pharmacological approach because there are no specific antidotes to these products. When PCP is inhaled, the intoxication can last for a few minutes or several hours. If PCP is used repeatedly, the individual can lose consciousness; high concentrations can cause heart failure or death. Some of the products can replace oxygen in the body, and the individual can suffocate. Each of these side effects needs to be treated separately. The permanent health effects caused by the use of these inhalants can include hearing loss, peripheral neuropathies (numbness, tingling) or spasms of arms and legs, CNS or brain damage, and bone marrow damage, which results in blood problems. Kidney and liver damage can also occur.

11. Nursing Assessment

Patients who abuse drugs require a careful and complete assessment that includes measurement of vital signs (temperature, blood pressure, heart rate, and respiratory rate). Pupil size is inspected, and the skin is examined for needle marks and abscesses. The patient's nutrition, elimination, and sleep patterns are noted as well. It is important to determine whether the patient has a past medical history of drug use, drug abuse, and related drug illnesses such as HIV, cellulitis, endocarditis, and pneumonia or other respiratory problems.

The following are commonly used nursing diagnoses for drug abuse patients:

- Knowledge deficit related to denial of problem
- Ineffective individual coping related to lack of support system
- Risk for violence to oneself or others related to drug use
- Altered health maintenance related to drug dependence
- Ineffective management of therapeutic regimen

The plan of care for a patient who abuses drugs will depend on the reason for hospitalization. The physical response to drug use should be monitored, and any infections or disease states must be treated. The plan should also include treatment for the abuse in a supportive and rehabilitative setting. This may include counseling, psychotherapy sessions, and medications to overcome the withdrawal symptoms.

Nursing implementation may focus on managing the patient's acute intoxication and withdrawal and then monitoring the effectiveness of therapy to treat the patient's substance abuse problem.

Evaluation of the effectiveness of the treatment centers on how successfully the patient detoxifies and withdraws from the drug and refrains from repeated abuse of the same substance. It is important for nurses to realize that overcoming a drug addiction is a long and sometimes lifetime task. Patients may experience many relapses along the way, and the process can seem frustrating and hopeless. However, the nurse should remain nonjudgmental and objective when caring for substance abuse patients.

Summary

Substance abuse is one of the most widely misunderstood areas of pharmacology.

Substance abuse is the indiscriminant misuse of medication that results in a physical and/or psychological dependence on the drug. A person is considered addicted to a drug if, over a 6-month period, she/he develops a dependence on the drug, experiences withdrawal symptoms when the drug is no longer administered, and requires increased doses of the drug to experience the same therapeutic effect.

An addicted person also has an uncontrollable urge to use the drug and to self-medicate, which can interfere with the activities of daily life, and continues to depend on the drug despite the negative consequence of using it.

Drug abusers exhibit common behavioral patterns such as an inability to maintain a normal routine, have poor hygiene, and experience strained family and social relationships. Most importantly, they are frequently in denial that they have a problem.

Healthcare professionals are especially prone to drug abuse because drugs can enhance performance during long work shifts, drugs are easily accessible to them, and they know how to self-medicate. Furthermore, healthcare providers are reluctant to reveal their own abuse of drugs because this would place their license and livelihood in jeopardy.

There are tests available to determine whether a person has taken drugs; however, those tests are not foolproof. There is a chance that the results will be a false positive or false negative.

Commonly abused drugs fall into one of five groups. These are heroin, cocaine, cannabis, hallucinogens, and inhalants. Although many of the drugs that are in these groups are illegal in the United States, some of them are legal in other countries.

1. **Tolerance to a drug occurs when**
   (a) a drug is no longer effective.
   (b) a person becomes addicted to a drug.
   (c) a higher dose is required to achieve the same therapeutic effect.
   (d) none of the above applies.

2. **A patient undergoing withdrawal from hashish is treated by**
   (a) administering a lower dose of hashish.
   (b) administering a sedative.
   (c) doing nothing.
   (d) prescribing exercise.

3. **When a patient is withdrawing from LSD, the healthcare provider should**
   (a) provide massive doses of tranquilizers.
   (b) restrain the patient.
   (c) talk down the patient.
   (d) isolate the patient.

4. **A patient who only takes prescription drugs cannot become dependent on the drug.**
   (a) True
   (b) False

5. **Some drugs increase a person's performance.**
   (a) True
   (b) False

6. **Psilocybin is**
   (a) extracted from Mexican mushrooms.
   (b) extracted from coca leaves.
   (c) extracted from coca resins.
   (d) extracted from the stalk of the coca plant.

7. **Prolonged exposure to a drug increases the excretion of the drug from the body.**
   (a) True
   (b) False

8. A licensed practitioner can help prevent a patient from becoming dependent on a drug by

   (a) using a prescribed management routine.
   (b) limiting treatment to one month.
   (c) providing the patient with psychological counseling.
   (d) doing all of the above

9. A healthcare professional is ethically expected to report another healthcare professional if there is a suspicion of drug abuse.

   (a) True
   (b) False

10. Some healthcare providers use drugs for recreational purposes.

    (a) True
    (b) False

chapter **6**

Route of Administration

The patient has the right to receive the proper medication and have that medication administered using the best route to achieve the desired therapeutic effect. Selection of the route is based on the form in which the medication is given to the patient.

The best route depends on a number of factors that include the nature of the medication and the patient's condition. In this chapter you'll learn the routes and how to administer medication using each route.

1. Medication and Routes

The last time that you had a headache and took an aspirin, you were using the oral route to get rid of your headache. The oral route is just 1 of 11 different routes that are used to administer medication.

As the term implies, the *oral* route means that the patient ingests the medication. Sublingual and buccal are two other routes that also involve the patient's mouth but instead of ingesting the medication, the medication is absorbed within the oral cavity from beneath the tongue (*sublingual*) or between the cheek and the gum (*buccal*).

You probably rubbed hydrocortisone on an insect bite to relieve itching. Itching subsides as the skin absorbs the hydrocortisone. This is the *topical* route. Medication is also absorbed by the skin using the *transdermal* route, which is commonly known as the "patch."

Medication that you place in your eyes, ears, or nose is administered using the *instillation* route in the form of drops, ointment, and sprays. Patients with lung problems sometimes receive medication using the *inhalation* route. Medication is delivered using an inhaler that changes liquid medication into a spray.

Patients who have upper gastrointestinal (GI) disturbances might have a tube inserted via the nasal passage into the stomach (nasogastric tube) or a tube inserted directly into the stomach through the skin and stomach wall (gastrostomy tube) that is used to bypass the upper GI tract and provides a direct path to the stomach. Both tubes can be used to introduce medication into the patient.

The suppository route is used to administer medication through the rectum and the vagina. A route that few patients look forward to is the parenteral route because medication is given using injections or directly into the vein, the intravenous (IV) routes.

Oral Route

Oral medications are in the form of tablets, capsules, and liquids, and most are absorbed in the small intestine and have a peak time of 1–3 hours. Tablets can be divided using a tablet cutter into half or quarters to reduce the dosage that is given to the patient. Some tablets can also be crushed so that the medication can be mixed with food such as applesauce. Capsules must be taken whole because they are enteric-coated, thus preventing release of the medication until it reaches the intestines. Some capsules contain timed-release medication.

Here are the precautions that must be taken when the oral route is prescribed:

- No oral medication is given to patients who are vomiting, who lack a gag reflex, or who are in an unresponsive state.

- Oral medication should not be mixed with large amounts of food or liquid because it can alter the effectiveness of the medication. Food and liquid might interfere with the patient's ability to absorb the medication depending on the drug. In that case the medication should be given while the patient's stomach is empty.

Liquid Medication

Liquid medication is administered in one of three forms: elixirs, emulsion, or suspensions. An *elixir* is a sweet, pleasant-smelling solution of alcohol and water used as a vehicle for medicine. Robitussin, a commonly used cough preparation, is an elixir. An *emulsion* is a suspension of small globules of one liquid in a second liquid with which the first one will not mix, such as milk fats in milk. A *suspension* is a preparation of finely divided, undissolved particles dispersed in a liquid, such as bismuth subsalicylate (Pepto-Bismol).

The following are guidelines for administering liquid medication:

- Dilute, shake, or stir the medication only if required (follow the directions on the label).
- Read the meniscus at the lowest fluid mark to determine the dose while pouring the liquid. This is best done at eye level.
- Refrigerate open or reconstituted (mixed) liquid medication as per the medication label. Date and label the time when the medication was opened or reconstituted.

Sublingual and Buccal Medication

These medications are quickly absorbed into the circulatory system because the tissues beneath the tongue and between the cheek and the gum consist of a thin layer of epithelium cells and a vast network of capillaries. Nitroglycerin can be administered sublingually.

Here are guidelines for administering sublingual or buccal medication:

- Do not permit the patient to ingest food or liquid if the medication is administered sublingually (under the tongue) or buccally (between the cheek and the gum) until the medication is completely absorbed.
- Sublingual medication such as nitroglycerin can be administered to a nonresponsive patient because it dissolves quickly with minimal chance of aspiration.

Transdermal Route

The transdermal route is commonly referred to as "the patch" because the medication is contained in a patch that is absorbed through the skin. An increasing number of drugs are administered by this route. These include cardiovascular medication such as nitroglycerin, neoplastic drugs (cancer), and hormones (estrogen and birth control medications). In addition, analgesics (fentanyl), medications used to treat allergic reactions, and smoking cessation drugs such as Nicotrol are also administered through the transdermal route.

Transdermal patches provide a consistent blood level and less absorption problems in the gastrointestinal tract that are commonly experienced by patients who take oral medications.

The following are guidelines for administering transdermal medication:

- Check the prescriber's order.
- Don't cut the patch in half.
- Remove the patch before applying another one.

- Apply the patch onto the specified area of the body. Nitroglycerin is placed on the chest or upper arm. The nicotine patch is applied to the trunk or upper arm. Fentanyl is positioned on the chest, flank, or upper arm.
- Alternate the sites of the patch on the patient's body.
- Wear gloves when administering the patch because the nurse can easily absorb the medication, which can cause an undesirable reaction.
- Place the patch on a clean, dry, hairless area where the skin is intact.
- Some transdermal medication is available in a tube with an accompanying pad of paper patches. The paper has measurement lines on it, and the medication is squeezed onto the paper in the amount ordered (eg, nitroglycerin ½ in.). Label the patch with the date and time of administration and your initials.

Topical Route

The *topical* route refers to applying medication to the skin for a local effect. There are three ways to administer topical medication: with a glove, with a tongue blade, or with a cotton-tipped applicator. Never apply topical medication with an ungloved hand because medication may be absorbed into your body as well as into the patient's body.

Here are guidelines for administering a topical medication:

- Check the prescriber's order.
- Use a clean or sterile technique if you are applying the medication to skin that is broken or burned.
- Stroke the medication firmly onto the skin.
- Ensure that the patient is comfortable when you apply medication to painful areas of the skin.
- Do not use a light, feathery touch when administrating medication to an area that is pruritic (itchy) because this increases the itch.

Instillation Route

Instillations are liquid medications that are administered to the eyes and ears as drops, ointment, or sprays. You will need to take special precautions when administering an instillation to avoid spreading the disease.

Here's what you need to do to administer installations in the eye:

- Check the prescriber's order.
- Wash your hands and then apply clean gloves. You do not need sterile gloves.
- Position the patient so that she/he is looking toward the ceiling.

- Gently pull down the skin below the infected eye to expose the conjunctival sac.
- If you are administering eyedrops, then
  - Administer the prescribed number of drops into the center of the conjunctival sac.
  - Do not touch the eyelids or the eyelashes with the dropper.
  - Release the skin and gently press the lacrimal duct (inner corner of the eye) with sterile cotton balls or tissues for 1–2 minutes. This prevents the systemic absorption of the medication through the lacrimal canal.
- If you are applying eye ointment, then
  - Squeeze about a ½ in. of ointment onto the conjunctival sac.
  - Tell the patient that she/he might experience blurred vision temporarily.
- Instruct the patient to keep her/his eyes closed for 1–2 minutes.
- Avoid placing medication on the cornea because this can cause discomfort and possibly damage the cornea.

Here's what you need to do to administer eardrops:

- Check the prescriber's order.
- Wash your hands and then apply clean gloves.
- Make sure that the medication is at room temperature.
- Position the patient so that her/his head is tilted slightly toward the unaffected side.
- Straighten the external ear canal by pulling the auricle up and back for a patient who is ≥3 years of age and down and back for a patient who is <3 years of age. (**Hint:** Children are shorter than adults, so you pull down.)
- Instill the prescribed number of drops into the ear.
- Do not touch the ear with the dropper, to avoid contaminating the dropper.
- The patient should remain with her/his head tilted for 2–3 minutes.

Here are some guidelines for administering nose drops and sprays:

- Check the prescriber's order.
- Ask the patient to blow her/his nose.
- For nose drops, do the following:
  - Position the patient's head back if the infection is in the frontal sinus.
  - Position the patient's head to the affected side if the infection is in the ethmoid sinus.

- Administer the prescribed number of drops.
- Tilt the patient's head backward for 5 minutes after administering drops.
- For nose sprays, do the following:
  - Tell the patient to close the unaffected nostril.
  - Ask the patient to tilt her/his head to the side of the closed nostril.
  - Spray the medication.
  - Ask the patient to hold her/his breath or open the closed nostril and breathe through it per the medication instructions.

Inhalation Route

The *inhalation* route is used to have the patient inhale the medication using an inhaler. This is a common route used to administer bronchodilators to patients with breathing problems such as asthma, pneumonia, and chronic obstructive pulmonary disease (COPD).

The medication enters the lower respiratory tract, where it is rapidly absorbed in the bronchioles, providing the patient relief from bronchospasms, wheezing, asthma, or allergic reactions.

Inhalation is used to deliver antibiotics, steroids, and mucolytic agents (drugs that thin secretions, making it easier to clear the bronchi). The patient can experience side effects such as tremors, nausea, tachycardia, palpitations, nervousness, and dysrhythmias (see Chapter 14).

There are two commonly used inhalers: the handheld nebulizer and the handheld metered-dose device. The handheld nebulizer changes liquid medication into a fine spray. The handheld metered-dose device is a small, metal container about 5–6 in. high, with a pushbutton spray device on the top to release the medication.

Inhalers are not a very efficient way of delivering medications to the lungs because only 9% of the medication reaches the lungs. The efficiency increases by using a spacer, which delivers 21% of the medication to the lungs. The *spacer* is a funnel-like device that attaches to the mouthpiece of the metered-dose inhaler (MDI). The medication is released into the spacer, and then the patient inhales slowly and deeply to get the drug into the airway.

Here are some guidelines for administering medication using an inhaler:

- Check the prescriber's order.
- Position the patient in a semi- or high-Fowler position (with the patient sitting at a 45–90° angle relative to the legs).
- Teach the patient to wait for 2 minutes between puffs of an MDI if the prescriber orders more than one puff.

- The patient should rinse her/his mouth with water and expectorate (spit) following inhalation of steroids because steroid inhalants promote oral fungal infections.

Nasogastric and Gastrostomy Tube Route

Nasogastric and gastrostomy tubes are used for patients who are unable to swallow or ingest anything orally. The nasogastric tube is passed through the nose and into the stomach opening with direct access to the stomach, through which medication can be administered to the patient. The *nasogastric tube* is also used as a temporary feeding tube and to remove stomach contents. The *gastrostomy tube* is inserted through the skin and directly into the stomach and is used primarily as a permanent feeding tube that can also be used to administer medication.

Here are guidelines for administering medication through the nasogastric or gastrostomy tube:

- Check the prescriber's order.
- Be sure that the tube is in the proper position by employing one of two methods:
  - Attach the syringe to the free end of the nasogastric tube; inject one or more 20-mL bursts of air into the tube.
  - Aspirate the gastric contents and check the pH with test paper. If it is less than or equal to 5.5, the tube is in the stomach.
- Remove the plunger from a syringe and pour medication into the syringe.
- Close the clamp on the nasogastric or gastrostomy tube.
- Attach the syringe to the nasogastric or gastrostomy tube.
- Open the clamp, pour the medication into the syringe, and hold the tube up, allowing the medication to flow down the tube.
- Flush the tube with 30–50 mL of water.
- Close the clamp and remove the syringe.

Suppository Route

Suppositories are used to administer medication via the rectum or the vagina, depending on the nature of the patient's condition or the type of medication. Rectal suppositories are the preferred route to administer medication when the patient's upper GI tract is not functioning properly or when the medication has an offensive taste or foul odor. It is also used when digestive enzymes change the chemical integrity of the medication.

The rectum promotes absorption of the medication because it contains many capillaries and can produce a high blood concentration of the medication.

Here are some guidelines for administering a suppository rectally:

- Check the prescriber's order.
- Provide the patient privacy.
- Position the patient in the Sims position (lying on left side).
- Wash your hands and then apply clean gloves.
- Lubricate the suppository, if necessary.
- Ask the patient to breathe through her/his mouth. This relaxes the anal sphincter.
- Insert the suppository.
- Ask the patient to remain in the Sims position for 20 minutes.

When administering a suppository vaginally, follow this procedure:

- Check the prescriber's order.
- Wash your hands and then apply clean gloves.
- Place the patient in the lithotomy position (on back with legs flexed at the knees).
- Insert the suppository using an applicator.
- Clean the vaginal area after the suppository is inserted.

Parenteral Route

In the *parenteral* route, medication is injected into the patient using a syringe. There are four commonly used parenteral routes: intradermal (ID), subcutaneous (SC), intramuscular (IM), and intravenous (IV).

The choice of which parenteral routes to use is determined by the prescriber according to the nature of the medication, the desired onset of the therapeutic effect, and the patient's needs. For example, the test for tuberculosis is performed by injecting the purified protein derivative intradermally, which is under the skin. Insulin is injected subcutaneously, although regular insulin can also be administered intravenously. Medications administered intravenously have a more rapid onset of therapeutic effect than other parenteral routes. Vaccinations, some antibiotics, and other medications are injected intramuscularly.

Intradermal

Intradermal injections are given in hairless areas of the body that are lightly pigmented and thinly keratinized so that the nurse can observe any reaction to the medication. The following areas are suitable for intradermal injections:

- Inner aspect of forearm or scapular area of back
- Upper chest
- Medial thigh sites

Medication injected intradermally has a localized effect because it does not enter the bloodstream. It usually causes a wheal (blister) to appear at the injection site. Injections are given using a 26–27-gauge needle and a 1-mL syringe calibrated in 0.01-mL increments. The typical injection is between 0.01 and 0.1 mL.

Here's how to administer medication intradermally:

- Check the prescriber's medication order.
- Wash your hands and then put on clean gloves.
- Properly identify the patient.
- Cleanse the area of the site in a circular motion using alcohol or betadine, depending on the medication and agency policy.
- Hold the skin taut.
- Position the bevel up and insert the needle at a 10–15° angle. You should be able to see the outline of the needle through the skin.
- Inject slowly to form a wheal.
- Slowly remove the needle.
- Do not massage the area.
- Mark the site with a pen.
- Tell the patient not to wash the mark until a healthcare provider assesses the site for a reaction 48–72 hours after the injection.
- Assess the patient within 48–72 hours. If the patient is allergic to the medication, then the diameter of the wheal should increase. If the patient is tested for tuberculosis, the reaction should be measured in millimeters of the induration (palpable, raised, hardened area or swelling), not the redness.

Subcutaneous

Subcutaneous injection is suitable for medications that need to be absorbed slowly to produce a sustained effect, such as insulin and heparin. Subcutaneous medications are absorbed through capillaries, and the onset of the medication is slower than that with intramuscular and intravenous routes.

Choose an injection site that has an adequate fat pad. To prevent lypodystrophy, sites must be rotated if injections are given frequently. *Lypodystrophy* is a loss of the fat area under the skin, causing ineffective absorption of insulin.

Suitable injection sites are the abdomen, the upper hips, the upper back, the lateral upper arms, and the lateral thighs.

Subcutaneous injections are given using a 25–27-gauge needle that is ½ or ⅝ in. in length and with a 1–3-mL syringe calibrated to 0.5–1.5 mL. However, syringes used for insulin are measured in syringe measurement units and not milliliters (mL).

Here's how to administer medication subcutaneously:

- Check the prescriber's medication order.
- Wash your hands and then put on clean gloves.
- Properly identify the patient.
- Cleanse the area of the site in a circular motion using alcohol, betadine, or soap and water as per agency policy.
- Pinch the skin.
- Insert the needle at 45–90° angle (45° is preferred if the patient has a small amount of subcutaneous tissue).
- Release the skin.
- Inject the medication slowly.
- Quickly remove the needle.
- Gently massage the area unless heparin is injected.
- Apply a bandaid as necessary.

Intramuscular

Intramuscular injections are used so that the medication is rapidly absorbed into the patient's body. The absorption rate depends on the patient's circulatory state. For most medications, usually no more than 3 mL of medication is injected for an adult or a child. Some medications such as those used in chemotherapy may be more effective in doses of ≤5 mL.

Choose an injection site according to the size of the muscle with a minimum number of nerves and blood vessels in the area. These sites are suitable:

- Ventrogluteal (hip)
- Dorsogluteal (buttocks)
- Deltoid (upper arm)
- Vastus lateralis (front of thigh)

See Table 6–1 for more details.

Intramuscular injections use a 20–23-gauge needle that is 1–1½ in. in length and a 1–3-mL syringe that is calibrated to 0.5–1.5 mL.

TABLE 6–1 Injection Sites	
Injection Site	**Description**
Ventrogluteal	• Relatively free of major nerves and vascular branches.
	• Well-defined bony anatomic landmarks.
	• For IM or Z-track injections.
	• Locate the site by placing the heel of your hand on the greater trochanter of the femur with the thumb pointed toward the umbilicus. The index finger marks the anterosuperior iliac spine. The middle finger traces the iliac crest curvature. The space between the index and middle fingers is the injection site.
Dorsogluteal	• Good site for IM and Z-track injections.
	• Danger to major nerves and vascular structures near site.
	• Easy to give subcutaneously by mistake when trying to give an IM because the fat is often very thick.
Deltoid	• Preferred site for vaccines.
	• Easily accessible.
	• Muscle mass is small compared to other sites.
	• Use a ⅝ in. to 1.5 in. long needle.
	• Locate the acromion process of the scapula and the deltoid. Measure 2 to 3 fingers below the acromion process on the lateral midline of the arm to identify the proper site. Inject at a 90° angle.
Vastus lateralis	• Preferred site for infants younger than 7 months.
	• It has a relatively large muscle mass.
	• Free from major nerves and vascular branches.
	• Site is a hand's breadth below the greater trochanter and above the knee.
	• Inject at a 45° angle toward the knee.

Here's how to administer medication intramuscularly:

- Check the prescriber's medication order.
- Wash your hands and then put on clean gloves.
- Properly identify the patient.
- Cleanse the area of the site in a circular motion, using alcohol or betadine according to the agency guidelines.
- Flatten the skin at the injection site using your thumb and index finger.
- Insert the needle at a 90° angle into the muscle between your thumb and index finger.

- Release the skin.
- Slowly inject the medication.
- Quickly remove the needle.
- Gently massage the area (unless this is contraindicated by the medication).

2. Z-Track Injection Technique

The Z-track inject technique is used to prevent medication from leaking back into the subcutaneous tissue after it has been injected into the patient. This technique is used whenever the medication—such as dextran (iron)—might cause a visible and permanent skin discoloration. The gluteal muscle is the preferred site for a Z-track injection.

Here's how to administer medication using the Z-track technique:

- Check the prescriber's medication order.
- Wash your hands and then put on clean gloves.
- Properly identify the patient.
- Cleanse the area of the site in a circular motion using alcohol or betadine as per the agency guidelines.
- Pull the skin to one side and hold it.
- Insert the needle at a 90° angle.
- Inject the medication as you hold the skin to one side.
- Withdraw the needle.
- Release the skin.

3. Tips for Minimizing Pain

Receiving medication via injection is a painful process for the patient. However, you can minimize the discomfort by following these tips:

- Encourage the patient to relax. The more they tense their muscles, the more the injection hurts.
- Replace the needle with a new one after you withdraw medication from a vial or if the medication is irritating.
- Position the patient on her/his side—with knees flexed if you are using the ventrogluteal site. Position the patient flat on the abdomen with toes turned inward if you are using the dorsogluteal site. Use the same technique if the patient prefers to stand.

- Do not inject into sensitive or hardened tissues.
- Compress tissues at the injection site.
- You can prevent the antiseptic (eg, alcohol wipe) from clinging to the needle during the injection by waiting for the antiseptic to dry before injecting the medication.
- Dart the needle to reduce puncture pain.
- Inject the medication slowly.
- Withdraw the needle quickly and in a straight line.
- Use the Z-track technique.
- Ask the patient to cough on the count of 3. Inject the medication when the patient coughs.

Intravenous

Intravenous injections are used to provide rapid onset for a medication because the medication is directly injected into the circulatory system [this is referred to as *IV push* (IVP)]. Intravenous tubing can be placed in the cephalic or cubital vein of the arm or the dorsal vein of the hand. However, cubital veins should be avoided except in emergency situations because cubital veins are used for withdrawing blood specimens for laboratory testing. Start an IV at the hand and then work toward the cubital vein.

Intravenous injections use a 21–23-gauge needle that is 1–1½ in. in length. Use the wider-bore needle for viscous (thicker) drugs. IV lines are inserted with a butterfly needle or with an angiocatheter that ranges from 14 gauge for whole blood or fractions of blood to 23 gauge for rapid infusion. Medication may be administered directly into the vein with a syringe, injected into an intermittent catheter inserted into the patient's vein, or injected into IV fluids such as 5% dextrose in water (D_5W) and delivered as an IV drip called a "piggyback."

Here's how to administer medication IV:

- Check the prescriber's medication order.
- Wash your hands and then put on clean gloves.
- Properly identify the patient.
- Cleanse the area of the site in a circular motion using alcohol or betadine according to the agency guidelines.
- Apply a tourniquet above the site.
- Insert the butterfly needle or catheter into the vein until blood returns through the needle or catheter.

- Remove the tourniquet.
- Stabilize the needle or catheter.
- Dress the site according to your healthcare agency's policy.
- Monitor the flow rate of the IV fluid, distal pulses, skin color [redness (infection)], skin temperature, insertion site for infiltration (swelling), and side effects of the medication as the action of the medication occurs rapidly.
- Follow agency policy regarding the addition of medications to the fluid in the bottle or bag, piggyback technique, and IV push.

Summary

Medication is given to a patient using one of several routes depending on the nature of the medication and the patient's condition. The prescriber selects the route, which is written in the medication order.

The oral route is used for tablets, capsules, liquids, suspensions, and elixirs. Do not use this route if the patient cannot swallow or is not conscious or alert.

The sublingual and buccal routes are used for rapid absorption of medication because blood vessels are close to the surface of the tongue and gums. The transdermal route is used for medication that can be absorbed through the skin by the use of a patch. The topical route is used to apply medication locally. The instillation route is used to administer medication through drops and sprays. Medication is directed to the lungs by using the inhalation route where the patient uses an inhaler.

If the patient experiences disruption of the upper GI tract, then the prescriber will order a nasogastric or gastrostomy tube. The nasogastric tube is inserted through the nose and into the stomach. The gastrostomy tube is inserted through the skin and directly into the stomach. Either of these tubes can be used to deliver medication to the patient.

The suppository route is used to absorb medication directly into the rectum or vagina. The parenteral route is used to inject medication directly into the dermal or subcutaneous tissue, muscle, or veins.

QUIZ

1. A patient who is administered medication sublingually
   (a) has upper GI problems.
   (b) should ingest food or liquid to facilitate absorption of the medication.
   (c) shouldn't eat or drink until the medication is absorbed.
   (d) do none of the above.

2. If the dose of a transdermal patch is more than the prescriber's medication order
   (a) cut the patch to an appropriate length.
   (b) contact the prescriber.
   (c) do nothing.
   (d) give the patient the patch anyway.

3. When giving eardrops to a 2-year-old child
   (a) pull the earlobe downward and back.
   (b) pull the earlobe upward and back.
   (c) pull the earlobe upward and forward.
   (d) pull the earlobe downward and forward.

4. A rectal suppository can be used if the patient cannot absorb medication in the upper GI tract.
   (a) True
   (b) False

5. The inner aspect of the forearm is the good site for an intradermal injection.
   (a) True
   (b) False

6. The Z-track injection method is used
   (a) to prevent medication from leaking back onto the tissue.
   (b) to prevent dislodging of the needle.
   (c) to ease the pain of the injection.
   (d) for none of the above.

7. Withdrawing a needle slowly decreases the pain of an injection.
   (a) True
   (b) False

8. A piggyback is inserted
   (a) into the IV tube.
   (b) into the patient's arm.
   (c) into the patient's leg.
   (d) into none of the above.

9. The nurse should massage the site after giving a heparin injection.
   (a) True
   (b) False

10. Pinch the skin when giving an insulin injection.
    (a) True
    (b) False

Dose Calculations

Calculating the proper dose of medication is a critical aspect of administering medicine to a patient. Although the prescriber specifies a dose in the medication order, the dose prescribed may not be the same as the dose that is on hand, requiring the nurse to calculate a comparable dose on the basis of available medication.

With intravenous (IV) medications, the prescriber might order a dose to be infused into the patient over a specific amount of time. The nurse must use this information to calculate the drip rate, which is used to set the IV so that medication can be administered at the proper rate.

Some medication orders prescribe a dose according to the patient's weight. The nurse is responsible for weighing the patient and then applying a formula to calculate the actual dose.

This chapter teaches you how to perform on-hand calculations, IV calculations, and weight calculations in order to determine the correct amount of medication to administer.

1. The Metric System and Medication

Medication is prescribed in measurements of the metric system. Some students become anxious at just the mention of calculations. If you feel anxious and panicky, relax. We'll show you the easy way to perform these calculations.

Unit	Purpose	Equivalents
Gram	Weight	1 kilogram (kg) = 1000 grams (g)
		1 gram (g) = 1000 milligrams (mg)
		1 milligram = 1000 micrograms (mcg)
		1 kilometer = 1000 liters
Liter	Volume	1 liter (L) = 1000 milliliters (mL) = 1000 cubic centimeters (cc)
		1 milliliter (mL) = 1 cubic centimeter (cc)

TABLE 7–1   Units and Their Equivalents

Medication calculation requires you to know how to multiply and divide. You'll also need to know six metric measurements and five household measurements (ounces, teaspoons, tablespoons, cups, and drops).

Let's begin with the metric system. The metric system uses grams to measure weight and liters to measure volume as shown in Table 7–1. Prefixes are used to indicate the number of grams and liters. Table 7–2 shows the commonly used prefixes that you'll see when calculating medication.

Each prefix indicates the value. The prefix is placed before the unit of measure such as 1 kilogram or 1 milliliter. Look up kilo in Table 7–2. The factor is 1000, which is larger than a gram or a liter. Therefore, you multiply the gram or liter by 1000. Thus, a kilogram is 1000 grams and a kiloliter is 1000 liters. The important point to remember is that the prefix of the measure implies the size of the measurement.

Household Measurements

Household measurements are used for liquid medications that are given to patients in the home setting. An example is two teaspoons of cough medication. Nurses encounter household measurements when providing home healthcare services and when determining a patient's fluid intake and output in the hospital setting. Nurses need to

TABLE 7–2   Prefixes Used in Medication

Unit	Purpose	Equivalents
Kilo	1000	One thousand times
Centi	0.01	One hundredth part of
Milli	0.001	One thousandth part of
Micro	0.000001	One millionth part of

TABLE 7–3 Commonly Used Conversion Factors for Household and Metric Measurement	
Household System	Metric System
Weight	
2.2 pounds (lb)	1 kilogram (kg)
Volume	
1 ounce	30 mL = 30 cc
16 ounces	500 mL = 500 cc
32 ounces	1000 mL = 1000 cc
1 liter	1000 mL = 1000 cc
Household Measurement	
60 drops (gtt)	1 teaspoon (tsp)
1 teaspoon (tsp)	5 mL = 5 cc
1 tablespoon (tbs)	15 mL = 15 cc
2 tablespoons (tbs)	1 ounce = 30 mL = 30 cc

instruct patients about these measurements at home and gain feedback indicating whether the patient or caretaker understands how to measure the medication. Nurses also use pounds when calculating a dose that is based on a patient's weight. Patients should use measuring spoons for medication administration at home and avoid using tableware.

Patients are usually more comfortable self-administering medication if the dose is in household measurements. However, medication is recorded using metric measurements. Therefore, a nurse must be able to convert household measurements to metric measurements.

Let's say that the patient drinks an 8-ounce (oz) glass of orange juice. The nurse must convert that to milliliters (mL) or cubic centimeters (cc) in order to record the intake volume in the patient's fluid input and output chart. (Remember that 1 mL = 1 cc.)

Table 7–3 contains commonly used conversion factors for household measurement and metric measurement.

2. Converting Metric Units

Let's take a look at how to convert units of the metric system. You'll need to learn how to convert from one metric unit to another (eg, from grams to milligrams) in order to arrive at like units when calculating a dose. For example, if the dose available is in milligrams and the prescriber's medication order specifies grams, you'll need to convert grams to milligrams before calculating the dose.

Converting from one metric unit to another metric unit isn't difficult if you remember these three rules:

1. Determine whether the desired measurement is larger or smaller than the given measurement. Remember that gram, liter, and meter are larger units and milligram, milliliter, and millimeter are smaller units.

2. If you are converting from a smaller unit to a larger unit, then you multiply by moving the decimal three places to the left.

3. If you are converting from a larger unit to a smaller unit, then you divide by moving the decimal three places to the right.

Suppose that the medication order is 300 mg and you need to convert this to grams. A milligram is smaller than a gram. You are converting from a smaller unit (a milligram) to a larger unit (a gram). Therefore, you divide by moving the decimal three places to the left, as shown here:

$$300 \text{ mg} \div 1000 = 0.3 \text{ g}$$

If the prescriber ordered 0.9 grams and the dose that you need is in milligrams, you are converting from a larger unit (a gram) to a smaller unit (a milligram). Therefore, you multiply by moving the decimal three places to the right, as shown here:

$$0.9 \text{ g} \times 1000 = 900 \text{ mg}$$

One of the most common conversions that you'll perform is converting milliliters into cubic centimeters. This is also the easiest conversion because one milliliter (mL) is equal to 1 cubic centimeter (cc).

Always place a zero to the left of the decimal point when the quantity is not a whole number. This avoids errors when reading the number.

Incorrect: .9
Correct: 0.9

Converting Household Units into Metric Units

Sometimes you (the nurse) may need to convert between household and metric units when you calculate a patient's input and output volume and when you provide home healthcare to a patient. There, you'll use a teaspoon, tablespoon, or cups measured in ounces to administer medication.

When converting from milliliters or cubic centimeters to ounces, divide by 30, as shown here [remember that 30 cc (30 mL) = 1 oz]:

$$240 \text{ mL} \div 30 = 8 \text{ oz}$$
$$60 \text{ cc} \div 30 = 2 \text{ oz}$$

When converting from ounces to milliliters or cubic centimeters, multiple by 30, as shown here:

$$2 \text{ oz} \times 30 = 60 \text{ mL}$$
$$4 \text{ oz} \times 30 = 120 \text{ mL}$$

When converting from pounds to kilograms, divide by 2.2, as shown here: Remember 2.2 lbs = 1 kilogram

$$22 \text{ lbs} \div 2.2 = 10 \text{ kilograms}$$

When converting from kilograms to pounds, multiple by 2.2, as shown here:

$$63 \text{ kg} \times 2.2 = 138.6 \text{ pounds}$$

3. Formulas for Calculating the Desired Dose

In the ideal world, the prescriber will write a medication prescription at a dose that is available in the hospital. For example, the medication prescription is for a 15-mg tablet of Inderal and the hospital has on hand a 15-mg tablet of Inderal.

In the real world, the dose specified in the medical prescription may not be available. The hospital might have 10-mg tablets of Inderal and not the 15-mg tablets prescribed. Instead of asking the prescriber to change the medication order, the nurse calculates the proper medication to give the patient according to the medication order and the dose that is on hand.

In this example, the nurse calculates that the patient should receive 1.5 tablets of Inderal. This means that the nurse must divide one tablet into halves.

There are two methods nurses can use to calculate the desired dose. These are the *formula method* or the *ratio-and-proportion method*. Either method will produce same result. When applying either method, make sure that all the terms are expressed in the same units before calculating the desired dose. For example, the medication order might be in grams and the dose on hand might be in milligrams. You will need to convert the grams to milligrams before calculating the desired dose to give. Always convert to the unit of the "have" dose.

The formula method uses the following formula to determine the correct dose:

$$\frac{D}{H} \times V = \text{A quantity (desired dose divided by dose you have}$$
$$\text{multiplied by vehicle of drug you have equals}$$
$$\text{the amount calculated to be given to the patient)}$$

D = desired dose

H = dose you have

V = vehicle you have (tablets or liquids)

A = amount calculated to be given to the patient

Ratio-and-proportion method:

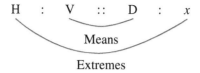

H = drug on hand (available)
V = vehicle or drug form (tablet, capsule, liquid)
D = desired dose (as prescribed)
x = unknown amount to give
:: = "as" or "equal to."
Multiply the means and the extremes. Solve for x; x is the divisor.
Example: Give 500 mg of ampicillin sodium by mouth when the dose on hand is in capsules containing 250 mg:

500 mg divided by 250 mg multiplied by 1 capsule = 2 capsules

Formula method:

$$\frac{500\text{ mg}}{250\text{ mg}} \times \frac{\text{capsule}}{1} = 2\text{ capsules}$$

Example: Give 375 mg of ampicillin when it is supplied as 250 mg/5 mL:

375 mg divided by 250 mg multiplied by 5 mL = 7.5 mL

Example: Diltiazem (Cardizem) 60 mg PO b.i.d. On hand are 30-mg tablets.

$$\frac{60\text{ mg}}{30\text{ mg}} \times \text{tablet} = 2\text{ tablets}$$

Ratio-and-proportion method:
Prescribed: Amoxicillin 100 mg PO q.i.d.
Available: Amoxil (amoxicillin) 80 mL

250 : 5 mL :: 100 mg : x mL

Means
Extremes

$250x = 500$
$x = 2$ mL
Answer: Amoxicillin 100 mg = 2 mL.
Prescribed: Aspirin/ASA grains x, q4h, PRN for headache.
Available: Aspirin 325 mg/tablet.

a. Convert to one system and unit of measure. Change grains to milligrams.

b.

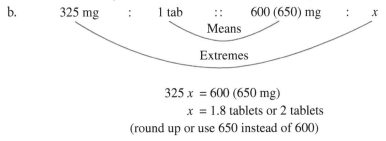

$$325\,x = 600\,(650\text{ mg})$$
$$x = 1.8\text{ tablets or 2 tablets}$$
(round up or use 650 instead of 600)

Be sure to label all the terms in the formula with the appropriate unit. This will help to prevent errors. For example, use mg following a value in the formula if the value is in milligrams.

4. Parenteral Medications

Parenteral medication is a medication that is administered to a patient by an injection or by an IV flow. The dose for an injection is calculated using the formula method or the ratio-and-proportion method that was described earlier in this chapter.

For example, the prescriber might order Demerol (meperidine hydrochloride) 45 mg IM PRN to alleviate the patient's pain. The Demerol label states 75 mg/mL. This is the dose that you have. The nurse must calculate the number of milliliters that should be administered to the patient.

Using the basic formula $\left(\dfrac{\text{D}}{\text{H}} \times \text{V} = \text{A}\right)$ here's the calculation:

$$\frac{45\text{ mg}}{75\text{ mg}} \times \frac{1\text{ mL}}{1} = \text{A}$$

$$\frac{45}{75} \times \frac{1\text{ mL}}{1} = \text{A}$$

$$\frac{45\text{ mL}}{75} = 0.6\text{ mL}$$

Calculating the IV Flow Rate for Continuous or Intermittent (Piggyback) Infusions

The *IV flow rate* is the number of drops of the IV fluid that the patient receives in a minute. The intravenous order directs the nurse to administer a specific volume of fluid to the patient over a specific time period. It is the nurse's responsibility to calculate the number of drops per minute that is necessary to infuse the IV fluid into the patient over the prescribed time period.

In order to calculate the drip rate, you need to know the following:

- The volume of fluid that is to be infused. This is found in the medication order in milliliters (mL) or cubic centimeters (cc).
- The amount of time over which the infusion is to take place.
- The drip factor, which is specified on the IV tubing that is used for the infusion.

Here's how to calculate the drip rate. It is important to remember that although we use milliliters in the following examples, you can substitute cubic centimeters (cc) for milliliters (mL) if cc is specified in the order. Always express gtt/min (drops per minute) in whole numbers. Always carry out to the tenth and then round to the nearest whole number. If a volumetric pump is used to deliver the IV fluid, then you'll need to use cc per hour.

Total fluid multiplied by drip factor and divided by the infusion time in minutes.

Medical prescription: 250 mL 5% D/W to infusion over 10 hours. Drip factor 60.

Total fluid = 250 mL (cc)

Drip factor = 60 gtt/min

Infusion time in minutes = 600 min

$$\frac{250 \text{ mL} \times 60 \text{ gtt/min}}{600 \text{ min}} = \frac{15{,}000 \text{ mL}}{600 \text{ min}} = 25 \text{ gtt/min}$$

Heparin Infusion

Heparin is a medication that inhibits the formation of platelets and can be administered either as a subcutaneous injection or as a continuous intravenous infusion. The proper dose of heparin is always calculated using either the formula method or the ratio-and-proportion method.

Example: Medical prescription: heparin 7500 units SC.

Available heparin 10,000 units per milliliter.

Using the formula method, we obtain the following:

$$\frac{7500 \text{ units}}{10{,}000 \text{ units}} \times \text{mL} = 0.75 \text{ mL}$$

Summary

The dose specified in a medication order may not be the same dose for the medication that you have on hand. Therefore, you must calculate a new dose that is proportional to the prescribed dose.

All doses are calculated using the metric system. You must be able to convert within the metric system and convert between household and metric measurements because patients are likely to self-medicate using household measurement—such as a teaspoon—rather than using metric measurements.

Converting between metric units is performed by moving the decimal to the left or right depending on whether you are moving from a smaller metric unit to a larger metric unit or vice versa. Converting between household and metric measurements is achieved by multiplying or dividing using a conversion factor. This depends on whether you are converting from household to metric measurements or vice versa.

Two methods are used to calculate a dose: the formula method and the ratio-and-proportion method. Both use the on-hand dose of a medication to determine the desired dose on the basis of the medication prescription.

The formula method and the ratio-and-proportion method are also used to calculate parenteral medications. Alternatively, parenteral medication can be administered through a vein as either a bolus or an infusion. If infusing through an intravenous line, the nurse must calculate the number of drops per minute that the IV should run to deliver the amount of medication ordered.

We'll leave the topic of preparing medications and explore medications that are available in nature in the form of herbs. You'll learn about herbal therapy in the next chapter.

QUIZ

1. **Prescribed: Duricef (cefadroxil) 0.4G PO q.i.d. On hand: Duricef 200 mg capsules. How many capsules do you need?**
   - (a) 1 capsule
   - (b) 2 capsules
   - (c) 5 capsules
   - (d) 20 capsules

2. **Prescribed: Ceclor (cefaclor–oral) 150 mg. On hand: Ceclor 300-mg tablets. How many tablets do you need?**
   - (a) 30 tablets
   - (b) 5 tablets
   - (c) 50 tablets
   - (d) 0.5 tablets

3. Prescribed: 1000 mL of 0.9% normal saline (NS) intravenously every 8 hours. The intravenous tubing delivers 15 gtt/mL. How many gtt/min (drops per minute) will be infused?

   (a) 31 gtt/min
   (b) 44 gtt/min
   (c) 25 gtt/min
   (d) 28 gtt/min

4. Prescribed: Diabenese (chlorpropamide) 600 mg. On hand: Diabenese 300-mg tablets. You need 2 tablets.

   (a) True
   (b) False

5. Ordered: 1 liter of NS q7h. Available 1 liter of NS and IV tubing with a drip factor of 10. You would regulate the IV at 23.8 gtt/min.

   (a) True
   (b) False

6. Prescribed: Heparin 1000 units/hr intravenously. Available: Heparin 25,000 units/hr in 250 cc D_5W. What volume should be administered to give the correct dose?

   (a) 0.10 mL/hr
   (b) 1.0 mL/hr
   (c) 10 mL/hr
   (d) None of the above

7. Prescribed: 1 liter of D_5W q8h. Available: 1 liter of D_5W and IV tubing 10 gtt/mL. You regulate the IV at 20.8 gtt/min.

   (a) True
   (b) False

8. Prescribed: 1000 mL of IV fluid q12h. Available: 1000 mL of IV fluid and micro-drip tubing. How many drops per minute will you regulate the IV?

   (a) 83 gtt/min
   (b) 83.3 gtt/min
   (c) 8.33 gtt/min
   (d) 0.833 gtt/min

9. Prescribed is Prilosec (omeprazole) 4.4 mg/kg for a child who weighs 88 lb. Available is Prilosec 50 mg/5 mL. You would give the child 1.76 mL.

   (a) True
   (b) False

10. Prescribed is Ceclor 2 mg/kg for a child who weighs 20 lb. Available is Ceclor 20 mg/2 mL. You would administer 1.8 mL.

    (a) True
    (b) False

chapter **8**

Herbal Therapy

Ever wonder how people survived centuries ago when there wasn't a local pharmacy and the local physician was several days' travel away? They used plants—called *herbs*—as medicine to treat the common cold, infections, diseases of the GI tract, and anything else that ailed them.

Today, herbal therapy has made a comeback as an alternative to prescription medication and over-the-counter (OTC) remedies. Herbs continue to elicit a therapeutic effect on patients. However, patients who use herbal therapies are exposed to risk. There is no quality standard for herbal therapy, and many herbs can cause adverse reactions when combined with prescription and OTC medication.

In this chapter, you'll learn about the therapeutic effect of herbal therapies and about the nursing process that should be implemented to prevent patients from developing adverse reactions to herbal therapy when combined with conventional therapy.

1. Inside Herbal Therapy

In recent years, herbal therapies have gained popularity as multi-million-dollar businesses have capitalized on the therapeutic properties of natural herbs and the fact that herbs are exempt from the government regulations imposed on the pharmaceutical industry.

Herbs are plants or parts of plants that have a proven therapeutic effect. These were the "original" medicines. Even today, physicians in many countries prescribe herbs as the first choice for combating certain diseases.

However, herbs are not typically prescribed in the United States for a number of reasons. Few pharmacy schools offer courses in botanical remedies, and some nursing pharmaceutical courses focus more on misuse of herbal therapies than their proper use. Probably the leading reason why herbs are not prescribed is that health insurance in the United States does not pay for these therapies.

Herbal therapies cannot be patented, which is a likely reason why the pharmaceutical industry has not pushed the government and the medical community to use herbal therapies as treatment for diseases and symptoms of diseases.

The US Food and Drug Administration (FDA) is not required to approve herbal therapies. This creates an open and unregulated market for herbal therapies that lacks quality standards found in the pharmaceutical industry.

In 1992, Congress instructed the National Institutes of Health to develop an Office of Alternative Medicine to support research studies of alternative therapies, including herbals.

Interestingly, herbs are the raw material of old and new pharmaceutical medication. For example, the herb foxglove is the source for digitalis, and the herb salicin is the source for aspirin. The breast-cancer-fighting drug Taxol (paclitaxel) comes from the Pacific yew tree.

Although the therapeutic effects of herbs have been well known for thousands of years, there seems to be a lack of uniform information about them that describes their use, dosage, side effects, and contraindications. This is the information that is available for all prescription and OTC pharmaceutical medications.

In addition, there are no qualitative monographs that provide guidelines for compounding and standards of purity for herbal medication. In other words, there is no well-defined measurement for purity and manufacturing of herbal medication as there is for prescription and OTC pharmaceutical medications.

An effort has been launched by the *United States Pharmacopeia* (USP), the World Health Organization (WHO), the *American Herbal Pharmacopeia* (AHP), and other agencies to develop herbal therapeutic monographs that provide this information for herbal therapies.

One in five people in the United States who have taken prescription medication also have taken herbal medications. Also, whereas herbal preparations can be therapeutic, the lack of quality standards and contraindication with prescribed and OTC medication exposes patients to potential toxicity and other adverse side effects.

2. Forms of Herbal Therapy

Herbs are plants or parts of plants that contain medicinal qualities. Some herbs can be taken as whole. One such herb is fresh aloe, which can be used topically to treat burns and minor cuts. Other herbs must be transformed into a form that is suitable for ingestion.

Herbs are living organisms that have a very short life after they are removed from their source of nutrition (ie, plucked from the ground). Enzymatic activity begins to cause the herb to decay immediately after it is harvested. Therefore, steps must be taken to preserve the herb by drying it in sunlight or by using another heat source. Drying removes moisture and lowers the enzymatic activity. This enables the herb to retain its therapeutic qualities for up to 6 months.

Extraction techniques are used to remove the therapeutic material from an herb. The most commonly used extraction technique is to first isolate the part of the herb that contains the therapeutic material and then soak that part in alcohol or water. This helps to produce a reliable dose.

Some extractions take the form of oils. Herbal oil is prepared by soaking the dried herb in olive oil or vegetable oil and heating it for an extended period of time. Oils promote the concentration of the therapeutic material and, if properly stored, extend the therapeutic life of the material for months.

Herbal therapies also are available in the form of salves. *Salves* are semisolid fatty preparations such as balms, creams, and ointments. They are prepared in a way similar to herbal oil preparation, except that once the dried herb is soaked in oil, melted wax is mixed with the oil. It is left to cool and harden to form the therapeutic balm, cream, or ointment.

Herbal tea is another popular form of herbal therapy. It is prepared by soaking fresh or dried herbs in boiling water. Once the herb blends with the water, the resulting tea can be stored in the refrigerator for later use as a drink, bath water additive, or applied topically in a compress to the skin.

Herbs are also available as tinctures. Chaparral tincture, for example, contains important ingredients that cannot be dissolved in water. Tinctures are also a convenient way to take herbs that do not require kitchen preparation. Disagreeable-tasting herbs can be swallowed more quickly, and their bitter flavor can be masked with juice. Tinctures are made by soaking fresh or dried herbs in water or alcohol, causing the water-soluble and fat-soluble components of the herb to concentrate. The concentrate is the desired form. Water is used for people who do not consume alcohol. Alcohol is used to preserve the herbal concentrate for a year.

Herbal capsules are another common form of herbal therapy. The herb is dried and pulverized into a powder that is placed inside the capsule. Some herbal capsules contain oil-soaked herbals or herbal juices.

Herbal tablets are similar to herbal capsules except the dried, pulverized herb is combined with stabilizers and binders and then compressed into a tablet. A *stabilizer* is an ingredient that ensures that the herb maintains its therapeutic effect. A *binder* is an ingredient that acts like glue to hold together the powdery mixture of herb and stabilizer.

Herbal therapy can also take the form of syrup. Syrups are made by drying the herb and soaking it in water or oil and then adding a sweetener to the mix. The sweetener is usually honey or sugar. The sweetened mixture is then heated until the syrup forms. Herbal syrups are used to treat colds, cough, and sore throat.

3. Hazards of Herbal Therapeutics

Herbal therapies have a therapeutic effect and provide acceptable interventions for certain diseases and their symptoms. However, the lack of standards in manufacturing and oversight by regulatory agencies expose patients to potential hazards.

Pharmaceuticals approved for distribution in the United States have undergone rigorous testing that identifies the purity and concentration of the active ingredient that delivers the therapeutic effect. This also identifies the toxic levels that can cause serious and potentially lethal toxic effects. In addition, testing also identifies the effect that a pharmaceutical has when combined with other prescribed or OTC medications.

Herbal therapies lack this testing for a number of reasons, including the high cost of these tests and the lack of regulation. Anyone can sell herbal therapy without the need to receive approval from a governmental agency or from the medical community.

A major concern is the effect of herbal therapy on the patient who is also taking prescribed medications. Medication interaction is always a risk. A prescriber should always ask what medication the patient is taking and review the patient's chart before prescribing another medication. Prescribers should also ask what OTC or herbal therapies and/or home remedies the patient is taking.

For example, a patient who takes cascara, a laxative for constipation, and senna—also a laxative—along with digoxin, which is used to treat an irregular heart rhythm, can develop a toxicity. Likewise, taking juniper, a diuretic that causes increased urination, and dandelion—also a diuretic—along with lithium, which is a commonly prescribed psychiatric medication, elevates the therapeutic effect of lithium and can result in a toxic level.

Another hazard is the route in which herbal therapy is administered. For example, comfrey is used as an ointment to relieve swelling that is associated with abrasions and sprains. However, internal use can cause liver damage. Some comfrey therapies are designed for internal use. One such use is treating a cough using comfrey as an expectorant.

The herbal dietary supplement ephedra, commonly known as ma huang, is used as an energy boost and for losing weight. Ephedrine and pseudoephedrine are components of ephedra that have a stimulant and bronchodilation effect. However, ephedra has the adverse effect of palpitations, which can result in stroke.

4. Herbal Therapy and the Nursing Process

In the assessment, nurses need to include a discussion about the patient's use of non-conventional therapeutic agents by name, dosage, frequency, side effects, and why the patient is taking this remedy. This assessment should include information about all prescription and OTC medications taken by the patient and why the patient is taking these drugs. Herbal medications, OTC medications, and prescribed medications can combine to create undesirable results and in some cases can have a toxic and dangerous effect on the patient. Many patients use home remedies that the healthcare community is not familiar with, and it is difficult to assess the effect that the remedy might have on the patient.

After assessing the patient, the nurse considers a nursing diagnosis that is related to herbal therapies. The following symptoms or conditions are significant:

- **Knowledge Deficit:** The patient may be unaware of the impact that herbal therapies have on the patient's health.
- **Altered Nutrition:** The patient may be unaware of how herbal therapies alter her/his nutritional balance.
- **Side Effects:** The patient might be experiencing nausea, diarrhea, headache, fatigue, and other symptoms that can actually be side effects of herbal therapies.
- **Toxicity:** The patient might be experiencing a toxic effect as a result of interactions of herbal therapies with prescribed medications.
- **Alteration in Skin Integrity:** The patient might have developed a reaction to the herbal therapy such as a rash.

After choosing a nursing diagnosis that is related to herbal therapy, the nurse plans for the proper intervention. The goals are as follows:

1. The patient will verbalize an understanding of the risks of herbal therapy.

2. The patient will verbalize an understanding of the interaction between herbal therapy and conventional therapy.

The nurse intervenes by doing the following:

- Monitoring the patient's response to conventional and herbal therapy, looking for adverse side effects.
- Consulting with dietitians and other healthcare specialists to ensure that the patient's nutrition remains balanced.
- Telling the patient to continue with the same brand of herbs and to notify the healthcare provider if there is a change in brand.
- Teaching the patient to
  - Understand the rationale for herbal therapy
  - Notify healthcare providers if she/he plans to substitute herbals for conventional therapies
  - Read all labels
  - Review the optimal storage for the herbal remedy
  - Know what foods increase or decrease the action of the herbs
  - Review the potential side effects, symptoms that require prompt reporting to the healthcare provider, and the correct preparation for use of herbals
- Evaluating the patient for the effectiveness of herbal remedies for alleviating symptoms and the patient's knowledge regarding the use of herbals.

5. The Do's and Don'ts Regarding the Use of Herbs

- Don't take them if pregnant or trying to become pregnant.
- Don't take if breastfeeding.
- Don't give to babies or young children.
- Don't take large quantities.
- Buy herbs with the plant and quantities listed on the package.
- Don't stop taking prescribed medication before contacting the healthcare provider.
- Keep herbs away from children.
- Use fresh herbs.
- Don't delay seeking healthcare if you experience adverse symptoms.
- Understand that herbs do not provide a miracle cure.

Make sure that the patient thinks of herbs as medicine that is less potent than conventional medication. However, adverse reactions can occur if conventional medication is taken with herbal therapy. For example, some conventional medication may act more rapidly than expected when combined with herbal therapy.

The patient should not take any herbal where the following information is not included on the packaging:

- Scientific name of the product and the part of the plant used in the preparation
- Manufacturer's name and address
- Batch and lot number
- Date of manufacture and expiration

6. Commonly Used Herbs

The following is a list of commonly used herbs and the ailments treated:

Ailment	Herb
Acne	Calendula, aloe, tea tree
Alcoholism	Evening primrose, kudzu
Allergy	Chamomile
Alzheimer's disease	Ginkgo biloba, rosemary
Angina	Hawthorn, garlic, willow, green tea
Anxiety and stress	Hops, kava, passionflower, valerian, chamomile, lavender
Arteriosclerosis	Garlic
Arthritis	Capsicum, ginger, turmeric, willow, cat's claw, devil's claw
Asthma	Coffee, ephedra, tea
Athlete's foot	Topical tea tree oil
Attention-deficit disorder	Evening primrose oil
Bad breath	Parsley
Boils	Tea tree oil, topical garlic, echinacea, eleutherococcus, ginseng, rhodiola
Bronchitis	Echinacea, pelargonium
Burns	Aloe
Cancer	Bilberry, blackberry, cocoa (dark chocolate), green tea, garlic, ginseng, maitake mushroom, pomegranate, raspberry, reishi mushroom

(Continued)

Ailment	Herb
Cankers	Goldenseal
Colds	Echinacea, andrographis, ginseng, coffee, licorice root (sore throat), tea (nasal and chest congestion)
Congestive heart failure	Hawthorn
Constipation	Apple, psyllium seed, senna
Cough	Eucalyptus
Depression	St. John's wort
Diabetes, type 2	Garlic, beans (navy, pinto, black, etc.), cinnamon, eleutherococcus, flaxseed, green tea
Diabetic ulcers	Comfrey
Diarrhea	Bilberry, raspberry
Diverticulitis	Peppermint
Dizziness	Ginger, ginkgo biloba
Earache	Echinacea
Eczema	Chamomile, topical borage seed oil, evening primrose oil
Fatigue	Cocoa (dark chocolate), coffee, eleutheroccocus, ginseng, rhodiola, tea
Flu	Echinacea, elderberry syrup (also see "Colds")
Gas	Fennel, dill
Giardia	Goldenseal
Gingivitis	Goldenseal, green tea
Hay fever	Stinging nettle, butterbur
Herpes	Topical lemon balm, topical comfrey, echinacea, garlic, ginseng
High blood pressure	Garlic, beans, cocoa (dark chocolate), hawthorn
High blood sugar	Fenugreek
High cholesterol	Apple, cinnamon, cocoa (dark chocolate), evening primrose oil, flaxseed, soy foods, green tea
Hot flashes	Red clover, soy, black cohosh
Impotence	Yohimbe
Indigestion	Chamomile, ginger, peppermint
Infection	Topical tea tree oil, astragalus, echinacea, eleutherococcus, garlic, ginseng, rhodiola
Insomnia	Kava, evening primrose, hops, lemon balm, valerian
Irregular heartbeat	Hawthorn
Irregularity	Senna, psyllium seed

(Continued)

Ailment	Herb
Irritable bowel syndrome	Chamomile, peppermint
Lower back pain	Thymol, carvacrol, white willow bark
Menstrual cramps	Kava, raspberry, chasteberry
Migraine	Feverfew, butterbur
Morning sickness	Ginger
Muscle pain	Capsicum, wintergreen
Nausea	Ginger
Premenstrual syndrome	Chasteberry, evening primrose
Ringing in the ears	Ginkgo biloba
Seasonal affective disorder	St. John's wort
Shingles	Capsicum
Sore throat	Licorice, marshmallow, mullein
Stuffy nose	Echinacea
Tonsillitis	Goldenseal, astragalus, echinacea
Toothache	Willow, clove oil
Ulcers	Aloe, licorice
Varicosities	Bilberry, horse chestnut
Yeast infection	Garlic, goldenseal, Pau D'arco

Summary

Herbal therapy is the use of plants called *herbs* to treat symptoms and diseases. The government and the medical community do not regulate herbal therapies. This results in a lack of standards for the manufacture and sale of herbal therapies. The quality, purity, dosage, and side effects may be different for the same herb.

There are different forms of herbal therapies. These are oils, balms, creams, ointments, teas, tinctures, capsules, tablets, and syrups. Although herbs are available in these forms, some herbs should be administered only externally and not used internally.

While herbal therapies provide patients with a therapeutic effect, they can also leave the patient exposed to hazards. When combined with conventional therapies, herbal therapies can produce a toxic effect or an adverse reaction.

The nurse should ask if the patient is taking herbal therapies and, if so, for what condition. The patient should be taught about herbal therapies, including their risks and benefits, and then given clear instructions on how to continue herbal therapies while undergoing conventional treatment—if approved by the patient's healthcare provider.

QUIZ

1. **Herbal therapies**
   (a) require FDA approval.
   (b) are safe to use to self-medicate as long as the patient isn't undergoing conventional therapy.
   (c) are industry-regulated.
   (d) are none of the above.

2. **The "herbal prozac" is**
   (a) sage.
   (b) St. John's wort.
   (c) psyllium.
   (d) Kava Kava.

3. **The patient should not take an herb unless which of the following information in on the package?**
   (a) Scientific name
   (b) Manufacturer's name and address
   (c) Batch and lot number
   (d) All of the above

4. **Chamomile should not be taken by a patient who is allergic to ragweed.**
   (a) True
   (b) False

5. **Peppermint relieves migraine headaches when rubbed on the forehead.**
   (a) True
   (b) False

6. **A patient who complains about palpitations and who is undergoing herbal therapy may be taking**
   (a) comfrey.
   (b) chamomile.
   (c) ma huang.
   (d) ginkgo biloba.

7. **Patients should never use herbal therapies.**
   (a) True
   (b) False

8. What herb has a therapeutic effect similar to that of Benadryl?

   (a) Ginseng

   (b) Zingiber

   (c) Valerian

   (d) None of the above

9. The nurse should instruct the patient on how to monitor for adverse side effects of herbal therapies.

   (a) True

   (b) False

10. Comfrey is an ointment used to relieve swelling associated with abrasions and sprains.

   (a) True

   (b) False

chapter 9

Vitamins and Minerals

Growing up, you may have been told it is important to eat a well-balanced meal so that you get the vitamins and minerals needed to build a strong, healthy body. As children, we probably considered this a ploy to finish our suppers.

Some patients may not eat a balanced diet for various reasons. Therefore, it is critical that you assess the patient for vitamin and mineral deficiencies and administer the prescribed therapy to restore the patient's nutritional balance.

In this chapter you'll learn about vitamins and minerals and how to assess patients for deficiencies. You'll also learn about vitamin therapy and mineral therapy and how to educate your patient about proper nutrition.

1. Vitamins

Vitamins are organic chemicals that are required for metabolic activities necessary for tissue growth and healing. Under normal conditions, only a small amount of vitamins—which are provided by a well-balanced diet—are necessary. However, larger amounts of vitamins may be needed for a patient who is pregnant, undergoing rapid growth, or has a debilitating illness.

Likewise, patients whose diets are not well balanced (such as some elderly people, alcoholics, children, and people on fad diets) might also develop vitamin deficiencies. That would require the patient to take vitamin supplements to ensure that there are sufficient vitamins to support her/his metabolism.

Expect to provide vitamin supplements for patients who have any of the following conditions:

- Conditions that inhibit absorption of food
- Diarrhea
- Infection and fever
- Inflammatory diseases
- Cancer
- Inability to use vitamins
- Undergoing hemodialysis
- Hyperthyroidism
- GI surgery
- Fad diets
- Pregnancy
- Growing children

Well-Balanced Diet

Many patients realize the importance of having a well-balanced diet. Few, however, know what constitutes a well-balanced diet. Patients can use the US Department of Agriculture (USDA) definition of a well-balanced diet as a guideline.

The USDA uses a food pyramid to illustrate the mixture of food groups that are necessary for receiving the proper amount of vitamins and minerals to maintain a healthy life. Recently the USDA revised its longstanding food pyramid to reflect the individual needs of people of a specific age, gender, and activity group. The previous food pyramid placed everyone in the same group, which is not realistic.

The revised food pyramid is organized into five color-coded groups, each with a general recommendation:

- **Grains:** Eat 3 oz of whole-grain bread, rice, cereal, crackers, or pasta (orange) daily.
- **Vegetables:** Eat more dark-green vegetables, orange vegetables, beans, and peas (green).
- **Fruits:** Eat fresh-frozen, dry, or canned fruit. Go easy on fruit juices (red).
- **Milk:** Eat calcium-rich foods. Choose lactose-free products (blue).
- **Meat and Beans.** Eat low-fat and lean meats and poultry. Bake it, broil it, grill it. Eat more fish, beans, peas, nuts, and seeds (purple).

However, the USDA has a website (http://www.mypyramid.gov/pyramid/index.html) that will calculate the desired portions for each group according to a person's age, gender, and the amount of exercise that the person performs daily.

In addition to the USDA, the National Academy of Sciences Food and Nutrition Board (http://www.iom.edu) publishes the US Recommended Dietary Allowance (RDA) for daily dose requirements of each vitamin (Table 9–1).

Types of Vitamins

There are two groups of vitamins: fat-soluble vitamins and water-soluble vitamins.

Fat-Soluble Vitamins

Fat-soluble vitamins are absorbed by the intestinal tract by the same metabolism as that in fat absorption. Any condition that interferes with the absorption of fats will also interfere with the absorption of fat-soluble vitamins. Fat-soluble vitamins are stored in the liver, fatty tissues, and muscle and remain in the body longer than water-soluble vitamins. Fat-soluble vitamins are excreted slowly in urine. (**Hint to remember:** ADEK = addicted to fat are fat soluble vitamins.)

The fat-soluble vitamins are described in the following paragraphs.

Vitamin A   Vitamin A (Acon, Aquasol) helps to maintain epithelial tissue, eyes, hair, and bone growth. It is also used for treatment of skin disorders such as acne. Vitamin A has a toxic effect if consumed in excess. For example, birth defects can occur if the patient ingests >6000 international units (IU) during pregnancy. It is important to keep in mind that vitamin A is stored in the liver for ≤2 years, which can result in inadvertent toxicity if the patient is administered large doses of vitamin A.

Vitamin D   Vitamin D, absorbed in the small intestine with the assistance of bile salts, is necessary for the intestines to absorb calcium. Vitamin D plays a major role in regulating the metabolism of calcium and phosphorus. There are two forms of vitamin D: D_2, called *ergocalciferol*; and D_3, called *cholecalciferol*. D_2 is a synthetic fortified form of vitamin D. D_3 is the natural form of vitamin D that is produced in the skin by ultraviolet sunlight. Once absorbed, vitamin D is converted into calcifediol in the liver and then converted to an activated form of calcifediol in the kidneys. The active form is a hormone that combines with parathyroid hormone (PTH) and calcitonin to regulate calcium and phosphorus metabolism in the body and stimulate the reabsorption of calcium and phosphorus by bone. When serum levels of calcium are low, more vitamin D is used to create the active form of calcifediol (25-hydroxycholecalciferol, also known as *calcidiol*). Low serum levels of calcium cause a decrease in the creation

TABLE 9–1 Recommended Daily Allowances (RDAs)

Vitamin	Food Sources	RDA
Fat Soluble		
A	Whole milk, butter, eggs, leafy green and yellow vegetables, fruits, liver	Male: 1000 µg or 5000 IU Female: 800 µg or 4000 IU Pregnancy: 1000 µg or 5000 IU Lactating: 1200 µg or 6000 IU
D	Fortified milk, egg yolk, tuna, salmon	Male and Female: 40–80 µg or 200–400 IU
E	Whole-grain cereals, wheat germ, vegetable oils, lettuce, sunflower seeds	Male: 10 mg/day; 15 IU Female: 8 mg/day; 12 IU Pregnancy: 10–12 mg/day
K	Leafy green vegetables, liver, cheese, egg yolk	Male: 70–80 µg/day Female: 60–65 µg/day Taking broad spectrum antibiotics: 140 µg/day Pregnancy: 65 µg/day
Water-Soluble		
C Ascorbic acid	Citrus fruits, tomatoes, leafy green vegetables, potatoes	Male and female: 60 mg/day Pregnancy: 70 mg/dL Lactating: 95 mg/dL
B_1 thiamine	Enriched breads and cereals, yeast, liver, pork, fish, milk	Male: 1.5 mg Female: 1.1 mg Pregnancy: 1.5 mg Lactating: 1.6 mg
B_2 riboflavin	Milk, enriched breads and cereals, liver, lean meats, eggs, leafy green vegetables	Male: 1.4–1.7 mg Female: 1.2–1.3 mg Pregnancy: 1.6 mg Lactating: 1.8 mg
B_3 niacin	Eggs, meat, liver, beans, peas, enriched bread and cereals	
B_6 pyridoxine	Lean meat, leafy green vegetables, whole-grain cereals, yeast, bananas	Male: 15–19 mg/day Female: 13–15 mg/day Pregnancy: 18 mg/day Lactating: 20 mg/day
B_{12}	Liver, kidney, fish, milk	Male and female: 3 µg/day Pregnancy: 4 µg/day
Folic Acid	Leafy green vegetables, yellow fruits and vegetables, yeast, meats	Male and female: 400 µg/day Pregnancy: 600–800 µg/day Lactating: 600–800 3 µg/day

Vitamin A	
Dose for treatment of deficiency	100,000–500,000 IU daily × 3 days; then 50,000 IU × 14 days
Maintenance	10,000–20,000 IU qd × 60 days
Pregnancy category	A; PB: UK; $t_{1/2}$: weeks–months
Deficiency conditions	Treats vitamin A deficiency, prevents nightblindness, treats skin disorders, promotes bone development
Side effects	Headache, fatigue, drowsiness, irritability, anorexia, vomiting, diarrhea, dry skin, visual changes
Adverse reactions	Evident only with toxicity; leukopenia, aplastic anemia, papilledema, increased intracranial pressure, hypervitaminosis A (loss of hair and peeling skin); excess dose during pregnancy can cause birth defects
Contraindications	Mineral oil, cholestyramine, alcohol, and antilipemic drugs decrease the absorption of vitamin A; it is excreted through the kidneys and feces

Abbreviations: PB = protein binding; UK = unknown; $t_{1/2}$ = half-life.

of the active form of calcifediol. Excess vitamin D is then excreted in bile, and a small amount is excreted in urine.

It's amazing how quickly adequate levels of vitamin D can be restored by sunlight. Just 6 days of casual sunlight exposure without sunscreen can make up for 49 days of

Vitamin D	
Dose for treatment of deficiency	Mild deficiency: 50–125 µg/dL Moderate to severe: 2.5–7.5 mg/day; 2500–7500 µg
Maintenance	Male and female: 40–80 µg; 200–400 IU
Pregnancy category	A
Deficiency conditions	Rickets, deficit of phosphorus and calcium in blood
Side effects	None significant
Adverse reactions	Excess of 40,000 IU results in hypervitaminosis D and may cause hypercalcemia (an elevated serum calcium level); early symptoms of toxicity are anorexia, nausea, and vomiting
Contraindications	Hypercalcemia, hypervitaminosis D, or renal osteodystrophy with hyperphosphatemia. Use with caution in patients with arteriosclerosis, hyperphosphatemia, hypersensitivity to vitamin D, and renal or cardiac impairment.

Vitamin E	
Dose for treatment of deficiency	Malabsorption: 30–100 mg/day Severe deficit: 1–2 mg/kg or 50–200 IU/kg daily
Maintenance	Male: 10 mg/day; 15 IU Female: 8 mg/day; 12 IU Pregnancy: 10–12 mg/day
Pregnancy category	A (C if used in doses above RDA)
Deficiency conditions	Breakdown of red blood cells
Side effects	None significant
Adverse reactions	Large doses may cause fatigue, weakness, nausea, GI upset, headache, and breast tenderness, and may prolong the prothrombin time (PT) (clotting time).
Contraindications	Patients taking warfarin (an anticoagulant) should have their pro thrombin (PT) monitored closely; iron and vitamin E should not be taken together because iron can interfere with the body's absorption and use of vitamin E

no sunlight exposure. Sunlight exposure is an easy, reliable way for most people to obtain vitamin D. Exposure of the hands, face, arms, and legs to sunlight 2–3 times a week will cause the skin to produce a sufficient amount of vitamin D.

Body fat acts like a type of storage battery for vitamin D. During periods of sunlight, vitamin D is stored in fatty fat and then released when sunlight is gone. Nevertheless, vitamin D deficiency is very common, especially in people living in Canada and the northern half of the United States. Vitamin D deficiency also occurs even in sunny climates, possibly because people tend to stay indoors more, cover up when going outside, or using sunscreens consistently sunny days to reduce skin cancer risk.

Vitamin E Vitamin E protects the heart and arteries and cellular components from being oxidized and protects red blood cells from hemolysis (rupture). If there is a sufficient balance of salts, pancreatic secretion, and fat, vitamin E is absorbed from the GI tract and stored in all tissues, especially in the liver, muscle, and fatty tissues. Seventy-five percent of excess vitamin E is excreted in the bile, and the remainder is excreted in urine.

Vitamin K Vitamin K is derived from dietary sources such as leafy green vegetables, liver, cheese, and egg yolk and is synthesized by intestinal flora. Vitamin K is required to synthesize prothrombin and clotting factors VII, IX, and X and is an antidote for oral overdose of the anticoagulant Coumadin (warfarin). There are four forms of

Vitamin K	
Dose for treatment of deficiency	5–15 mg/day (based on PT laboratory results)
Maintenance	Male: 70–80 µg/day Female: 60–65 µg/day If taking a broad-spectrum antibiotic: 140 µg/day Pregnancy: 65 µg/day
Pregnancy category	C
Deficiency conditions	Increased clotting time leading to increased bleeding and hemorrhage
Side effects	Occasional pain, soreness, and swelling at IM injection site; pruritic erythema (itchy redness) with repeated injections; flushed face, unusual taste
Adverse reactions	Rare: severe reaction immediately following IV administration (cramp-like pain, chest pain, dyspnea, facial flushing, dizziness, rapid/weak pulse, rash, profuse sweating, hypotension; may progress to shock, cardiac arrest)
Contraindications	Last few weeks of pregnancy and in neonates; use with caution: asthma and impaired hepatic function

vitamin K: K_1 (phytonadione), which is the active form; K_2 (menaquinone), which is synthesized by intestinal flora, but not commercially available; and K_3 (menadione) and K_4 (menadiol), both of which are produced synthetically. K_1 and K_2 are absorbed in the presence of bile salts. K_3 and K_4 are absorbed without bile salts. Vitamin K_1 prevents hemorrhage and is available as Mephyton, AquaMEPHYTON, and Konakion. Vitamin K_4 is available as Synkayvite. Vitamin K is absorbed in the intestines and is stored in the liver and in other tissues.

Water-Soluble Vitamins

Water-soluble vitamins are also known as the *B complex* because they were originally considered as only one vitamin. It was later discovered that these are separate vitamins. The water-soluble vitamins are described in the following paragraphs.

Vitamin C Vitamin C may be found in citrus fruits, tomatoes, leafy green vegetables, and potatoes and are used to metabolize carbohydrates and for synthesis of protein, lipids, and collagen. Vitamin C is also required for capillary endothelium and repair of tissues. Vitamin C aids in the absorption of iron and the metabolism of folic acid. Unlike fat-soluble vitamins, vitamin C is not stored in the body and is excreted in urine.

Vitamin C	
Dose for treatment of deficiency	Adult daily dose is 50–100 mg/kg; for severe deficit (scurvy) PO: IM, IV: 150–500 mg/day in one or two divided doses; 500–6000 mg/day for treatment of upper respiratory infections, cancer, or hypercholesterolemia
Maintenance	45–60 mg/day
Pregnancy category	C
Deficiency conditions	Prevents and treats C deficiency (scurvy); increases wound healing; for burns; sickle cell crisis; deep-vein thrombosis; megavitamin therapy (massive doses) of vitamins are not recommended as this can cause toxicity
Side effects	Headaches, fatigue, drowsiness, nausea, heartburn, vomiting, diarrhea; vitamin C with aspirin or sulfonamides may cause crystal formation in the urine (crystalluria); it can also cause a false-negative occult (blood) stool result and false-positive sugar result in the urine when tested by the Clinitest method
Adverse reactions	Kidney stones, crystalluria, hyperuricemia; massive doses can cause diarrhea and GI upset
Contraindications	Large doses can decrease the effect of oral anticoagulants; oral contraceptives can decrease C concentration in the body; smoking decreases serum levels of C; use with caution if renal calculi (kidney stones), gout, anemia, sickle cell disease, sideroblasts, or thalassemia are present
Drug-food interactions	Decrease ascorbic acid uptake taken with salicylates; may decrease effect of oral anticoagulants; may decrease elimination of aspirin

However, high serum levels of vitamin C can result from excessive doses and can be excreted without any change. Vitamin C is commercially available as Ascorbicap, Cecon, Cevalin, and Solucap C.

Vitamin B Complex Vitamin B complex consists of four vitamins: B_1 (thiamine), B_2 (riboflavin), B_3 (niacin), and B_6 (pyridoxine). B_1 is used to treat peripheral neuritis from alcoholism or beriberi. B_2 is used to manage dermatologic problems, such as scaly dermatitis, cracked corners of the mouth, and inflammation of the skin and tongue. B_3 is given in large doses to alleviate pellagra (dietary deficiency of niacin) and hyperlipidemia and may cause GI irritation and vasodilatation, resulting in a flushing sensation. B_6 is given to correct B_6 deficiency and helps alleviate symptoms of neuritis causes by isoniazid (INH) therapy for tuberculosis.

Vitamin B Complex	
Dose for treatment of deficiency	Thiamine: 30–60 mg/day Riboflavin: 5–25 mg/day Prophylactic: 3 mg/day Nicotinic acid or niacin: prevention, 5–20 mg/day Deficit: 50–100 mg/day Pellagra: 300–500 mg in 3 divided doses Hyperlipidemia: 1–2 g/day in 3 divided doses Pyridoxine: 25–100 mg/day Isoniazid therapy prophylaxis: 20–25 mg/day Peripheral neuritis: 50–200 mg/day
Maintenance	Thiamine: male, 1.5 mg; female, 1.1 mg Pregnancy: 1.5 mg Lactating: 1.6 mg Riboflavin: male, 1.4–1.7 mg; female, 1.2–1.3 mg Pregnancy: 1.6 mg Lactating: 1.8 mg Nicotinic acid or niacin: male, 15–19 mg/day; female, 13–15 mg/day Pregnancy: 18 mg/day Lactating: 20 mg/day Pyridoxine: male, 2.0 mg/day; female, 1.6 mg/day Pregnancy: 2.1 mg/day Lactating: 2.2 mg/day
Pregnancy category	A (C if dose is >RDA)
Deficiency conditions	Thiamine: sensory disturbances, retarded growth, fatigue, anorexia Riboflavin: visual defects such as blurred vision and photophobia, cheilosis, rash on nose; numbness of extremities Niacin or nicotinic acid: retarded growth, pellagra, headache, memory loss, anorexia, insomnia Pyridoxine: neuritis, convulsions, dermatitis, anemia, lymphopenia
Side effects	Thiamine: raised skin rash, pruritus, or wheezing after a large IV dose Riboflavin: orange-yellow discoloration in urine Niacin or nicotinic acid: flushing, pruritus, sensations of warmth; dizziness, arrhythmias, dry skin, hyperglycemia, myalgia, nausea, vomiting, diarrhea at high doses Pyridoxine: occasional—stinging at IM injection site; rare—headache, nausea, somnolence; high doses cause sensory neuropathy (paresthesia, unstable gait, clumsiness of hands)

(Continued)

Vitamin B Complex (Continued)	
Adverse reactions	Thiamine: rare anaphylaxis after a large IV dose
	Riboflavin: none known
	Niacin or nicotinic acid: cardiac arrythmias may occur rarely
	Pyridoxine: long-term megadoses may produce sensory neuropathy
	Thiamine: patients with renal dysfunction
Contraindications	Riboflavin: patients with renal dysfunction
	Niacin or nicotinic acid: hypersensitivity to niacin or tartrazine; active peptic ulcer, severe hypotension, hepatic dysfunction, arterial hemorrhaging
	Caution: diabetes mellitus, gallbladder disease, gout, history of jaundice or liver disease
	Pyridoxine: IV therapy in cardiac patients
	Caution: megadosage in pregnancy

Folic Acid (Folate, Vitamin B₉) Folic acid is essential for body growth and is needed to synthesize DNA. Folic acid is found in leafy green vegetables, yellow fruits and vegetables, yeast, and meat and is absorbed in the small intestine. The active form of folic acid, called *folate*, circulates to all tissues in the body. A third of folate is stored in the liver, and the remainder is stored in other tissues. Most folic acid is excreted in bile and a small amount is excreted in urine. Chronic alcoholism, poor nutrition, pregnancy, and diseases that disrupt absorption by the small intestine can lead to an inadequate amount of folic acid. This can disrupt cellular division. A patient with low folic acid has nausea and diarrhea and is anorexic and fatigued, and has stomatitis, alopecia, and blood dyscrasias (megaloblastic anemia, leukopenia, and thrombocytopenia). Symptoms seldom appear for 2–4 months after folic acid storage is depleted.

Vitamin B₁₂ Vitamin B₁₂ may be found in liver, kidney, fish, and fortified milk and helps convert folic acid into its active form. Vitamin B₁₂ is essential to DNA synthesis, promotes cellular division, and is required for hematopoiesis (development of red blood cells in bone marrow) and to maintain the integrity of the nervous system. Vitamin B₁₂ is absorbed in the intestine with the aid of an intrinsic factor produced by gastric parietal cells. Once absorbed, vitamin B₁₂ binds to the transcobalamin II protein and is then transferred to tissues. Vitamin B₁₂ is stored in the liver for ≤3 years, during which time it is slowly excreted in urine. Vitamin B₁₂ deficiency is common in patients who are strict vegetarians and in patients who have malabsorption syndromes (cancer, celiac disease), gastrectomy, Crohn's disease, and liver and kidney diseases.

Folic Acid	
Dose	1–2 mg/day
Maintenance	Male and female: 400 µg/day
	Pregnancy: 600–800 µg/day
	Lactating: 600–800 µg/day
Pregnancy category	A (C if >RDA)
Deficiency conditions	Decreased white blood cell (WBC) count and clotting factors, anemias, intestinal disturbances, depression
Side effects	None significant
Adverse reactions	High doses of folic acid can mask signs of B$_{12}$ deficiency, which is a risk in the elderly; patients taking phenytoin (Dilantin) for seizures should be cautious about taking folic acid because it can increase the risk of seizures
	During the first trimester of pregnancy, folic acid deficiency can affect the development of the central nervous system (CNS) of the fetus; this can lead to neural tube defects such as spina bifida (a defective closure of the bony structure of the spinal cord) or anencephaly (lack of brain mass formation)
Contraindications	Pernicious, aplastic, normocytic, refractory anemias

Vitamin B$_{12}$	
Dose	100 mg/dL × 14 days
	Pernicious anemia: 40–100 µg/day or 1000 µg/week × 3 weeks
Maintenance	Male and female: 3 µg/day
	Pregnancy: 4 µg/day
Pregnancy category	A (C if use doses >RDA)
Deficiency conditions	Pernicious anemia, hemolytic anemia, hyperthyroidism, bowel and pancreatic malignancies, gastrectomy, GI lesions, neurologic damage, malabsorption syndrome, metabolic disorders, renal disease, and certain bariatric procedures
Side effects	Occasional: diarrhea, itching
Adverse reactions	Rare allergic reaction; may produce peripheral vascular thrombosis, pulmonary edema, hypokalemia, congestive heart failure (CHF)
Contraindications	History of allergy to cobalimin; folate-deficient anemia, hereditary optic nerve atrophy

2. Vitamins and the Nursing Process

The nurse must assess the patient for signs and symptoms of vitamin deficiency before beginning vitamin therapy because vitamin therapy could result in a toxic effect if the patient does not have a vitamin deficiency. The physician may also order laboratory tests to determine whether a vitamin deficiency exists.

In addition, the patient must be assessed for debilitating diseases and GI disorders that may disrupt the absorption, metabolism, and excretion of vitamins used to treat vitamin deficiency.

For some patients, vitamin deficiency is caused by inadequate nutrient intake. Therefore, it is critical that the patient's diet be assessed to determine whether it is the cause of the deficiency. If so, then the nurse should educate the patient on the importance of maintaining a balanced diet.

In many cases, the nurse may reach one of the following diagnoses:

- Altered nutrition; less than body requirements
- Lack of knowledge related to proper nutrition
- Lack of knowledge related to vitamin use

On the basis of these diagnoses, the nurse should develop a plan for having the patient eat a well-balanced diet and take vitamin supplements as prescribed. The plan should also take into consideration the following interventions:

- Administer vitamins with food to promote absorption.
- Store vitamins in light-resistant container.
- Use a calibrated dropper for administration of liquid vitamins.
- Administer IM if patient is unable to take PO.

Teaching the patient is an important intervention because this gives the patient the knowledge to implement preemptive actions that will reduce the risk of vitamin deficiency in the future.

The nurse should teach the patient to do the following:

- Take prescribed amount of vitamin.
- Read labels carefully.
- Not use megavitamins over a prolonged period of time.
- Check expiration dates on containers before purchasing or taking them (potency is reduced after the expiration date).
- Not take vitamin A with mineral oil, which interferes with vitamin A absorption.
- Not take megadoses of vitamin C (ascorbic acid) to "cure a cold."

- Not take megadoses of vitamin C with aspirin or sulfonamides.
- Avoid excessive intake of alcoholic beverages, which can cause vitamin B-complex deficiencies.

The nurse should refer the patient to the USDA website (http://www.mypyramid.gov/pyramid/index.html) to calculate the desired portions for each food group on the basis of age, gender, and the amount of exercise that the patient performs daily. It is important that the patient understand that vitamin supplements are not necessary if she/he is healthy and eats properly.

The nurse should alert the patient to the signs and symptoms of hypervitaminosis. Hypervitaminosis A causes nausea, vomiting, headache, loss of hair, and cracked lips. Hypervitaminosis D causes anorexia, nausea, and vomiting.

The nurse should evaluate the patient for proper dietary intake and determine whether vitamin therapy is having a therapeutic effect.

3. Minerals

Minerals are inorganic compounds that are required by the body for metabolism and to form bones and teeth. Minerals are extracted from ingested food such as meats, eggs, vegetables, and fruits. There are five minerals that are critical to maintain a healthy body.

Iron

Iron (ferrous sulfate, gluconate, or fumarate) is used for the regeneration of hemoglobin. Iron deficiency causes anemia. The patient requires 5–20 mg/day of iron,

Iron	
Dose	Adult 50 mg/day
	Infant and child dose of iron, ages 6 months–2 years is 1.5/mg/kg
	Ferrous sulfate for therapeutic: 600–1200 mg/day in divided doses
Maintenance	Ferrous sulfate for prophylactic: 300–325 mg/day
Pregnancy category	A; PB = UK; $t_{1/2}$ UK
Treatment	Given to correct or control iron-deficiency anemia
Side effects	GI discomfort, nausea, vomiting, diarrhea, constipation, epigastric pain, elixir may stain teeth
Adverse reactions	Pallor, drowsiness
	Life-threatening: cardiovascular collapse, metabolic acidosis
Contraindications	Avoid a megadose in the first trimester because it might cause birth defects

Abbreviations: PB = protein-binding; UK = unknown; $t_{1/2}$ = half-life.

obtained from eating liver, lean meats, egg yolks, dried beans, green vegetables (such as spinach), and fruit.

Pregnant women require an increased amount of iron, but they need to avoid a megadose in the first trimester because this can cause birth defects. Larger doses of iron are necessary in the second and third trimesters. Iron is absorbed in the intestines, where it enters plasma as heme, or it is stored as ferritin in the liver, spleen, and bone marrow. Food, the antibiotic tetracycline, and antacids decrease absorption by ≤50% of iron. However, the patient should take iron with food to avoid GI discomfort. Vitamin C may slightly increase iron absorption. Iron toxicity is a serious cause of poisoning in children. Toxicity can develop with as few as 10 tablets of ferrous sulfate (3 g) taken at one time—and can be fatal within 12–48 hours.

Calcium

Calcium is a mineral that is an essential part of bones and teeth. The heart, nerves, and blood-clotting systems also need calcium to work. Calcium is used for treatment and prevention of low calcium levels and resulting bone conditions, including osteoporosis (weak bones due to low bone density), rickets (a condition in children involving softening of the bones), and osteomalacia (a softening of bones involving pain). Calcium is also used for premenstrual syndrome (PMS), leg cramps in pregnancy, high blood pressure in pregnancy (preeclampsia), and reducing the risk of colon and rectal cancers.

Calcium carbonate is used as an antacid for "heartburn." Calcium carbonate and calcium acetate are also used for reducing phosphate levels in people with kidney disease.

Calcium-rich foods include milk and dairy products, kale and broccoli, as well as the calcium-enriched citrus juices, mineral water, canned fish with bones, and soy products processed with calcium.

Calcium can interact with many prescription medications, but sometimes the effects can be minimized by taking calcium at a different time.

Copper

Copper is used in the formation of red blood cells and connective tissues. It is also a cofactor for many enzymes. Without copper, enzymes are unable to initiate metabolic reactions in the body. Copper is also a component in the production of the neurotransmitters norepinephrine and dopamine. Foods rich in copper are shellfish (crabs and oysters), liver, nuts, seeds (sunflower, sesame), legumes, and cocoa. It is absorbed in the intestines. A prolonged copper deficiency can result in anemia and cause changes in the skin and blood, including a decrease in the white blood count, intolerance to glucose, decrease in skin and hair pigmentation, and mental retardation if the patient is young. High levels of copper in serum can be an indication of Wilson's disease, which is an inborn error of metabolism that allows for large amounts of copper to accumulate in the liver, brain, cornea, or kidney.

Calcium	
Dose	Age 0–6 months, 1000 mg; 6–12 months, 1500 mg; 1–8 years, 2500 mg; 9–18 years, 3000 mg; 1950 years, 2500 mg; 51+ years, 2000 mg
Maintenance	1000–1300 mg/day of calcium
Pregnancy category	Not assigned to a pregnancy category; safe for use in pregnancy
Deficiency conditions	Inadequate intakes of dietary calcium from food and supplements produce no obvious symptoms in the short term; circulating blood levels of calcium are tightly regulated; hypocalcemia results primarily from medical problems or treatments, including renal failure, surgical removal of the stomach, and use of certain medications (such as diuretics); symptoms of hypocalcemia include numbness and tingling in the fingers, muscle cramps, convulsions, lethargy, poor appetite, and abnormal heart rhythms; if left untreated, calcium deficiency leads to death; over the long term, inadequate calcium intake causes osteopenia, which, if untreated, can lead to osteoporosis; the risk of bone fractures also increases, especially in older individuals; calcium deficiency can also cause rickets, although it is more commonly associated with vitamin D deficiency
Side effects	Calcium may cause gas, bloating, and constipation; symptoms of hypocalcemia include numbness and tingling in the fingers, muscle cramps, convulsions, lethargy, poor appetite, and abnormal heart rhythms; if left untreated, calcium deficiency leads to death
Adverse reactions	Hypercalcremia can cause renal insufficiency, vascular and soft-tissue calcification, hypercalciuria (high levels of calcium in the urine) and kidney stones; although very high calcium intake can cause hypercalcemia, it is most commonly associated with primary hyperparathyroidism or malignancy
Contraindications	Tumors that dissolve bone, incomplete or infrequent bowel movements, kidney stones, kidney disease, sarcoidosis, increased activity of the parathyroid gland, high amounts of calcium in the blood, extreme loss of body water

Copper	
Dose	1.5–3 mg/day
Maintenance	1.5–3 mg/day
Pregnancy category	A (C if >RDA dose)
Deficiency conditions	Anemia, decreased WBCs, glucose intolerance, decrease in skin and hair pigmentation, and mental retardation in the young
Side effects	None significant
Adverse reactions	Vomiting and diarrhea
Contraindications	None known

Zinc	
Dose	12–19 mg/day
Maintenance	12–19 mg/day
Pregnancy category	A (C if taken in doses >RDA)
Deficiency conditions	Growth retardation, diarrhea, vomiting, delayed puberty, weakness, dry skin, delay in wound healing
Side effects	None known
Adverse reactions	Anemia, increased low-density lipoprotein (LDL) cholesterol, muscle pain, fever, nausea, vomiting
Contraindications	Do not take with tetracycline

Zinc

Zinc stimulates the activity of over 100 enzymes for important functions in the body, which includes production of insulin and sperm and plays a key role in the immune system and in DNA synthesis. Zinc helps wounds heal and helps the patient maintain a sense of taste and smell. A dose of zinc larger than 150 mg can cause copper deficiency, decrease high-density lipoprotein (HDL) cholesterol, and weaken the patient's immune response. Zinc also inhibits tetracycline (antibiotic) absorption and therefore should not be taken with antibiotics. The patient should wait 2 hours after taking any antibiotic before taking zinc.

Chromium

Chromium is acquired from meats, whole-grain cereals, and brewer's yeast and plays a role in controlling non-insulin-dependent diabetes by normalizing blood glucose,

Chromium	
Dose	50–200 µg/day is considered within the normal range for anyone >6 years of age (there is no RDA)
Maintenance	50–200 µg/day is considered within the normal range for anyone >6 years of age (there is no RDA)
Pregnancy category	A
Deficiency conditions	Inability to properly use glucose
Side effects	None known
Adverse reactions	May cause hypoglycemic reaction in patients who are taking insulin or an oral hypoglycemic agent
Contraindications	Although contraindicated for diabetic patients, blood sugar levels should be monitored closely

Selenium	
Dose	40–75 µg (high doses for males and lower dose for females)
Maintenance	40–75 µg (high doses for males and lower dose for females)
Pregnancy category	A
Deficiency conditions	Heart disease
Side effects	Causes a garlic-like odor from the skin and breath in large doses
Adverse reactions	Disorders of nervous and digestive systems and loss of hair with doses >200 µg
Contraindications	None known

thereby increasing the effects of the body's insulin on cells. Chromium 50–200 µg/day is considered within the normal range for children aged >6 years old and adults.

Selenium

Selenium is a trace mineral that is a cofactor for antioxidant enzymes that protect protein and nucleic acids from damage caused by oxidation. Selenium is found in meats (especially liver), seafood, eggs, and dairy products. With a dose greater than 200 µg, selenium has a possible anticarcinogenic (anticancer) effect and may reduce the risk of lung, prostate, and colorectal cancer. However, such a dose might cause weakness, loss of hair, dermatitis, nausea, diarrhea, and abdominal pain.

Summary

Vitamins and minerals are required for the body to function properly. Each day we need to eat a balanced diet that supplies us with the sufficient amount of vitamins and minerals to remain healthy. Our diet should contain grains, vegetables, fruits, milk, meat, and beans. The portion of each varies depending on our age and gender. The USDA website publishes the Recommended Dietary Allowance (RDA) for daily dose requirement of each vitamin.

Vitamins are divided into two groups: fat-soluble and water-soluble. Fat-soluble vitamins can be stored in the body for ≤2 years. Water-soluble vitamins are used immediately and then excreted from the body in urine.

As part of the nursing process, assess the patient for vitamin deficiencies and determine what caused the deficiency. Some deficiencies are caused by changes in the body that affect absorption of vitamins. Other deficiencies are due to a poor or an unbalanced diet. After administering prescribed vitamin therapy, the patient should be educated about the importance of eating well-balanced meals and taking vitamin supplements if necessary.

Minerals are inorganic substances that the body uses for blood cells, tissues, and to stimulate enzymes to cause a catabolic reaction in the body.

In the next chapter, we'll examine the balancing act of fluids and electrolytes and how they maintain equilibrium. We'll also see how to use fluid and electrolyte therapies to restore the equilibrium if they become imbalanced.

QUIZ

1. Vitamins that are stored in the body are called
   (a) water-soluble.
   (b) fat-soluble.
   (c) storage vitamins.
   (d) none of the above.

2. What vitamin is converted into calcifediol in the liver?
   (a) Vitamin A
   (b) Vitamin E
   (c) Vitamin D
   (d) Vitamin C

3. What vitamin protects the heart and arteries and cellular components from being oxidized?
   (a) Vitamin A
   (b) Vitamin E
   (c) Vitamin D
   (d) Vitamin C

4. Vitamin K is synthesized by intestinal flora.
   (a) True
   (b) False

5. Vitamin C is used to metabolize carbohydrates.
   (a) True
   (b) False

6. **What vitamin is used to treat acne?**

    (a) Vitamin A
    (b) Vitamin E
    (c) Vitamin D
    (d) Vitamin C

7. **Fat-soluble vitamins are immediately excreted in urine shortly after they are absorbed.**

    (a) True
    (b) False

8. **What vitamin is given to help alleviate symptoms of neuritis caused by isoniazid therapy for tuberculosis?**

    (a) Vitamin A
    (b) Vitamin E
    (c) Vitamin D
    (d) None of the above

9. **Minerals are organic compounds synthesized in the liver.**

    (a) True
    (b) False

10. **Spinach is a source for iron.**

    (a) True
    (b) False

chapter 10

Fluid and Electrolyte Therapy

What would happen if your muscles no longer contracted? You couldn't eat and digest food and water. You would be unable to move and talk, and eventually your brain would be unable to function. Most importantly, your heart is a muscle, and it would simply stop beating.

In order for muscles to contract, the human body needs the proper balance between fluids and electrolytes both inside and outside of cells. *Electrolytes* are salts whose positive and negative charges generate the electrical impulse to contract muscles in the body.

Diseases and treatment of disease can cause fluids and electrolytes to become imbalanced and require the patient to receive medication to restore balance. In this chapter, you'll learn how to recognize the signs and symptoms of fluid and electrolyte imbalance and learn about therapeutic treatment that brings them back into balance.

1. Body Fluids

Water constitutes 60% of adult body weight. However, water makes up 45–55% of an older adult's body weight, and as much as 70–80% of an infant's weight is water. This places older adults and infants at high risk for fluid imbalance. Lean adults have a higher water content than heavy adults because adipose cells (cells containing fat) contain less water than other cells. Water is the solvent that contains salts, nutrients, and wastes that are solutes dissolved in the water and transported by the water throughout the body. Salts are electrolytes.

Body fluids are stored in intracellular and extracellular compartments. *Intracellular fluid* (ICF) is located inside the cell and constitutes 40% of body weight. *Extracellular fluid* (ECF) is divided into smaller compartments. These spaces between the cells are called the *interstitial space*. The space is occupied by plasma and lymph, transcellular fluid, and fluid in the bone and connective tissues. This makes up 20% of body weight. About a third is plasma, and two-thirds of extracellular fluid is located in the space between the cells. *Transcellular fluid* is also ECF but is found in the gastrointestinal (GI) tract, cerebrospinal space, aqueous humor, pleural space, synovial space, and peritoneal space. Although the volume of fluid in the transcellular space is small when compared with fluid volumes in intracellular and extracellular compartments, the increase or decrease in volume in transcellular spaces can have a dramatic effect on the fluid-electrolyte balance.

2. Electrolytes

An *electrolyte* is a substance that splits into ions when placed in water. An *ion* is an electrically charged particle that is either positively or negatively charged. A positively charged ion is called a *cation*, and a negatively charged ion is called an *anion*. The following are examples of cations and anions (see also Table 10–1):

- Sodium (Na^+), potassium (K^+), calcium (Ca^{2+}), and magnesium (Mg^{2+}) are electrolytes that are cations.
- Chloride (Cl^-), bicarbonate (HCO_3^-), phosphate (PO_4^-), and sulfate (SO_4^-) are electrolytes that are anions.

An electrolyte is measured as a millimole per liter (mmol/L). A *millimole* is the atomic weight of the electrolyte in milligrams. For example, the atomic weight of sodium is 23 mg. Therefore, 23 mg of sodium is measured as 1 mmol of sodium.

An electrolyte is stored either intracellularly (inside the cell) or extracellularly (outside the cell).

Intracellular electrolytes are mainly potassium, magnesium, and some calcium.

Extracellular electrolytes are mainly sodium and some calcium.

TABLE 10–1 Electrolytes

Electrolyte	Normal Range (mEq/L)*	Signs and Symptoms of Electrolyte Imbalance	Low Levels	High Levels
Calcium	4.5–5.5	Muscle spasm, weakness, twitching, or convulsions	Irregular heartbeat, confusion, blood pressure changes, or bone disorders	Weakness or twitching of the muscles, numbness, fatigue, irregular heartbeat and blood pressure changes
Chloride	97–107	Symptoms rare	Dehydration, fluid loss, or high levels of blood sodium; muscle twitching, irritability, increased urination, poor appetite	Excess fluid loss, high blood sugar, Kussmaul's breathing, dyspnea, intense thirst, weakness, tachypnea, hypertension, pitting edema, diminished cognitive ability, possible coma
Potassium	3.5–5.3	Muscle spasm, weakness, twitching, or convulsions	Irregular heartbeat, confusion, blood pressure changes, or bone disorders	Irregular heartbeat, confusion, blood pressure changes, or bone disorders
Magnesium	1.5–2.5	Muscle spasm, weakness, twitching, or convulsions	Irregular heartbeat, confusion, blood pressure changes, or bone disorders	Irregular heartbeat, confusion, blood pressure changes, or bone disorders
Sodium	136–145	Muscle spasm, weakness, twitching, or convulsions	Irregular heartbeat, confusion, blood pressure changes, or bone disorders	Irregular heartbeat, confusion, blood pressure changes, or bone disorders

*Normal values may vary slightly from laboratory to laboratory.

3. Fluid Concentration

Movement of electrolytes between compartments is based on the concentration of electrolytes, the gradients of the concentration, and the electrical charge. For example, there is a higher concentration of sodium outside than inside the cell. Therefore, the gradient is toward the inside of the cell.

Fluids move through the body continuously. As the heart pumps the blood, pressure is exerted on the vessels from outside the body, and muscles relax and contract to help the heart move the fluid through the vascular system. Osmotic pressure causes fluid to move into and out of the cells and the extracellular spaces. This is the pressure exerted by the flow of water through a semipermeable membrane separating two solutions with different solute concentrations. Osmotic pressure is determined by the concentration of the electrolytes and other solutes in water and is expressed as osmolarity or osmolality. The terms are used interchangeably.

Osmolality is the concentration of body fluids. *Tonicity* is the effect of fluid on cellular volume. Serum osmolality is a better indicator of the concentration of solutes in body fluids than tonicity; tonicity is used primarily as a measurement of the concentration of intravenous solutions.

There are three types of fluid concentration:

- **Isoosmolar:** This is a fluid that has the same concentration of solute particles as water.
- **Hypoosmolar:** This is a fluid that has a lower concentration of solute particles than water.
- **Hyperosmolar:** This is a fluid that has a higher concentration of solute particles than water.

Normal serum has an osmolality ranging between 275 and 295 mOsm/dg (milliosmoles per decigram). Fluid concentrations of <275 mOsm/dg and >295 mOsm/dg are hypoosmolar and hyperosmolar, respectively. Hypoosmolarity might be caused by a fluid excess. Fluid volume increases, and solute volumes usually decrease. Hyperosmolarity might be caused by a fluid deficit with an increase in solutes. The blood becomes more concentrated, and the fluid is pulled out of the body's organs. These patients might be dehydrated. The concentration of solutes is important when determining the proper replacement fluid for a patient whose fluids and electrolytes are imbalanced. Replacement fluids are replaced orally (by mouth or nasogastric tube) or parenterally with IV fluids (intravenously or subcutaneously).

4. Intravenous Fluids

The osmolality of many IV fluids is similar to serum osmolality, which is 290 mOsm/kg H_2O. There are three categories of IV fluids osmolality:

- **Isotonic:** This is in the isoosmolar range (240–340 mOsm/L), where the IV fluid concentration is the same as the intracellular fluid concentration (NaCl 0.9%, normal saline).
- **Hypotonic:** This is in the hypoosmolar range (<240 mOsm/L), where the IV fluid concentration is less than the intracellular fluid concentration (NaCl 0.45%, sodium chloride).
- **Hypertonic:** This is in the hyperosmolar range (>340 mOsm/L), where the IV fluid concentration is more than the intracellular fluid concentration (dextrose 5% in 0.45% saline).

Intravenous solutions are classified as crystalloids, colloids, or lipids.

Crystalloids

Crystalloids are used for replacement and maintenance of fluid balance therapy. These include dextrose, saline, and lactated Ringer's solution.

Colloids

Colloids are volume expanders that increase the patient's fluid volume. These include dextran, amino acids, hetastarch, and plasmanate:

- *Dextran* is not a substitute for whole blood because it does not have components that carry oxygen. Dextran 40 tends to interfere with platelet function, resulting in prolonged bleeding times.

- *Amino acids* provide protein, calories, and fluid for the body. It is helpful for patients who are old and malnourished and for those with hypoproteinemia resulting from other causes.

- *Hetastarch* is a nonantigenic agent used to treat or prevent shock following serious injury or surgery, or for burn patients when blood is not available for transfusion. This, also, is not a substitute for whole blood. In an isotonic solution (310 mOsm/L), hetastarch decreases platelet and hematocrit counts and must not be used for patients who have bleeding disorders, congestive heart failure (CHF), or renal dysfunction.

- *Plasmanate* is a protein-containing fluid that is derived from human plasma and is used to treat shock that results from burns, crushing injuries, abdominal emergencies, or any emergency where there is a loss of plasma, but not red blood cells. Plasmanate is nonantigenic and must not be given to patients who have anemia, increased blood volume, or congestive heart failure.

Lipids

Lipids are a fat emulsion that is given when IV therapy extends for longer than 5 days. This is used for prolonged parenteral nutrition to provide essential fatty acids.

5. Blood and Blood Products

Blood and blood products consist of whole blood, packed red blood cells, plasma, and albumin. Whole blood consists of all cellular and plasma components of blood. Whole blood should be used to treat severe cases of anemia—not mild cases of anemia—because one unit of whole blood elevates hemoglobin by 0.5–1.0 g. (By comparison, a unit of packed red bloods elevates the hematocrit—the percentage of serum occupied by red blood cells—by three points.) Packed red blood cells are whole blood without plasma and are used to decrease circulatory overload and thereby the risk of reaction to antigens contained in plasma.

6. Fluid Replacement

The amount of water that a patient requires each day depends on the patient's age and the nature of the patient's medical condition. Water constitutes 30 mL/kg of body weight. A patient who weighs 70 kg has 2100 mL of water (70 kg × 30 mL/kg). In other words, a patient who weighs 150 lb weighs 68 kg (150 lb/2.2 = 68.18 kg) and contains 2240 mL of water.

Each day the patient loses the following amounts of water:

- 400–500 mL of water through evaporation from the skin
- 400–500 mL of water through breathing
- 100–200 mL of water in feces
- 1000–1200 mL of water in urine

This means that each day the patient must take in 1900–2400 mL of fluid in order to maintain fluid-electrolyte balance. However, disease and the treatment of disease can increase the patient's output of water, requiring that the patient increase the intake of water.

For example, a patient with a fever loses as much as 15% more water than the normal daily water loss, or between 2185 and 2760 mL of water.

Fluid Replacement and the Nursing Process

When a patient is experiencing the loss of fluid, the nurse should do the following:

- Establish baseline vital signs and weight.
- Review laboratory (lab) results and report elevations in the hematocrit and blood urea nitrogen (BUN). An elevation of both values could indicate that the patient is dehydrated. If the BUN is >60 mg/dL, renal impairment may be the cause.
- Measure urine output. An output that is <30 mL/hr or 600 mL/day should be reported. Normal urine output should be >35 mL/hr or 1000–1200 mL/day.
- Review the lab results for urine specific gravity (SG). Normal range is 1.005–1.030. If the SG is greater than 1.030, dehydration may be the cause.

- Verify that the proper osmolality levels of the IV fluids are ordered. If there is continuous use of one type of IV fluid such as 5% dextrose in water (D5W), hypoosmolality of body fluid could occur.

Potential nursing diagnoses for a patient who is receiving fluid volume replacement therapy are described as follows:

- Risk for fluid volume excess, which can occur when the patient is given too much replacement fluid, fluid is infused too rapidly, or the volume is excessive in proportion to the patient's physical size or condition
- Risk for fluid volume deficit related to inadequate fluid intake
- Altered tissue perfusion, related to decreased blood circulation or inadequate fluid replacement

Before beginning fluid replacement therapy, goals should include the following:

- The patient will not develop fluid volume deficit or excess as a result of IV fluid replacement.
- The patient will remain hydrated.
- Vital signs and urine output will remain within normal ranges.

When fluid replacement therapy is in progress, the nurse should monitor the following:

- Vital signs
- Fluid intake and output
- Daily weight
- Signs and symptoms of fluid volume excess (overload), which include cough, dyspnea (difficulty breathing), jugular vein distention (JVD) (neck vein engorgement), and moist rales (abnormal breath sounds)
- Signs and symptoms of fluid volume deficit (dehydration), which include thirst, dry mucous membranes, poor skin turgor, decreased urine output, tachycardia, and slight decrease in systolic blood pressure
- Lab results, especially BUN, hemoglobin, and hematocrit
- Types of IV fluids being infused
- IV site for infiltration or phlebitis

The patient should be taught the following:

- How to recognize signs and symptoms of fluid volume excess and fluid volume deficit
- How to measure fluid intake and output
- How to weigh her/himself

The nurse must frequently evaluate the patient's

- Urine output (normal limits)
- Breath sounds (normal limits)
- Lab results (normal limits)
- Vital signs (normal limits)
- Weight (not increased)
- Skin turgor (normal)
- IV site (should not be red, swollen, hot, or hard)
- IV patency (should be flowing as per the set drip rate)

Potassium

Potassium is an electrolyte cation that is more prevalent inside cells than it is in extracellular fluid. It is used to transmit and conduct neurological impulses and to maintain cardiac rhythm. Potassium is also used to contract skeletal and smooth muscles.

In order for a muscle to contract, the concentration of potassium inside the cell must move out and be replaced by sodium, which is the prevalent electrolyte outside the cell (see Sodium section, below). These electrolytes reverse position when the muscle repolarizes. The concentrations of potassium and sodium are maintained by the sodium-potassium pump found in cell membranes. The sodium-potassium pump uses adenosine triphosphate (ATP) to pump potassium back into the cell and to pump sodium out of the cell.

Potassium regulates intracellular osmolality and promotes cell growth. It moves into cells as new tissues form and leaves cells when tissues break down. Patients receive potassium from their diets and excrete potassium in urine (90%) and feces (8%).

Serum potassium is measured to determine whether the patient's potassium content is within the normal range. The normal serum potassium is 3.5–5.3 milliequivalents per liter (mEq/L). **Caution:** A serum potassium level of <2.5 or >7.0 mEq/L can induce cardiac arrest. Conditions such as kidney disease can cause potassium to become imbalanced. When this happens, the patient will exhibit specific signs and symptoms and the serum potassium will be outside the normal range.

Hyperkalemia *Hyperkalemia* occurs when a patient has a serum potassium level of >5.3 mEq/L. A number of factors can cause this condition, including the following:

- Impaired renal excretion (most common)
- Massive intake of potassium

- Medications such as potassium-sparing diuretics Aldactone (spironolactone) and Dyrenium (triamterene) and angiotensin-converting enzyme (ACE) inhibitors Vasotec (enalapril) and Prinivil (lisinopril), which reduce the kidney's ability to secrete potassium.

The nurse should monitor a patient for the signs and symptoms of hyperkalemia, the more common of which are as follows:

- Nausea

- Cold skin; grayish pallor

- Hypotension

- Mental confusion and irritability

- Abdominal cramps

- Oliguria (decreased urine output)

- Tachycardia (fast pulse) and later bradycardia (slow pulse)

- Muscle weakness, ranging from mild to flaccid paralysis

- Numbness or tingling in the extremities

- Peaked T waves on the EKG

The nurse must respond quickly once signs and symptoms of hyperkalemia develop as the patient may be at risk for seizures, injury related to muscle weakness, and cardiac arrhythmias. Here is what needs to be done:

- Restrict intake of potassium-rich foods.

- Administer diuretics and ion-exchange resins such as Kayexalate (sodium polystyrene sulfonate; used as a retention enema) as directed to increase the elimination of potassium.

- In critical cases, order dialysis therapy to remove potassium.

- Administer insulin and glucose parenterally to force potassium back inside cells.

- Administer sodium bicarbonate intravenously to correct the acidosis (elevate pH).

- Administer calcium gluconate intravenously to decrease the irritability of the heart; it does not promote potassium loss.

Hypokalemia *Hypokalemia* occurs when a patient has a serum potassium level of <3.5 mEq/L. A number of factors can cause this condition, including the following:

- Diarrhea

- Vomiting

- Fistulas
- Nasogastric suctioning
- Diuretic agents
- Hyperaldosteronism
- Magnesium depletion
- Diaphoresis
- Dialysis
- Increased insulin
- Alkalosis
- Stress (increases epinephrine)
- Starvation
- Low potassium in diet

The patient may have the following signs and symptoms when experiencing hypokalemia:

- Leg cramps
- Muscle weakness
- Vomiting
- Fatigue
- Decreased reflexes
- Polyuria
- Irregular pulse
- Bradycardia

The patient may also exhibit an abnormal EKG that shows any of the following anomalies:

- Depressed ST segment
- Flattened T wave
- Presence of U wave
- Premature ventricular contractions

The nurse must respond with the following interventions if the patient is at risk for injury related to muscle weakness and cardiac arrhythmias:

- Increase dietary intake of potassium.
- Teach the patient how to prevent hypokalemia by maintaining an adequate dietary intake of potassium. These include fruits, fruit juices, vegetables, or

potassium supplements. Bananas and dried fruits are higher in potassium than oranges and fruit juices.

- Administer potassium chloride supplements (Table 10–2) orally (onset may begin after 30 minutes) or IV. Use a central IV line for rapid infusion in critical conditions. Instruct the patient to take the medication with at least a half glass of fluid (juice or water) because potassium is extremely irritating to the gastric and intestinal mucosa.

- Teach patients the signs and symptoms of hypokalemia and to contact the healthcare provider if any of these are experienced.

Caution: This deficit cannot be corrected rapidly. The infusion should not exceed 10–20 mEq/hr, or the patient may experience hyperkalemia and can experience cardiac arrest. Be aware that infusions containing potassium may cause pain at the IV insertion site. If urine output is <30 mL/hr, notify the prescriber. Infusions should not

TABLE 10–2 Potassium Supplements	
Potassium Supplements	**Description**
10% potassium chloride	20 mEq/15 mL oral
20% potassium chloride	40 mEq/16 mL oral
10% Kaochlor	Oral
Potassium triplex (potassium actetate, bicarbonate, citrate)	Oral, rarely used
Kaon (potassium gluconate)	Enteric-coated tablet. Maintenance: 20 mEq in 1–2 divided dose
Kaon-Cl (potassium chloride)	Enteric-coated tablet. Maintenance: 20 mEq in 1–2 divided dose
Slow-K (potassium chloride)	Enteric-coated tablet. Maintenance: 8 mEq
Kaochlor (potassium chloride)	Correction: 40–80 mEq in 3–4 divided doses
K-Lyte (potassium bicarbonate)	Effervescent tablet. Correction: 40–80 mEq in 3–4 divided doses
K-Lyte/Cl (potassium chloride)	Effervescent tablet. Correction: 40–80 mEq in 3–4 divided doses
K-Dur (potassium chloride)	Effervescent tablet. Correction: 40–80 mEq in 3–4 divided doses
Micro-K (potassium chloride)	Effervescent tablet. Correction: 40–80 mEq in 3–4 divided doses
Potassium chloride	Clear liquid in multi-dose vial or ampule: 2 mEq/mL
Potassium chloride	IV: 20–40 mEq diluted in 1 L of IV solution

contain more than 60 mEq/L of potassium chloride (KCl). The preferred amount to add to 1000 mL of IV solution is 40 mEq/L.

Warning: *Never* give potassium as an IV push or IV bolus, as this will cause immediate cardiac arrest, which is not reversible with cardiopulmonary resuscitation. Potassium must be diluted in IV fluids as stated above. Do not give potassium if the patient suffers from renal insufficiency, renal failure, or Addison's disease. Do not give potassium if the patient has hyperkalemia, severe dehydration, or acidosis, or takes potassium-sparing diuretics. Use with caution with patients who have cardiac disorders or burns.

Sodium

Sodium is the major cation in extracellular fluid found in tissue spaces and vessels. Sodium plays an important role in the regeneration and transmission of nerve impulses and affects water distribution inside and outside cells. It is part of the sodium-potassium pump that causes cellular activity. When it shifts into the cell, depolarization (contraction) occurs; when it shifts out of the cell, potassium goes back into the cell and repolarization (relaxation) occurs. Sodium also combines readily in the body with chloride (Cl) or bicarbonate (HCO_3) to promote acid-base balance (pH).

The patient receives sodium when food is absorbed in the GI tract. Typically, a patient takes in more sodium than the daily requirement. The kidneys regulate the sodium balance by retaining urine when the sodium concentration is low and excreting urine when the sodium concentration is high. Most excess sodium is excreted in urine, although sodium also leaves the patient by way of perspiration and in feces.

The *serum sodium level*, which is the ratio of sodium to water, indicates the sodium level in a patient's body. Sodium is measured in milliequivalents per liter (mEq/L). The normal range of serum sodium is 135–145 mEq/L.

A patient's serum sodium level moves out of the normal range when she/he is retaining too much or too little water, has a high or low concentrations of sodium, or a combination of both. A patient is *hypernatremic* or *hyponatremic* when there is a high or low sodium concentration, respectively.

Hypernatremia *Hypernatremia* occurs when the patient's serum sodium concentration is >145 mEq/L. This occurs for one of two reasons: when the patient's (1) sodium concentration has increased while the volume of water remains unchanged or (2) water volume has decreased while the sodium concentration remains unchanged.

Regardless of what happened, the patient experiences *hyperosmolality*, which is a higher-than-normal concentration of sodium. This causes water to shift out of cells and into extracellular space, resulting in cellular dehydration. A patient who is alert and can drink water to quench a thirst is at less risk for hypernatremia. However, a patient whose consciousness is impaired or who cannot swallow, such as a frail elderly patient, is at risk for hypernatremia.

Hypernatremia is caused by one or more of the following conditions:

- Inadequate water intake
- Inability of the hypothalamus gland to synthesize antidiuretic hormone (ADH) (which the kidneys require to regulate sodium)
- Inability of the pituitary gland to release ADH
- Inability of the kidneys to respond to ADH
- Excess sodium (such as from a hypertonic IV solution)
- Inappropriate use of sodium-containing drugs
- Ingestion of excessive amounts of sodium such as seawater

The nurse can intervene by doing one or more of the following:

- Replacing water using an IV of 5% dextrose in water or a hypotonic saline solution as ordered
- Lowering the serum sodium level slowly to avoid the risk of cerebral edema (brain swelling)
- Restricting sodium intake
- Monitoring the patient's weight
- Assessing extremities for edema (swelling)
- Monitoring breath sounds and respiratory effort for signs of heart failure

The nurse must be alert to recognize the following signs and symptoms of hypernatremia:

- Agitation
- Restlessness
- Weakness
- Seizures
- Twitching
- Coma
- Intense thirst
- Dry swollen tongue
- Edematous (swollen) extremities

The nurse should educate the patient to do the following:

- Avoid foods rich in sodium such as canned foods, lunch meats, ham, pork, pickles, potato chips, and pretzels, and to refrain from adding salt to foods when cooking or at the table
- Read all labels on food products
- Monitor her/his weight daily (for cardiac patients)
- Look for signs of swollen feet (tight shoes) and hands (tight rings)
- Notify healthcare provider if any respiratory distress occurs

Hyponatremia   *Hyponatremia* occurs when the patient's serum sodium is <135 mEq/L. This can result from (1) an increased water volume while the sodium concentration remains normal or (2) a loss in sodium while the water volume remains normal.

Hyponatremia is caused by one or more of the following conditions:

- Profuse sweating on a hot day or after running a marathon
- Inappropriate administration of a hypotonic IV solution (sodium loss)
- The result of major trauma or after surgery (sodium loss)
- Excessive ingestion of water (water gain)
- Syndrome of inappropriate antidiuretic hormone (SIADH), which causes abnormal water retention (sodium loss) or Addison's disease
- Loss of sodium from the GI tract as a result of diarrhea and vomiting (sodium loss)
- The use of potent diuretics (losing water and salt together)
- Burns and wound drainage (sodium loss)
- Intake of too much water caused by polydipsia (excessive thirst)

The nurse must recognize the following symptoms of hyponatremia:

- Fatigue
- Headache
- Muscle cramps
- Nausea
- Seizures
- Coma

Hyponatremia is treated by the following measures:

- Treating the underlying cause
- Administering hypertonic saline solution IV such as dextrose 5% in saline to restore the serum sodium level
- Replacing fluid loss with commercially available electrolytic fluids

The nurse should monitor the following factors:

- Vital signs
- Fluid intake and output
- Serum sodium levels
- Dietary sodium intake
- Breath sounds and signs of respiratory distress

The nurse should educate the patient to do the following:

- Not drink excessive amounts of pure water on a hot day or after extreme exercise. Fluid replacement should be an electrolyte solution such as commercial preparations that include sodium.
- Monitor her/himself for signs and symptoms of hyponatremia [for patients taking a potent diuretic such as furosemide (Lasix) or a thiazide diuretic such as hydrochlorothiazide (HydroDiuril)].
- Report any signs of respiratory distress to the healthcare provider.

Calcium

Calcium is found in equal proportions in intracellular fluid and extracellular fluid. It is combined with phosphate in bone and with protein (albumin) in the serum. A patient receives calcium from ingesting calcium-containing food. Calcium plays a critical role in transmission of nerve impulses, blood clotting, muscle contraction, and the formation of teeth and bone.

There are three forms of calcium in serum that can fluctuate among forms depending on changes to the serum pH and/or serum protein (albumin) levels:

1. Free ionized form, which is the biologically active form. Half of the patient's total calcium is in the free ionized form.
2. Protein-bound, which binds primarily with albumin.
3. Complex form, which is where calcium is combined with phosphate, citrate, or carbonate.

The normal serum calcium ranges between 8.5 and 10.5 mg/dL. This reflects the calcium level for all three forms of calcium. However, ionized calcium (iC) levels are sometimes reported separately (4–5 mg/dL).

There is a balance between calcium and phosphorus. As serum calcium increases, serum phosphorus decreases. Conversely, as serum calcium decreases, serum phosphorus increases. The level of calcium is regulated by the parathyroid hormone (PTH), calcitonin, and vitamin D.

TABLE 10−3 Medications That Increase and Decrease Serum Calcium	
Decreases Serum Calcium	**Increases Serum Calcium**
Magnesium sulfate	Calcium salts
Propylthiouracil (propacil)	Vitamin D
Colchicines	IV lipids
Pliamythin	Kayexalate androgens
Neomycin	Diuretics (Thiazides, Chlorthalidone, Hygroten)
Acetazolamide	
Aspirin	
Anticonvulsants	
Glutethimide	
Estrogens	
Aminoglycosides (gentamicin, amikacin, tobramycin)	
Phosphate preparations: oral, enema, and IV (sodium phosphate, potassium phosphate)	
Corticosteroids (cortisone, prednisone)	
Loop diuretics (furosemide [Lasix])	

Low serum calcium causes an increase in the production of PTH. PTH moves calcium out of bone and into the serum. It increases the absorption of calcium from the GI tract. PTH also increases the reabsorption of calcium in the kidneys.

Calcitonin is produced by the thyroid gland. Production is increased when there is a high serum calcium level. Calcitonin reverses the action of PTH by increasing the absorption of calcium by bone, decreases calcium absorption in the GI tract, and causes an increase in urine to excrete calcium (see Table 10–3).

Dairy products are the major source of dietary calcium. Eggs, green leafy vegetables, broccoli, legumes, nuts, and whole grains provide smaller amounts. Only about 10–30% of the calcium in foods is actually absorbed in the body. Calcium is absorbed in the small intestine. Absorption is influenced by the amount of vitamin D available and the levels of calcium already present in the body.

Hypercalcemia *Hypercalcemia* is a condition when the serum calcium level is higher than 10.5 mg/dL indicating a higher-than-normal concentration of calcium. This usually produces a low serum phosphorus level.

Hypercalcemia can be caused by any of the following conditions:

- Renal failure

- Immobility

- Cancer

- Hyperparathyroidism

- Excess intake of calcium supplements [such as in Tums (an antacid used for heartburn relief that contains 500 mg of calcium carbonate) and other medications to prevent and treat osteoporosis]

- Overuse of antacids for GI disturbances

- Prolonged diarrhea

- Excessive use of diuretics

The nurse should be alert to identify the following signs and symptoms of hypercalcemia:

- Mild hypercalcemia, which may manifest no signs and symptoms

- Nausea

- Vomiting

- Constipation

- Anorexia

- Abdominal pain

- Polyuria (frequent urination)

- Polydipsia (extreme thirst)

- Decreased memory

- Personality changes or mood swings

- Confusion

- Depressed reflexes

- Muscular weakness

- Bone pain

- Fractures (which may occur when calcium supply is diminished or depleted in bone, which may be due to cancer, osteoporosis, and other disorders)

- Kidney stones

- Hypertension

- Cardiac arrhythmias

- Coma

Treatment is based on the calcium level. The calcium level may need to be lowered quickly because severe hypercalcemia can be life-threatening.

Treat the underlying cause if known.

- If kidney function is adequate, then
  - Administer isotonic saline IV to hydrate the patient.
  - Make sure that the patient drinks 3000–4000 mL of fluid, to ensure excretion of the calcium in urine.
  - Administer furosemide (Lasix) or ethacrynic acid (Edecrin) loop diuretics after adequate fluid intake is established.
- Administer synthetic calcitonin to lower serum calcium concentration.
- Administer plicamycin (Mithracin) to increase absorption of calcium in bone.
- Provide a low-calcium diet.
- Make sure the patient performs weight-bearing activities.
- Take safety measure to protect the patient who experiences neuromuscular effects.

Hemodialysis is the most effective method to lower calcium levels in severe cases when kidney function is not normal.

Hypocalcemia *Hypocalcemia* occurs when the serum calcium level is <8.5 mg/dL, indicating a lower-than-normal concentration of calcium. This usually produces a high serum phosphorus level. Too little calcium intake causes decrease or depletion of calcium in bone. Fractures (broken bones) may occur if a calcium deficit persists because of calcium loss from the bones (demineralization).

The causes of hypocalcemia are as follows:

- Hypoparathyroidism
- Thyroid or neck surgery where the parathyroid gland is removed or injured
- Hypomagnesium caused by alcoholism
- Ingestion of phosphates
- Inadequate intake of dietary calcium and/or vitamin D

Patients who experience hypocalcemia may have the following symptoms:

- Depression
- Memory loss
- Confusion
- Hallucinations

- Numbness and tingling in the face, around the mouth, and in the hands and feet
- Muscle spasms in the face, around the mouth, and in the hands and feet
- Hyperreflexia
- Ventricular tachycardia

Patients with hypocalcemia can be treated as follows:

- Calcium preparations can be given PO in tablet, capsule, or powder form or IV. If given IV, then mix with 5% dextrose in water. Do not mix with a saline solution because sodium encourages the loss of calcium.
- Administer parenteral calcium. **Caution:** Tissue infiltration leads to necrosis and sloughing. Calcium increases the action of digoxin and can result in cardiac arrest. Do not add calcium to bicarbonate or phosphorus because this can lead to formation of precipitates.
- Administer the following medication IV if ordered:
  - Calcium chloride IV 10 mL
  - Calcium gluceptate 5 mL
  - Calcium gluconate 10 mL
- Administer the following medication PO if ordered:
  - Calcium carbonate (Os-cal, Tums, Caltrate, Megacal) 650–1500-mg tablets
  - Calcium gluconate (Kalcinate) 500–1000 mg tablets
  - Calcium lactate 325–650 mg tablets
  - Calcium citrate 950-mg tablets
- Take safety precautions because the patient is at risk for tetany and seizures.
- Tell the patient to refrain from alcohol and caffeine ingestion because these substances inhibit calcium absorption.
- Increase dietary calcium to 1500 mg/day by instructing the patient to eat green leafy vegetables and fresh oysters and milk products.
- Administer vitamin D.
- Have the patient undergo regular exercises to decrease bone loss.

Patient education should include information about dietary sources of calcium, the need to maintain physical activity to avoid bone loss, avoiding overuse of antacids, and chronic use of laxatives. Patients should be taught to use fruits and fiber to improve bowel elimination, and to take oral supplements with meals or after meals to increase absorption.

Magnesium

Magnesium is a sister cation to potassium and is higher in intracellular fluid (ICF) content. If there is a loss of potassium, there is also a loss of magnesium. Magnesium is the coenzyme that metabolizes carbohydrates and proteins and is involved in metabolizing nucleic acids within the cell. Magnesium also plays a key role in neuromuscular excitability. The patient acquires magnesium by ingesting magnesium-rich food, which is absorbed in the GI tract and then excreted in urine.

There is a close relationship between magnesium, potassium, and calcium. PTH (see "Calcium" section), which regulates calcium, also influences the magnesium balance. Typically, you will assess serum magnesium, calcium, and potassium together. The normal serum magnesium level is between 1.5 and 2.5 mEq/L.

Hypermagnesemia *Hypermagnesemia* is a condition experienced by a patient whose serum magnesium level is >2.5 mEq/L. The major cause of hypermagnesia is an excessive intake of magnesium salts in laxatives such as magnesium sulfate, milk of magnesia, and magnesium citrate. Antacids such as Maalox, Mylanta, and DiGel can also cause hypermagnesemia. Patients who take lithium (antipsychotic medication) are also at risk for hypermagnesemia.

The following are signs and symptoms of hypermagnesemia:

- Lethargy
- Drowsiness
- Weakness
- Paralysis
- Cardiac (ventricular) arrhythmias
- Heart block
- Loss of deep-tendon reflexes
- Hypotension

Hypomagnesemia *Hypomagnesemia* occurs when the serum magnesium level is <1.5 mEq/L. This can be caused by long-term administration of saline infusions, which can result in the loss of magnesium and calcium. Diuretic agents, certain antibiotics, laxatives, and steroids are drug groups that promote magnesium loss. Hypomagnesemia also enhances the action of digitalis and can cause digitalis toxicity.

Patients who have hypomagnesemia may exhibit no signs and symptoms until the serum level approaches 1.0 mEq/L. Signs of severe hypomagnesemia include tetany-like symptoms caused by hyperexcitability (tremors, twitching of the face), ventricular tachycardia that leads to ventricular fibrillation, and hypertension.

Treatment for hypomagnesemia includes the following:

- Administering intravenous magnesium sulfate in solution slowly. Use an infusion pump to prevent rapid infusion that might result in cardiac arrest.
- Monitoring signs of magnesium toxicity such as hot flushed skin, anxiety, lethargy, hypotension, and laryngeal stridor.
- Monitoring EKG and pulse.
- Taking safety precautions for patients who are at risk for seizures and mental confusion.
- Increasing the dietary sources of magnesium, including nuts, whole grains, cornmeal, spinach, bananas, and oranges.

Keep calcium gluconate available for emergency reversal of hypermagnesemia as a result of overcorrecting hypomagnesemia.

Phosphorus

Phosphate is the primary anion inside the cell and plays a key role in the function of red blood cells, muscles, and the nervous system. Phosphate is also involved in acid–base buffering and is involved with metabolizing carbohydrates, proteins, and fats. Most of the body's phosphate (about 85%) is found in bones; the remainder is stored in tissues throughout the body.

Phosphorus is acquired by eating phosphorus-rich foods. Phosphorus is absorbed in the GI tract and excreted in urine and a small amount in feces. It is converted to phosphate in the body.

Both phosphate and calcium levels are regulated by parathyroid hormone (PTH). The amount of phosphate in the blood affects the level of calcium in the blood. Both levels are usually measured at the same time. As the serum calcium concentration increases, the concentration of serum phosphorus decreases; conversely, as serum phosphorus increases, serum calcium decreases. The normal range of serum phosphorus is between 2.5 and 4.5 mg/dL.

The kidneys regulate the amount of phosphate in the blood. Abnormally high levels of serum phosphate are usually caused by kidney malfunction.

Hyperphosphatemia

Hyperphosphatemia is a condition exhibited by a patient whose serum phosphate is >4.5 mg/dL. The following conditions cause hyperphosphatemia:

- Kidney disease
- Underactive parathyroid glands
- Acromegaly

- Rhabdomyolysis
- Healing fractures
- Untreated diabetic ketoacidosis
- Certain bone diseases
- Excessive ingestion of phosphate-containing laxatives
- Excessive drinking of milk
- Chemotherapy for neoplastic disease
- Excessive intake of vitamin D
- Decrease in magnesium levels as in alcoholism
- Increased phosphate levels during the last trimester of pregnancy

Unlike hyperkalemia and hypermagnesemia, acute hyperphosphatemia causes few sudden problems. The major effect is to cause hypocalcemia and tetany if serum phosphate rises too rapidly. Calcium can be deposited in the tissues in hyperphosphatemia.

The treatment for acute hyperphosphatemia is administration of phosphate binding salts, calcium, magnesium, and aluminum, although aluminum is avoided in renal failure.

Patients who have hyperphosphatemia show the following signs and symptoms:

- Muscle problems
- Hyperreflexia
- Soft-tissue calcification
- Nausea
- Vomiting
- Hypocalcemia
- Tachycardia
- Anorexia
- Tetany

Treatment for hyperphosphatemia can include the following measures:

- Restricting foods and drinks (carbonated soda) high in phosphate
- Treating the underlying cause
- Instituting seizure precautions
- Administering sevelamer hydrochloride (Renagel)
- Administering calcium supplements

Hypophosphatemia *Hypophosphatemia* occurs when the serum phosphate falls below 2.5 mg/dL and is caused by any of the following conditions:

- Inadequate intake
- Diuresis
- Dialysis
- Alcoholism
- Steroids
- Overuse of phosphate-binding antacids

The nurse should monitor the patient for the following signs and symptoms of hypophosphatemia:

- Bone and muscle pain
- Muscle weakness
- Rhabdomyolysis
- Confusion
- Osteomalacia
- Coma

Hypophosphatemia can be treated as follows:

- Administering phosphate supplements such as Neutra-Phos (a powder formulation of sodium and potassium phosphate) PO
- Administering sodium phosphate IV
- Administering potassium phosphate IV

Nursing interventions should include the following:

- Assessing vital signs
- Assessing changes in metal status
- Instituting seizure precautions
- Monitoring blood levels

Summary

The human body contains fluids (water) and salts called *electrolytes*, which are positively and negatively charged particles that generate electrical impulses that, among other things, cause muscles to contract.

Fluids and electrolytes are stored in two compartments: intracellularly (inside the cell) and extracellularly (outside the cell). The amount of electrolytes in fluid is called a *concentration*. There are three types of fluid concentration: isoosmolar (same concentration), hypoosmolar (low concentration), and hyperosmolar (high concentration). These concentrations are used to describe IV solutions as isotonic (isoosmolar), hypotonic (hypoosmolar), and hypertonic (hyperosmolar).

There are five key electrolytes: potassium, sodium, calcium, magnesium, and phosphorus. Collectively, they must remain in balance for the body to function properly. Diseases and their treatments are two factors that can cause fluids and electrolytes to become imbalanced. The healthcare professional must quickly identify the signs and symptoms of the imbalance and then take steps to restore the balance between electrolytes and fluids.

QUIZ

1. A decrease in serum potassium is called
   (a) hyperkalemia.
   (b) hypokalemia.
   (c) hypernatremia.
   (d) none of the above.

2. What is determined by the concentration of electrolytes and other solutes in water?
   (a) osmotic pressure
   (b) protein fluid
   (c) potassium fluid
   (d) calcium fluid

3. Electrolytes are found in
   (a) intracellular fluid.
   (b) interstitial fluid.
   (c) intravascular fluid.
   (d) all of the above.

4. Sodium and chloride are most prevalent outside the cell.
   (a) True
   (b) False

5. The concentration of a hypotonic intravenous solution has the same concentration as intracellular fluid.

   (a) True

   (b) False

6. Which of the following is a volume expander?

   (a) Blood and blood products

   (b) Lipids

   (c) Colloids

   (d) All of the above.

7. Potassium is necessary for conduction of nerve impulses:

   (a) True

   (b) False

8. Insulin and glucose administered parenterally

   (a) forces potassium out of the cell.

   (b) forces potassium into the cell.

   (c) corrects the acidosis balance.

   (d) does none of the above.

9. Vitamin D increases absorption of calcium in the GI tract.

   (a) True

   (b) False

10. The calcium balance can be affected by medications taken by the patient.

   (a) True

   (b) False

11

Nutritional Support Therapies

You probably ignored your mother when she told you to eat your vegetables so that you could grow big and strong. Yet today you're probably eating more nutritional foods—foods that you wouldn't touch when you were a child—because you've learned that certain foods provide the balanced nutrition needed to keep us healthy.

You might wonder how a chapter on nutrition slipped into a book on pharmacology. Nutrients are given to patients who are at risk for malnutrition caused by disease and even caused by treatments given to cure diseases. Nutrients are also given to strengthen the patient following a trauma such as surgery.

In this chapter, you'll learn about nutritional support therapies, how to prepare them, how to administer them, and how to avoid any complications that they might cause.

1. Nutrition

Nutrition is a three-step process that gives the body materials needed to make it grow and function. The process begins when food is ingested. Chemical reactions in the body then break down food into molecules that enter the bloodstream and are distributed to different parts of the body where they are used to sustain life.

Some nutrients are used for cell growth and cellular functions. Other nutrients become involved in enzymatic activities and carbohydrate-fat-protein synthesis. Nutrients are used to contract muscles and help wounds to heal. They also play a critical role in the integrity of the gastrointestinal (GI) tract and in the immune system.

Think of nutrients as fuel for your car. Fuel is used as you drive your car. The same is true about your body. Your body uses nutrients to go about daily activities; and just like your car, your body can continue to operate without a full complement of nutrients—that is, without a full tank of gas. A healthy, well-nourished person has a nutritional level sufficient to last 14 days before signs of malnutrition begin to appear. In other words, your full tank of gas will last 14 days.

However, there comes a point when your performance sputters—the level of nutrients falls below the level needed to sustain your daily activity. You simply run out of fuel and become fatigued and irritable, and exhibit an abnormal appearance.

This is referred to as a *nutritional deficit*. A nutritional deficit can occur from a number of situations. The most obvious is not adhering to a balanced, nutritional diet. However, there are less apparent reasons that cause a nutritional deficit. These are surgery, trauma, malignancy, and other illnesses that break down (*catabolize*) the body.

The effect of a nutritional deficit can be dramatic. The body needs nutrients to recover from trauma and disease. A nutritional deficit prolongs healing, and severe cases can prevent total recovery. Critically ill patients have sufficient nutrients to sustain them for a few days to a week before they begin to show signs of nutritional deficit.

Healthcare professionals provide nutritional support therapy for patients who are at risk for nutritional deficit. Nutritional support therapy replaces nutrients that the patient has lost and thereby provides the patient with the fuel needed for a full recovery.

A nutritional deficit is called a *negative nitrogen balance*, which means that the patient lacks sufficient nitrogen to fight infectious disease. *Nitrogen balance* is a measure of nitrogen input minus nitrogen output: Nitrogen balance = (nitrogen intake – nitrogen loss). Sources of nitrogen intake include meat, dairy, eggs, nuts and legumes, and grains and cereals. Examples of nitrogen loss include urine, feces, sweat, hair, and skin. Healthcare professionals treat patients who are at risk for negative nitrogen balance by providing them with nutrients before the imbalance occurs. A common misnomer is that dextrose 5% in water (D_5W), normal saline, and lactated Ringer's solution provide nutrients to the patient. However, these intravenous fluids are not forms of nutrients. These are electrolytes and fluids.

Nutritional Support

Nutrients are given to a patient via an enteral or parenteral route. Using the enteral route, food is administered by mouth or by a feeding tube that is directly inserted into the GI tract—usually into the stomach or small intestine. A feeding tube is used whenever the patient cannot swallow.

The *parenteral route* is the use of high-calorie nutrients administered through large veins such as the subclavian vein in a process called *total parenteral nutrition* (TPN) or *hyperalimentation*. The parenteral route is the least preferred because the process is 3 times more expensive than enteral administration without a significantly improved benefit. Furthermore, using the parenteral route increases the patient's chance of infection at the incision site and does not promote GI function, liver function, or weight gain.

Enteral Nutrition

Enteral feeding is the preferred method of providing nutritional support to a patient. However, the patient must have adequate GI tract function to enable digestion and absorption of the food and elimination of the waste product.

It is important to determine whether the patient has adequate GI motility and small-bowel function. Otherwise, the patient may experience uncontrolled vomiting and become at high risk for aspiration should the intestine be obstructed. Decreased bowel sounds are common in critically ill patients. They may also have a decrease or absence of gastric emptying. Nurses should ausculate carefully for bowel sounds and understand what the different sounds represent. It is also important to determine whether the patient is having regular bowel movements and is flatulent (able to pass gas). Finally, an assessment should include questions about abdominal pain and discomfort.

Several methods are used for enteral feeding:

- **Oral:** This is the preferred method as it enables the natural ingestion of food.
- **Nasogastric (NG) Tube:** This is the most commonly employed method. It consists in placement of a tube that passes through the nose and down the esophagus, ending shortly below the xiphoid process. This procedure is used for short-term therapy.
- **Gastrostomy:** In this method, a feeding tube is placed in a hole in the abdomen leading to the stomach. This procedure is used for long-term therapy.
- **Nasoduodenal:** In this method, a tube is inserted through the nose and passed down the esophagus, ending in the duodenum.
- **Nasojejunal:** In this method, a tube is passed through the nose and down the esophagus, ending in the small intestine.
- **Jejunostomy:** In this method, a feeding tube is placed in a hole in the abdomen leading to the small intestine.

Various mixtures are given to patients who are receiving nutritional support therapy that is based on the nutrient, caloric values, and osmolality that the patient requires. These mixtures belong to one of the following groups:

- **Blenderized:** This mixture type consists of liquids that are individually prepared according to the nutritional needs of the patient and can include baby food with added liquid.

- **Polymeric:** This mixture type is divided into two subgroups:

  1. **Milk-Based**: Powder mixed with milk or water is given in large amounts to provide complete nutritional requirements and can be used as a nutritional supplement in smaller amounts.

  2. **Lactose-Free:** Liquid is used for replacement feedings and consists of 50% carbohydrates, 15% protein, 15% fat, and 20% other nutrients in an isotonic solution (300–340 mOsm/kg H_2O). This provides 1 calorie per milliliter of feeding. This group includes Ensure, Isocal, and Osmolite.

- **Elemental:** Also known as *monomeric*, this mixture type is the most expensive enteral solution. It is useful for partial GI tract dysfunction and is available in both liquid and powder forms. Elemental nutrients are rapidly absorbed in the small intestines.

Regardless of the group, these solutions consist of the following:

- Carbohydrates in the form of dextrose, sucrose, and lactose. These are simple sugars that are absorbed quickly. The solution may also contain the carbohydrates starch and dextrin.

- Protein in the form of intact proteins, hydrolyzed proteins, or free amino acids.

- Fat in the form of corn oil, soybean oil, or safflower oil.

Enteral feedings are administered as follows:

- Bolus, 250–400 mL 4–6 times each day. Each bolus may take about 10 minutes to administer. A patient who cannot tolerate the large amount of solution given in a short timeframe may experience nausea, vomiting, aspiration, abdominal cramping, and diarrhea. This method is appropriate if the patient is ambulatory and relatively healthy.

- Intermittent drip or infusion, 300–400 mL given 3–6 hours over 30–60 minutes by gravity drip or infusion pump.

- Continuous drip or cyclic infusion, 50–125 mL infused per hour at a slow rate over a 24-hour period using an infusion pump such as a Kangaroo set. This method is used for treating critically ill patients and for patients who have an indwelling feeding tube in the small intestine or stomach.

Enteral feedings expose the patient to the following possible complications:

- **Dehydration:** In this case, an insufficient amount of water is given to the patient or a hyperosmolar solution is given, which draws water from the cells to maintain serum isoomolality.

- **Aspiration:** In this scenario the patient is fed while in a supine position or is unresponsive. This can be prevented by raising the head of the bed 30° and checking for gastric residuals by gently aspirating the stomach contents before the next feeding.

- **Diarrhea:** This is a major complication due to rapid administration of feeding, a high-calorie solution, malnutrition, GI bacteria (*Clostridium difficile*), and medications such as antibiotics and magnesium-containing drugs such as antacids and sorbitol. Sorbitol is used as a filler for certain drugs. Drugs in the form of oral liquids are hypersomolar and pull water from the cells and into the GI tract, resulting in diarrhea. Decreasing the infusion rate, diluting the solution, changing the solution, discontinuing the medication, or increasing the daily water intake helps to manage diarrhea.

Table 11–1 lists various preparations employed for enteral feeding.

Administering medications through the NG tube is discussed in Chapter 6; the drug must be in liquid form or dissolved into a liquid and must be properly diluted; it is usually given as a bolus and followed by water. Liquid medications should be diluted with water to reduce the osmolality to 500 mOsm/kg H_2O (mildly hypertonic) to decrease GI intolerance.

The procedure for calculating the correct dilution of enteral medications is as follows:

1. Calculate the drug order to determine the volume of the drug:

$$D \times V \text{ or } H : V :: D : x$$

   D = desired dose: dose ordered
   H = have available [on-hand dose; dose on label of container (bottle, vial, or ampule)]
   V = vehicle; form and amount in which the drug is available (tablet, capsule, or liquid)

2. Determine the osmolality of the drug (after consulting the drug literature or a pharmacist if needed) and liquid dilution. Use 500 mOsm as a constant value for the desired osmolality:

$$(\text{Known mOsm}) \times (\text{volume of drug}) = (\text{total volume of liquid at desired mOsm})$$

TABLE 11–1 Commonly Used Preparations for Enteral Feeding		
Category	Supplement	Comment
Blenderized	Compleat B (Sandox) Formula 2 (Cutter) Vitaneed (Sherwood)	Blended natural foods Ready to use
Polymeric milk-based	Meritene (Sandox) Instant Breakfast (Carnation) Sustacal Power (Mead Johnson)	Provides nutrients that are intact Pleasant-tasting oral supplement
Lactose-free	Ensure, Jevity, Osmolite (Ross) Sustacal Liquid, Isocal, Ultracal (Mead Johnson) Fibersource, Resource (Sandox) Entrition, Nutren (Clintec) Attain, Comply (Sherwood)	Used as oral supplement, tube feeding, or meal replacement Ready to use Meets daily intake of vitamins and minerals
Elemental (monomeric) formulas	Vital HN (Ross) Vivonex T.E.N. (Sandox) Criticare HN (Mead Johnson) Trayasorb (Clintec) Peptamen (Clintec) Reabilan (O'Brian)	Partially digested nutrients for feeding tube Required reconstitution except for Peptamen, Reabilan, and Criticare

3. Determine the volume of water for dilution:

(Total volume of liquid) – (volume of drug) = (volume of H_2O for dilution)

Example: acetaminophen 650 mg, q6h, PRN for pain
Have (on hand): acetaminophen elixir 65 mg/mL
Average mOsm/kg = 5400

1. $D \times V = 650 \text{ mg} \times 1 \text{ mL} = 10 \text{ mL}$
   $H \quad 65 \text{ mg}$

$$H \quad : \quad V \quad :: \quad D \quad : \quad x$$
$$65 \text{ mg} \quad : \quad 1 \text{ mL} \quad :: \quad 650 \text{ mg} \quad : \quad x \text{ mL}$$
$$65x = 650$$
$$x = 10 \text{ mL of acetaminophen}$$

2. Determine the osmolality of the drug:

$$[\text{Known mOsm (5400)}] \times [\text{volume of drug (10)}] = (5400 \times 10) = 108 \text{ mL of liquid}$$
$$\text{desired mOsm (500)} = 500$$

3. Determine the liquid volume:

[Total volume of liquid (108 mL)] × [volume of drug (10 mL = 98 mL
of water for dilution]

2. Nursing Process

General Nutrition

Assessment

Guidelines for assessing the general nutrition requirements of patients are as follows:

- Assess the tape around the nasogastric tube.
- Assess the signs and symptoms of intolerance to feedings.
- Assess the food intake and output levels.
- Assess the bowel sounds.
- Review the baseline laboratory values.

Nursing Diagnoses

The nurse should be aware of the following risks:

- Risk for fluid volume deficit
- Risk for diarrhea related to tube feedings
- Potential for loss of skin integrity related to diarrhea
- Risk for aspiration

Planning

The nurse should ensure the following conditions:

- That the patient will receive adequate nutritional support
- That side effects will be managed
- That no skin breakdown will occur
- That the patient will not aspirate

Interventions

The nurse should perform the following measures or ensure the following conditions:

- Check tube placement.
- Check for gastric residual before intermittent or bolus feedings.
- Check continuous feedings for residual every 2–4 hours.

- Feeding should be at room temperature.
- Flush feeding tube placement should be based on method of delivery.
- Monitor side effects such as diarrhea.
- Dilute drug solutions appropriately.
- Monitor vital signs.
- Monitor hydration.
- Weigh the patient daily.
- Change feeding bag daily.

Education

The nurse should instruct the patient to report diarrhea, sore throat, or abdominal cramping.

Evaluation

The nurse should ensure the following conditions:

- That the patient will not lose weight
- That the patient will not experience skin breakdown (pressure-induced dermal ulceration)
- That the patient will not experience diarrhea, abdominal cramping, or distention
- That the patient will remain in a positive nitrogen balance
- That the patient will not become dehydrated

Parenteral Nutrition

Parenteral nutrition support is used for patients who have severe burns, disorders of the GI tract, acquired immunodeficiency syndrome (AIDS), or a debilitating disease such as metastatic cancer.

These patients receive an infusion of a solution that contains hyperosmolar glucose, amino acids, vitamins, electrolytes, minerals, and trace elements. This solution is prepared in the pharmacy. In addition, the patient might be given fat emulsion supplemental therapy to increase the number of calories ingested and to receive fat-soluble vitamins. The infusion is given through a central venous line such as the subclavian or internal jugular vein to prevent irritation to the peripheral veins.

The nurse must monitor the patient for signs of complications as a result of inserting the catheter and the infusion of the feeding.

Catheter insertion can cause the following conditions:

- Pneumothorax
- Hemothorax
- Hydrothorax

Parental nutrition infusion can cause the following conditions:

- Air embolism
- Infection
- Hyperglycemia
- Hypoglycemia
- Fluid overload

It is important that strict asepsis (gloves and masks) be used when changing the IV tubing and the dressing at the infusion site because parenteral nutrition solutions are an excellent medium for yeast and bacteria growth. The pharmacy uses a laminar airflow hood when preparing parenteral nutritional solutions to reduce this risk.

The nurse should monitor the patient carefully for hyperglycemia when initiating parenteral nutrition support because the pancreas needs time to adjust to the hypertonic dextrose solution, which is high in glucose. Sometimes hyperglycemia is temporary and dissipates once the pancreas makes the necessary adjustments.

However, hyperglycemia might persist if the infusion rate is too rapid. To prevent this from occurring, the nurse should begin with 1 liter of solution for the first 24 hours, and increase this by 500–1000 mL each day until a daily volume of 2500–3000 mL is reached.

The nurse should change the solution and tubing every 24 hours, and change the dressing every 48–72 hours or according to the agency policy.

Caution: The nurse should not suddenly interrupt parenteral nutrition support, because the patient can experience hypoglycemia. The support should be discontinued gradually by decreasing the infusion rate. However, hypoglycemia may occur despite these precautions.

3. The Nursing Process and Parenteral Nutritional Therapy

When administering parenteral nutritional therapy, the nurse should employ the procedure described in the following paragraphs.

Assessment

The nurse should assess the following variables:

- The patient's vital signs
- The patient's weight

- The patient's laboratory values
- The patient's intake and output levels

Nursing Diagnoses

The nurse should assess the patient's risk for the following problems:

- Fluid volume excess
- Fluid volume deficit
- Infection
- Respiratory complications
- Altered nutrition status

Planning

The nurse should ensure the following conditions:

- That the patient will
  - Satisfy her/his nutritional needs
  - Maintain her/his appropriate body weight
  - Maintain fluid volume balance
- That the patient will not
  - Develop infection at the insertion site or a systemic infection

Interventions

Further guidelines for the nurse are as follows:

- Maintain sepsis when changing the solution and dressing.
- Weigh the patient each day.
- Refrigerate the solution until time for use.
- Do not use the parenteral nutritional line to draw blood, give medication, or check central venous pressure.
- Monitor the following patient variables:
  - Vital signs
  - Weight
  - Lab values:
    - Intake and output
    - Catheter insertion site
  - Signs of hyperglycemia when therapy is started
  - Signs of hypoglycemia after therapy is discontinued

- Change
  - The solution as ordered
  - The tubing per agency policy
  - The dressing per agency policy

Education

The nurse should instruct the patient to do the following:

- To report any signs of complications or actual complications
- To be aware of the difference between a parenteral nutritional infusion and an IV infusion

Evaluation

The nurse should ensure the following:

- That the patient will not
  - Lose body weight
  - Develop fluid volume overload
  - Develop hyperglycemia
  - Develop dehydration
  - Develop an infection
- That the patient will
  - Maintain positive nitrogen balance

Summary

The body requires nutrients for cell growth, cellular functions, muscle contraction, wound healing, and other vital activities. Nutrients enter the body as food and are absorbed as chemical reactions that break down food into molecules that enter the bloodstream, where they are distributed throughout the body.

Surgery, trauma, malignancy, and other catabolic illnesses cause a nutritional imbalance that, if prolonged, can have a dramatic impact on the patient and could ultimately lead to death.

Healthcare professionals can restore or maintain the patient's nutritional balance by administering nutritional support therapy to replace nutrients that the patient lost. There are two types of nutritional support therapies: enteral and parenteral.

Enteral nutritional support therapy introduces nutrition into the patient by mouth or a feeding tube that is inserted directly in the stomach or small intestine.

Parenteral nutritional support therapy administers high-calorie nutrients through large veins such as the subclavian vein.

QUIZ

1. **Hyperalimentation is**

   (a) parenteral nutrition.

   (b) enteral nutrition.

   (c) a high saline concentration for parenteral nutrition therapy.

   (d) none of the above.

2. **Blenderized**

   (a) is a lactose-free liquid.

   (b) consists of liquids that are individually prepared according to the nutritional needs of the patient.

   (c) is powder mixed with milk.

   (d) is powder mixed with water.

3. **Nausea and vomiting may occur during enteral therapy if which of the following occurs?**

   (a) Large amounts of solution are infused too rapidly.

   (b) The solution is infused directly onto the patient's stomach.

   (c) The solution is infused very slowly.

   (d) The solution is mixed with water.

4. **Monomeric is the least expensive enteral solution.**

   (a) True

   (b) False

5. **Parenteral nutrition therapy is used for a severely burned patient.**

   (a) True

   (b) False

6. **Catheter insertion can cause**

   (a) pneumothorax.

   (b) hemothorax.

   (c) hydrothorax.

   (d) all of the above.

7. It is dangerous to suddenly interrupt parenteral nutrition therapy.

   (a) True

   (b) False

8. Nutrients play a role in

   (a) carbohydrate-fat-protein synthesis.

   (b) enzymatic activities.

   (c) the GI tract.

   (d) all of the above.

9. Healthy, well-nourished individuals have nutritional levels that sustain them for 14 days before they begin to show signs of malnutrition.

   (a) True

   (b) False

10. A nutritional deficit is called a negative nitrogen balance

   (a) True

   (b) False

12

Inflammation

Scratch your arm, and within minutes the site turns red and hurts. This is your body's inflammatory response to tissue injury. Fortunately, the pain usually goes away and the inflammation subsides relatively quickly and doesn't interfere with daily activities.

However, this isn't always the case—especially when the injury is severe, such as arthritis, gout, toothache, or other painful conditions, including menstrual cramps. For these conditions, medication is needed to decrease the inflammation so that your daily activities will not be interrupted.

In this chapter, you'll learn about inflammation and the medications that are prescribed to reduce the redness, swelling, warmth, and pain that is associated with inflammation.

1. An Inside Look at Inflammation

Inflammation is the body's protective response to injury to tissues. Stimulated nerve endings signal the brain that there is an injury. Injury causes the release of three chemicals that stimulate a vascular response that forces fluid and white blood cells to flow to the site of the injury:

- **Histamines:** This chemical works to bring more blood and lymph fluid to the site of the invasion.
- **Kinins:** These are blood plasma proteins that influence smooth-muscle contractions, increase blood flow throughout the body, increase the permeability of small capillaries, and stimulate pain receptors.

- **Prostaglandins:** These fatty acids work as chemical messengers. They do not move but work right in the cell where they are synthesized. They are synthesized in every cell in the body. These chemicals activate the inflammatory response and produce pain and fever. They are produced in response to the white blood cells that flow to the area of injured tissue.

The injured tissue becomes red, swollen, and warm and loses its normal function. These, along with pain, are the five cardinal signs of inflammation. It is important not to confuse inflammation and infection because they are not the same.

Only a small percentage of inflammation is caused by infection from microorganisms. Trauma, surgery, extreme heat or cold, electricity, and caustic chemicals cause most inflammation.

Inflammation occurs in two phases.

Vascular Phase

The *vascular phase* occurs 10–15 minutes after the tissue is injured. It is during this phase that blood vessels dilate and become more permeable, enabling fluid and white blood cells to leave the plasma and flow to the injured tissue. This blood vessel dilation is termed *vasodilation*.

Delayed Phase

The *delayed phase* occurs when the injured tissue is infiltrated by white blood cells. White blood cells (also called *leukocytes* or *immune cells*) are components found in the blood. They are also found in the spleen, the lymphatic system, and other tissues. They help defend the body against infectious disease and foreign material as part of the immune system. The three main types of leukocytes (white blood cells) are granulocytes (neutrophils, basophils, and eosinophils), lymphocytes [B cells, T cells, and natural-killer (NK) cells], and monocytes.

2. Combating Inflammation

Although inflammation is a natural response to injury, this process can be uncomfortable for a patient, especially when there is fever, pain, and swelling. Anti-inflammatory medication can be given to reduce the inflammatory process and bring comfort to the patient.

Anti-inflammatory medication stops the production of prostaglandins, resulting in a decrease in the inflammatory process. There are three categories of anti-inflammatory medication:

1. *Analgesic*—pain-relieving medication

2. *Antipyretic*—fever-reducing medication

3. *Anticoagulant*—medication that inhibits platelet aggregation (grouping to form a clot)

Many anti-inflammatory medications fall within all three categories. Aspirin is one of them, and is the oldest and least expensive anti-inflammatory medication available and, along with acetaminophen and ibuprofen, is the first choice for relieving headaches.

Corticosteroids, such as prednisone, are frequently used as anti-inflammatory agents. This group of drugs can control inflammation by suppressing or preventing many of the components of the inflammatory process at the injured site.

There are other anti-inflammatory medications that are not chemically the same as corticosteroid medication. These are referred to as *nonsteroidal anti-inflammatory drugs* (NSAIDs). NSAIDs are appropriate for reducing swelling, pain, and stiffness.

There are eight groups of NSAIDs:

1. Salicylates (related to aspirin)

2. Parachlorobenzoic acid derivatives or indoles

3. Pyrazolone derivatives

4. Propionic acid derivatives

5. Fenamates

6. Oxicams

7. Phenylacetic acids

8. Selective COX-2 inhibitors

3. Common Types of Arthritis

Osteoarthritis or degenerative joint disease affects 86% of persons over 70 years of age, although symptoms may start in the fifth or sixth decade of life. This common form of arthritis is the result of deformation or mismatched joint surfaces, rather than an inflammatory disease. Symptoms include joint stiffness, which usually lasts only a few minutes after initiation of movement and may be accompanied by an aching pain in weight-bearing joints. Early disease stages may respond to local heat and nonprescription analgesics. Later stages may require orthopedic or other interventions.

Rheumatoid arthritis usually occurs between 30 and 70 years of age and more frequently in women than in men. Early symptoms may include feelings of fatigue and weakness, joint pain and stiffness, and joint swelling several weeks later. Joints are inflamed (warm, red, swollen) and often are limited in range of motion. This is a progressive disease that leads to joint deformity. Aspirin and aspirin-type products (NSAIDs) and disease-modifying antirheumatic drugs (DMARDs) are usually necessary to reduce the inflammation around the joints and inhibit the progression of the disease. Heat therapy, weight control, and exercise may also be helpful.

A list of drugs utilized in the treatment of arthritis is provided in the Appendix. Detailed tables show doses, recommendations, expectations, side effects, contraindications, and more; more information is available on the book's website (the URL is listed in the Appendix).

Gout has been called the "disease of kings" because in the past, royalty consumed rich foods and drank wine and alcohol and suffered from gout. However, it is not just for the "rich and famous." Gout is an inflammatory condition that attacks joints, tendons, and other tissues. The most common site of acute gouty inflammation is at the joint of the big toe. It may also be referred to as *gouty arthritis*. It is characterized by a uric acid metabolism disorder and a defect in purine (products of certain proteins) metabolism, resulting in an increase in urates (uric acid salts) and an accumulation of uric acid (hyperuricemia) or an ineffective clearance of uric acid in the kidneys. Uric acid solubility is poor in acid urine, and urate crystals may form, causing urate calculi (stones). Gout may appear as bumps or *tophi* in the subcutaneous tissue of earlobes, elbows, hands, and the base of the large toe. The complications of untreated or prolonged periods of gout include tophi, gouty arthritis, urinary calculi, and gouty nephropathy.

Fluid intake should be increased during an antigout drug regimen, and the urine should be alkaline. Foods rich in purine, including wine, alcohol, organ meats, sardines, salmon, and gravy, should be avoided.

A list of drugs utilized in the treatment of gout is provided in the Appendix. Detailed tables show doses, recommendations, expectations, side effects, and contraindications; more information is available on the book's website.

Summary

Inflammation is the body's response to tissue injuries. The body releases histamines, kinins, and prostaglandins that force fluid and white blood cells to the site of the injury to stimulate nerve endings and clean the area so that it can heal.

The site of the injury becomes red, swollen, and warm and loses its normal function. This happens in two phases: (1) in the *vascular* phase, blood vessels dilate and become permeable to enable fluid and white blood cells to leave the vessel; (2) in the *delayed* phase, white blood cells infiltrate the tissue.

Anti-inflammatory medication reduces the inflammatory process, which may allow the patient to perform normal daily activities while the tissue heals. There are three categories of anti-inflammatory medications: *analgesic*, to relieve pain; *antipyretic*, to reduce fever; and *anticoagulant*, to inhibit blood clotting.

Aspirin and other anti-inflammatory medications are called *nonsteroidal anti-inflammatory drugs* (NSAIDs). There are eight groups of NSAIDs: salicylates, para(chlorobenzoic acid) derivatives, pyrazolone derivatives, propionic acid derivatives, fenamates, oxicams, phenylacetic acids, and selective COX-2 inhibitors. Corticosteroids are also used as anti-inflammatory medication.

You learned in this chapter that inflammation is not an infection, although inflammation frequently occurs when a patient becomes infected with a microorganism. Inflammation occurs in response to tissue injury, whether it is from an injury or an acute or chronic disease such as rheumatoid arthritis or gout. You'll learn about infection and fever and antimicrobial medication in the next chapter.

QUIZ

1. **What stimulates nerve endings at the site of an injury?**
   (a) Hypothermic response
   (b) Infection response
   (c) Inflammatory response
   (d) None of the above

2. **During what phase of the inflammation response do WBCs infiltrate the injured tissue?**
   (a) Anti-inflammatory phase
   (b) Vascular phase
   (c) Delayed phase
   (d) All of the above

3. **Which of the following relieves pain?**
   (a) Analgesic
   (b) Antipyretic
   (c) Anticoagulant
   (d) All of the above

4. **Anti-inflammatory medication stops the production of prostaglandins, resulting in a decrease in the inflammatory process.**
   (a) True
   (b) False

5. Tinnitus is a side effect of salicylates.

   (a) True
   (b) False

6. The vascular phase occurs

   (a) 10–15 minutes before the tissue is injured.
   (b) 10–15 minutes after the tissue is injured.
   (c) 10–15 minutes before the tissue heals.
   (d) during none of the above.

7. DMARDs may arrest the progression of rheumatoid arthritis.

   (a) True
   (b) False

8. Which of the following is a sign of inflammation?

   (a) Redness
   (b) Warmth
   (c) Swelling (edema)
   (d) All of the above

9. A large percentage of inflammation is caused by infection.

   (a) True
   (b) False

10. The choices of medications for relieving headaches are aspirin, acetaminophen, and ibuprofen.

    (a) True
    (b) False

chapter 13

Antimicrobials—Fighting Infection

Pharmacology conjures up images of a magic pill that a prescriber gives you to relieve your runny nose, headache, fever, and other symptoms that make it unbearable to perform daily activities. Sometimes those symptoms are from your body adjusting to irritants like pollen. At other times, symptoms are caused by malfunctioning parts of your body such as the pancreas in the case of diabetes.

There is a third cause of symptoms—invading microbials. You'll remember from your courses on anatomy, physiology, and microbiology that a *microbial* is a tiny organism—such as bacteria and viruses—that can enter your body and make you feel sick.

The immune system produces antibodies that seek out, attack, and kill microbials. However, this natural defense isn't sufficient for some patients who need to call in the cavalry. The "cavalry" is a medication that kills the invading microbial. You'll learn about antimicrobial medication in this chapter.

1. Microorganisms: A Small Formidable Opponent

There are millions of microorganisms around us—and in the human body. Some are harmless. Others, called *flora*, facilitate digestion. Then there are the harmful ones called *pathogens*—microorganisms that cause infections.

Pathogens enter the body in various ways, such as through a cut in the skin or in food that is ingested. Once a pathogen is inside the body, a race begins between the invading organism and the body's defenses. The body reacts with an inflammatory response that dilates blood vessels and renders them permeable. This allows fluid containing white blood cells to infiltrate the infected area. Nerve endings are stimulated and send a message to the brain that something is wrong.

A person knows when this happens because the infected area turns red, swollen, and painful. The infection might be a patch of tissue referred to as a local infection. Other infections affect an organ or entire system of the body, which is referred to as a *systemic infection* or *septecemia*. An infection can also affect multiple organs and systems. This is called *sepsis*.

You can learn more about microbials by reading *Microbiology Demystified*.

2. Medication: A Formidable Defender

A person's natural defense against bacteria is a phagocytic response. Cells in the body engulf a pathogen, basically eating it and removing the injured tissue. Often the body needs help from medications that can kill microbials. Such medications, called *antimicrobials*, are used to kill microorganisms. There are many types of antimicrobials; each is designed to kill specific microorganisms. The most familiar is an antibiotic, which kills bacteria. Antibiotics kill microbials—the good and the bad. For example, an antibiotic used to kill bacteria that causes a urinary tract infection (UTI) will also kill the flora in the intestine that are used to help digest food.

Patients are also treated with medications that alleviate the symptoms of inflammation but do not kill microbials. These are *prostaglandin inhibitors*.

Prostaglandins are chemical mediators that elicit the inflammatory response by vasodilatation, relaxing smooth muscle, making capillaries permeable, and sensitizing nerve cells to pain within the affected area. A prostaglandin inhibitor reduces the production of prostaglandins and thereby reduces the symptoms of inflammation.

Nonsteroidal anti-inflammatory drugs (NSAIDs) are aspirin and "aspirin-like drugs." Aspirin is the most commonly used prostaglandin inhibitor because it is an analgesic employed to relieve pain. It is also an *antipyretic*, as it lowers body temperature, and it is an *anticoagulant* that inhibits the formation of platelets.

Other NSAIDs are also prostaglandin inhibitors and are administered at lower doses than aspirin to exert the same analgesic effect. However, most NSAIDs have a lower anti-inflammatory effect than aspirin.

Antimicrobials—Stuff Microorganisms Die for

Two of the first antimicrobials developed were sulfonamides and penicillin. Sulfonamides are *bacteriostatic*, which means they arrest the growth of—but do not kill—bacteria. Penicillin, the first antibiotic developed, is a *bactericidal* and kills bacteria using lysis, which explodes the bacteria into parts. (**Tip:** A *static* agent stops growth, whereas a *cidal* agent kills living organisms or cells.)

Today there are many synthetic and semisynthetic antimicrobials on the market that prevent some bacteria from growing and kill other bacteria. For example, chloramphenicol is bacteriostatic and prevents most bacteria from growing while at the same time it is bactericidal and kills *Streptococcus pneumoniae* and *Haemophilus influenzae* in cerebrospinal fluid (CSF). Tetracycline is both bacteriostatic and bactericidal; in small concentrations it stops the growth of bacteria and in high concentration it kills bacteria.

Sulfonamides and penicillin are administered orally, topically as an ointment or cream, or parenterally, and are absorbed into the body and distributed by the circulatory system. In severe infections, they can be administered directly at the site of the infection, such as in the eye, or rubbed on the skin.

These medications work in four different ways:

1. They inhibit the bacteria from growing a cell wall (cell wall synthesis).

2. They disrupt or alter the permeability of the bacteria's membrane. The membrane is located within the cell wall and is used to allow entry of nutrients into the cell and to send waste out of the cell.

3. They inhibit the bacteria's ability to produce protein (protein synthesis). Medications that stop the growth of bacteria also interrupt the process of protein synthesis. Those that kill bacteria cause the bacteria to form defective proteins.

4. They inhibit the bacteria's capability to produce (synthesize) essential metabolites. A *metabolite* is a component necessary for bacteria's metabolism to function properly.

Medication used to stop the growth of microbials or kill them outright have side effects, some of which can adversely affect the patient. Some cause an allergic reaction, while others lead to an exaggerated immune response. Here are a few common ones that you will probably recognize:

- Rash
- Fever
- Urticaria (hives) with pruritus (itching)
- Chills, general erythema (redness)
- Anaphylaxis (circulatory collapse)

These side effects are usually treatable by using other medication such as the following:

- Antihistamines (Benadryl)
- Epinephrine (adrenalin)
- Steroids for anti-inflammatory response

3. Superinfections

Antibiotics are both beneficial and harmful. The benefit is obvious. Antibiotics kill bacteria; however, problems can arise. The normal microbial flora die along with the bacteria. This flora can be replaced by resistant bacteria, and superinfection can occur. This poses a greater risk when large doses of antibiotics are used, when two more antibiotics are used simultaneously, or when broad-spectrum drugs are administered. For example, the overuse of cephalosporins may cause *Pseudomonas* infection, and the overuse of tetracycline may cause *Candida albicans* infection. *Pseudomonas* and *C. albicans* are then considered to be a superinfection in response to the use of cephalosporins and tetracycline.

Resistance to the antibiotic is another potential problem. Culture and sensitivity studies should be performed on all infections in order to determine which antibiotics will work for the microorganism that is causing the infection. The test can be performed on blood or wound drainage to identify the bacteria and help identify which antibiotic(s) will be effective.

Some patients stop taking medication as soon as the symptoms of infection dissipate; however, the bacterium is still alive and actively growing. As a result, the patient has a relapse and is again prescribed the antibiotic.

Other times, the healthcare professional may underprescribe an antibiotic by giving the patient a lower-than-effective dose, or may order the antibiotic for a short period of time. At first this seems like a logical way to prevent the bacterium from becoming resistant to the antibiotic. However, a low dose might fail to completely kill the bacterium, resulting in a recurrence of symptoms that requires additional doses of antibiotics. It is very important to choose the right antibiotic, in the right dose, for the right amount of time.

4. Preparing to Administer Antimicrobial Medication

Antimicrobial medication requires the nurse to follow the same general administration procedures that are required for any type of medication. The most critical step is to determine whether the patient has allergies to drugs, food, environmental stimuli, and/or a family history of allergies to antibiotics. There is also a high incidence of cross-sensitivity between some antibiotics such as penicillin and cephalosporins. Always display allergies in red and clearly write them on the patient's record. Even if the patient's record indicates an absence of allergies, always ask the patient each time that you administer the antimicrobial medication.

Always have emergency medications such as epinephrine, Benadryl, and steroids accessible to be administered in order to counteract any adverse side effect of the antimicrobial medication. Be sure to carefully monitor the patient for 30 minutes after administering the medication to determine whether the patient experiences an adverse reaction.

During treatment, you will need to monitor the therapeutic effect of the medication by monitoring the signs and symptoms of the disease and by obtaining the patient's white blood cell (WBC) count. Although you can monitor the antimicrobial serum level to determine whether the medication has achieved a therapeutic level, this is done only in cases where the therapeutic range is narrow, resulting in possible toxicities (ie, vancomycin ototoxicity).

It is important to administer antimicrobials at the times described in the prescriber's order in order to maintain a therapeutic blood level of the medication. Otherwise, this can lead to undertreatment or ineffective treatment if not maintained. Sometimes a double dose of an antibiotic is administered as the first dose to quickly achieve a therapeutic level. This is called a *loading dose*.

Intramuscular injections of antibiotics should be given deep inside the muscle, and sites should be rotated if two or more injections are prescribed. Stop orders and the need for renewal orders will depend on the healthcare agency policy. However, antibiotic orders usually remain valid for 72 hours only, until the results of a culture-sensitivity test can be obtained. Antibiotic prescriptions are seldom renewed. This is an effort to limit the opportunity for the microbial to become resistant to the medication.

In severe cases, aggressive treatment is necessary to control the growth and destroy the microbial quickly. To do this, the medication is administered parenterally in an IV dose that is diluted in a neutral solution (pH 7.0–7.2) such as normal saline (NS) or isotonic sodium chloride or 5% dextrose and water (D_5W). Antibiotics should not be mixed together or administered at the same time. They can be administered as a piggyback infusion. Information on the recommended time intervals between the infusions of different antibiotics should be obtained from the pharmacy or the drug insert in the package.

The following nursing diagnoses are common for patients who are taking antibiotics:

- Risk of infection related to treatment failure or superinfection
- Risk of fever related to treatment failure or superinfection
- Risk of fluid volume deficit related to adverse GI reaction such as anorexia, nausea/vomiting/diarrhea, and complications of allergic reaction

These patients are also at risk for developing the following collaborative problems:

- Sepsis
- Ototoxicity (ears)

- Blood dyscrasias
- Nephrotoxicity (kidneys)

It is critical that the patient be given information on the management of her/his condition. These instructions include the following:

- Take all the medication even after the symptoms subside.
- Do not take medication that is left over from a previous illness. (The medication may not treat the patient's condition or may have lost its therapeutic capabilities.)
- Do not take a medication that has been prescribed for another person even if it's for the same condition.
- Do not share drinks, food, and utensils with others until the healthcare provider determines that the patient is no longer infected by the microbial. Sharing may enable the microbial to spread to other people.
- Recognize the expected effects, side effects, and adverse reactions that might occur as a result of taking the medication. Also provide a telephone number in case the patient has any questions about these effects.
- Wear a MedicAlert bracelet if the patient has allergies to medication.

Penicillin

Penicillin is derived from molds that are sometimes visible on bread and fruit. It was discovered in 1940 and remains the most effective—and least toxic—antimicrobial drug. Penicillin weakens the cell wall of a bacterium, resulting in the rupture and destruction of a cell, which is called *lysis*.

Penicillin is most active against Gram-positive bacteria and some Gram-negative bacteria. However, it is not active against bacteria that contain enzymes that destroy penicillin.

There are four types of penicillin:

1. Basic (natural)
2. Penicillinase-resistant (resistant to β-lactamase inactivation)
3. Aminopenicillins (broad-spectrum)
4. Extended-spectrum

Besides route, dose, and time, drugs are also characterized by Pregnancy Category, protein-binding degree, and half-life. Pregnancy Category indicates whether the drug has been tested on pregnant women and how safe it might be if used during pregnancy. Although the FDA has stopped using pregnancy category designations, most prescribers still adhere to them. Penicillin is categorized by its usefulness against bacterial enzymes capable of destroying the drug. Four different classifications of antibiotics exist that contain the β-lactam ring and are more active against Gram-negative cell wall organisms, decreasing its susceptibility to enzymes that inactivate the antibiotic. *Protein binding* refers to binding of a drug to plasma proteins. When a drug is bound to a protein, it is not available for therapeutic use. The *percent* of protein binding is the amount of drug that cannot be used until it is released, at which time the free drug or the non-protein-bound amount of the drug is excreted from the body. The *half-life* is the amount of time for half (or 50%) of the drug to be eliminated from the body.

The category appears at the top of the table if the value of the category applies to all the drugs in a table; otherwise the category appears beneath the name of the drug in the table.

Several precautions must be taken when administering penicillin. If penicillin is given PO, avoid giving this medication an hour before and an hour after the patient has eaten. However, food has no effect on amoxicillin, amoxicillin/clavulanate, and bacampicillin. Give penicillin with a full glass of water, and not with acidic fruit juices.

If penicillin is administered IV, give it slowly because it contains a large amount of potassium that can cause heart failure in patients with renal insufficiency.

Before penicillin is administered, the patient must be assessed for a number of conditions. One of the most important conditions is allergies. An allergic reaction to penicillin can range anywhere from a mild rash to anaphylactic shock and death.

Furthermore, do not administer penicillin to patients who have any of the following conditions:

- A tendency to bleed
- Ulcerative colitis and any other GI disorder or disease
- Mononucleosis (a skin rash may develop with use of ampicillin or bacampicillin)
- A low-salt diet (parenteral carbenicillin and ticarcillin have high sodium content)
- Impaired renal function (a lower dose may be given in such cases)

After penicillin is administered, monitor the patient for the following conditions:

- Serum electrolytes for hyperkalemia (elevated potassium) and/or hypernatremia (elevated sodium)
- Unusual weight loss (especially in the elderly)
- Vital signs
- WBC
- Cultures
- Prothrombin time (PT) (bleeding times)

Descriptions of medication throughout this chapter use the following abbreviations:

PB	Protein binding	IV	Intravenous
$t_{1/2}$	Half-life	IM	Intramuscular
UK	Unknown	A	Adult
PO	By mouth	C	Child

Basic (natural) penicillin
Pregnancy Category: B
Protein binding: 65%
Half-life: 30 minutes

Route	Dose	Time
Penicillin G		
PO	200,000–500,000	Every 4–6 hours
IV	1–5 µ	Every 4–6 hours
IM	1.2–2.4 µ units	Single dose
Penicillin V (take on empty stomach)		
PO	125–500 mg	Every 8 hours

Penicillinase-resistant penicillin
Pregnancy Category: B
Half-life: 0.5–1 hour

Route	Dose	Time
Cloxacillin (Tegopen) Protein binding: 90%		
PO		Every 6 hours
IV	250–500 mg	Every 4–6 hours
Dicloxacillin (Dynapen) Protein binding: 90%		
PO	125–250 mg	Every 6 hours
Methicillin (Staphcillin) Protein binding: 25–40%		
IV	1 g	Every 6 hours
IM	1 g	Every 4–6 hours
Nafcillin (Unipen) Protein binding: 90%		
PO	250 mg–1 g	Every 4–6 hours
IV	0.5–1.5 g	Every 4 hours
IM	500 mg	Every 4–6 hours

Penicillinase-resistant penicillin (*Continued*)		
Pregnancy Category: B		
Half-life: 0.5–1 hour		
Oxacillin (Prostaphlin)		
Protein binding: 95%		
PO	0.5–1 g	Every 4–6 hours
IV	250–1 g	Every 6 hours
IM	250–1 g	Every 4–6 hours

Aminopenicillins (broad-spectrum) penicillin		
Pregnancy Category: B		
Route	Dose	Time
Amoxicillin (Amoxil)		
Protein binding: 20%		
Half-life: 1–1.3 hours		
PO	250–500 mg	Every 8 hours
Amoxicillin + potassium clavulanate (Augmentin, Clavulin)		
Protein binding: 25%		
Half-life: 1–1.5 hours		
PO	5000 mg	Every 8 hours
Ampicillin (Polycillin, Omnipen)		
Protein binding: 15–28%		
Half-life: 1–2 hours		
PO	250–500 mg	Every 6 hours
IV	250–500 mg	Every 8 hours
IM	250–500 mg	Every 8 hours
Ampicillin and sulbactam (Unasyn)		
Protein binding: 28–38%		
Half-life: 1–2 hours		
IV	1.5–3 g	Every 6 hours
IM	1.5–3 g	Every 6 hours
Bacampicillin (Spectrobid)		
Protein binding: 17–20%		
Half-life: 1 hour		
PO	499–800 mg	Every 12 hours

Extended-spectrum penicillin Pregnancy Category: B		
Route	Dose	Time
Carbenicillin (Geocillin) Protein binding: 50% Half-life: 1–1.5 hours		
PO	0.5–1 g	Every 6 hours
IV	50–83.3 mg/kg	Every 4 hours
IM	50–83.3 mg/kg	Every 4 hours
Mezlocillin (Mezlin) Protein binding: 30–40% Half-life: 0.5–1 hour		
IV	33.3–58.3 mg/kg	Every 4 hours
IM	33.3–58.3 mg/kg	Every 4 hours
Piperacillin (Pipracil) Protein binding: 16–22% Half-life: 0.6–1.5 hours		
IV	3–4 g	Every 4–6 hours
IM	3–4 g	Every 4–6 hours
Piperacillin + tazobactam (Zosyn, Tazocin) Protein binding: UK Half-life: 0.7–1.2 hours		
IV	3.375–4 .5 g	Every 6–8 hours
Ticarcillin (Ticar) Pregnancy Category: C Protein binding: 45–65% Half-life: 0.5–1.5 hours		
IV	1–4 g	Every 6 hours
IM	1 g	Every 6 hours
Ticarcillin + clavulanate (timentin) Protein binding: 45–65% Half-life: 1–1.5 hours		
IV	33.3–50 mg	Every 4 hours

Penicillin and Drug-Drug Interactions

Penicillin can produce adverse effects if it is administered in conjunction with other drugs. This can occur when giving penicillin with an antihypertensive drug such as Captopril [an angiotensin-converting enzyme (ACE) inhibitor], potassium-sparing diuretics such as Aldactone, potassium-containing drugs, or potassium supplements such as Kay Ciel. The combination of drugs may increase the patient's potassium level (hyperkalemia) and therefore require that the patient's serum potassium levels be carefully monitored while the patient receives penicillin.

There is an increased risk for bleeding with administration of high doses of parenteral carbenicillin or ticarcillin as these drugs inhibit platelet aggregation. These penicillins also increase the risk for severe bleeding if given with thrombolytic agents such as tissue plasminogen activator (TPA).

The absorption of penicillin G when taken PO may be decreased if taken with cholestyramine (Questran) or colestipol (Colestid). Similarly, the use of penicillin might decrease the effectiveness of estrogen contained in contraceptives.

Two other drugs affected by penicillin are methotrexate (Folex) and probenecid (Benemid). There is a decrease in the body's ability to clear methotrexate when penicillin is present. There can be a buildup of methotrexate, resulting in toxicity.

Probenecid decreases renal secretion of penicillin, resulting in an increase in the serum level of penicillin.

5. Penicillin, Nursing Diagnosis, and Collaborative Problems

A patient who is receiving penicillin may experience one or more conditions that require intervention. Here are some nursing diagnoses that are common for patients receiving penicillin:

- Altered protection against infection related to reduction in normal flora (superinfection)
- Altered bowel elimination pattern related to antibiotic-associated pseudomembranous colitis
- Fluid volume deficit related to nausea, vomiting, and/or diarrhea
- Impaired skin integrity related to side effects or allergic reaction
- Allergic response
- Hepatotoxicity (toxicity affecting the liver)
- Leukopenia (a decrease in the number of circulating WBCs)
- Neutropenia (abnormal decrease in the number of neutrophils, which are the most common type of WBCs)
- Thrombocytopenia (decreased number of platelets in the blood)
- Mental disturbances
- Seizures
- Cross-sensitivity to cephalosporins, cephamycins, griseofulvin, or penicillamine

- Abdominal cramps
- Diarrhea
- Darkened or discolored tongue
- Sore mouth

Penicillin and Patient Education

The patient must be instructed to monitor her/his temperature to ensure that the infection is subsiding. Generally, healthy patients can expect to see some improvement in the infection within 48 hours. They should be instructed to return to or contact the prescriber if symptoms worsen or do not improve somewhat in 48 hours. Patients with diabetes, immunosuppressed conditions such as AIDS, or certain cancers might not respond as quickly to antibiotic therapy.

In addition to information described for generic antibiotics, female patients should be informed that penicillin can interfere with the effectiveness of birth control pills that contain estrogen. It is recommended that females use alternative forms of birth control while being treated with penicillin.

6. Cephalosporins

The cephalosporin family of medications is a chemically modified version of penicillin that stops growth and kills a broad spectrum of bacteria by making it impossible for bacteria to create a cell wall. There are four generations of cephalosporins.

Cephalosporin can be prescribed for patients who are allergic to penicillin. However, about 10% of those patients might also be allergic to cephalosporins. Do not administer cephalosporins to patients who have had a serious reaction to penicillin such as anaphylaxis.

Prescribers use cephalosporins to combat a wide variety of infections and typically use these as a prophylaxis to prevent a bacterial infection to occur during or after surgery.

Cephalosporins also have side effects that include diarrhea, abdominal cramps or distress, oral and/or vaginal candidiasis, rash, pruritus, redness, or edema. There is also an increase in bleeding and bruising with four commonly prescribed cephalosporins: cefamandole, cefmetazole, cefoperazone, and cefotetan.

The patient assessment for cephalosporins is the same as that for penicillin. However, pay particular attention to any previous bleeding disorder reported by the patient because cephalosporins can exacerbate this condition.

Before administering cephalosporins, assess for allergies, vital signs, and urine output. Check laboratory results, especially those that indicate renal and liver function such as BUN, serum creatinine, aspartate aminotransferase (AST), alanine amino-transferase (ALT), alkaline phosphatase (ALP), and bilirubin. Also check bleeding time [prothrombin time (PT) and partial thromboplastin time (PTT)] and WBC count. Obtain a tissue or blood specimen for a culture-sensitivity test, if possible, to determine whether cephalosporins are the right antibiotic.

Administer cephalosporins using the same methods as used for penicillin. If given IM, it should be injected deeply into a large muscle mass. This decreases pain, indura-tion (becoming hard), and a sterile abscess.

The patient should be provided with the same instructions as those to a patient who is receiving penicillin (see "Penicillin and Patient Education" section, above).

Cephalosporins and Drug-Drug Interactions

Alcohol should be avoided by patients taking certain cephalosporins (cefamandole, cefoperazone, or moxalactam) because this combination might cause adverse side effects, including the following:

- Stomach pain
- Nausea
- Vomiting
- Headaches
- Hypotension
- Tachycardia (rapid heart rate)
- Difficulty breathing
- Sweating
- Flushed face

Some medications include alcohol, and the patient should be advised to check the labels carefully if taking one of these cephalosporins.

Besides alcohol, some cephalosporins (cefamandole, cefmetazole, cefoperazone, or cefotetan) expose the patient to an increased risk for hemorrhaging if administered with anticoagulants such as coumarin, indanedione, or heparin, and with clot-busting drugs such as thrombolytics. The same adverse reaction might occur if the patient takes NSAIDs, especially aspirin, or sulfinpyrazone (Anturane) while on cephalosporins.

Probenecid (Benemid) may extend the half-life of cephalosporins and can result in toxicity. However, cephalosporins and probenecid are sometimes given together to treat sexually transmitted diseases when a high serum level and prolonged level of cephalo-sporins are desirable.

A patient who is undergoing treatment with cephalosporins might experience other problems, namely, a fever and rash brought about by hypersensitivity, an allergic reaction such as anaphylaxis, Stevens-Johnson syndrome, renal dysfunction, serum sickness-like reaction, or seizures.

7. Cephalosporins, Nursing Diagnosis, and Collaborative Problems

Here are the common nursing diagnoses that are related to a patient who is receiving cephalosporins:

- Altered bowel elimination pattern related to antibiotic-associated pseudomembranous colitis
- Risk for superinfection
- Altered protection related to hypoprothrombinemia and superinfection

First generation: effective against Gram-positive bacteria Pregnancy Category: B		
Route	Dose	Time
Cefadroxil (Duricef) Protein binding: 20% Half-life: 0.5–2 hours		
PO	500 mg	Every 12 hours
Cefazolin (Ancef, Kefzol) Protein binding: 75–85% Half-life: 0.5–2.5 hours		
IV	0.25–1.5 g	Every 6–8 hours
IM	1 g	Presurgery
Cephalexin (Keflex) Protein binding: 65–80% Half-life: 0.5–1 hour		
PO	250–500 mg	Every 6 hours
Cephalothin (Keflin) Protein binding: 10–15% Half-life: 0.5–1.2 hours		
IM/IV	0.5–1 g	Every 4–6 hours
Cephapirin (Cefadyl) Protein binding 40–50% Half-life: 0.5–1 hour		
IM /IV	0.5–1 g	Every 4–6 hours

First generation: effective against Gram-positive bacteria (*Continued*)		
Pregnancy Category: B		
Cephradine (Velosef, Anspor)		
Protein binding: 20%		
Half-life: 1–2 hours		
PO	250–500 mg	Every 8 hours
IM/IV	0.5–1 g	Every 6 hours

Second generation: increased activity against Gram (–) microorganisms		
Pregnancy Category: B		
Route	Dose	Time
Cefaclor (Ceclor)		
Protein binding: 25%		
Half-life 0.5–2 hours		
PO	250–500 mg	Every 8 hours
IM/IV	500 g	Every 6 hours
Cefamandole (Mandol)		
Protein binding: 60–75%		
Half-life: 0.5–1 hour		
IM/IV	500 mg	Every 6–8 hours
Cefmetazole (Zefazone)		
Protein binding: 68%		
Half-life: 2.5–3 hours		
IV	2 g	Every 12 hours
Cefonicid (Monocid)		
Protein binding: 98%		
Half-life: 0.5–1.2 hours		
IM/IV	0.5–1 g	Every 24 hours
Cefotetan (Cefotan)		
Protein binding: 85%		
Half-life: 3–5 hours		
IM /IV	102 g	Every 12 hours
Cefoxitin (Mefoxin)		
Protein binding: 70%		
Half-life: 0.75–1 hour		
IV	102 g	Every 6–8 hours
Cefprozil (Cefzil)		
Protein binding: 99%		
Half-life: 1–2 hours		

Second generation: increased activity against Gram (−) microorganisms (*Continued*) Pregnancy Category: B		
PO	500 mg	Every 12 hours
Cefurozine (Ceftin, Zinacef) Protein binding: 50% Half-life: 1.5–2 hours		
PO	250–500 mg	Every 12 hours
IM/IV	0.75–1.5 g	Every 8 hours
Loracarbef (Lorabid) Protein binding: UK Half-life: 1 hour		
PO	200–400 mg	Every 12 hours

Third generation: more active against Gram (−); ceftazidime and cefoperazone are also effective against *Pseudomonas aeruginosa* (Gram −) and β-lactamase-producing microbial strains; less effective against Gram (+) cocci Pregnancy Category: B		
Route	Dose	Time
Cefixime (suprax) Protein binding: 65% Half-life: 2.5–4 hours		
PO	200 mg	Every 12 hours
Cefoperazone (Cefobid) Protein binding: 70–80% Half-life: 2.5 hours		
IV	1–2 g	Every 12 hours
Cefotaxime (Claforan) Protein binding: 30–40% Half-life: 1–1.5–3 hours		
IV	1–2 g	Every 12 hours
Cefpodoxime (Vantin, Proxetil) Protein binding: 20–40% Half-life: 2–3 hours		
PO	200 mg	Every 12 hours
Ceftazidime (Fortaz) Protein binding: 10–17% Half-life: 1–2 hours		
IM/IV	0.5–2 g	Every 8–12 hours

Third generation: more active against Gram (–); ceftazidime and cefoperazone are also effective against *Pseudomonas aeruginosa* (Gram –) and β-lactamase-producing microbial strains; less effective against Gram (+) cocci (*Continued*) Pregnancy Category: B		
Ceftibuten (Cedax) Protein binding: UK Half-life: 1.5–3 hours		
PO	400 mg	Once per day
Ceftriaxone (Recephin) Protein binding: 85–95% Half-life: 8 hours		
IV	1–2 g	Every 24 hours
Ceftizoxime (Cefizox) Protein binding: 30–60% Half-life: 2 hours		
IM/IV	500 mg	Every 8–12 hours
Cefdinir (Omnicef) Protein binding: UK Half-life: 1.7 hours		
PO	300 or 600 mg/day	Every 12 hours

Fourth generation: cefepime same as third generation + more resistant to β-lactamases Pregnancy Category: B		
Route	Dose	Time
Cefepime (Maxipime) Protein binding: UK Half-life 0.5–2 hours		
IM/IV	0.5–1 g	Every 12 hours

Macrolide Antibiotics

Macrolide antibiotics are used to combat Gram-positive and Gram-negative bacteria. As you may recall from microbiology, the Gram stain is used as a method to identify a bacterium. If after staining, the bacterium appears purple, then it is assumed to be Gram-positive; if pink, Gram-negative. There is one exception: If the bacteria are either purple or pink, then a macrolide antibiotic is effective against the bacteria.

The exception is with troleandomycin, which is a macrolide antibiotic. Troleandomycin is used to fight *Streptococcus pneumoniae* and *Streptococcuus pyogenes*.

Macrolide antibiotics are bacteriostatic; that is, they inhibit reproduction of bacteria, but do not kill the bacteria. By inhibiting reproduction, macrolide antibiotics control the bacterial growth, giving the body's own immune system—or other medication—time to kill the bacteria.

Prescribers give patients macrolide antibiotics to fight soft-tissue infections, skin infections, and infections of the respiratory system and gastrointestinal tract.

Macrolide antibiotics have some side effects that adversely affect the patient. The most common side effects are nausea, vomiting, stomach pain, and cramps. These occur with azithromycin, clarithromycin, erythromycin, and dirithromycin. Troleandomycin causes stomach cramps and discomfort.

Before receiving macrolides, the patient is assessed using the same techniques as described for other antibiotics. However, caution must be used when prescribing macrolides to patients who have liver disease. Those with a history of cardiac arrhythmias should not take erythromycin.

The patient should be advised to take macrolides with a full glass of water either 1 hour before or 2 hours after meals to avoid gastric distress. Some patients are intolerant to certain marcrolides when taken orally. In these cases, enteric-coated or delayed-release capsules are appropriate to prescribe.

If marcolides are administered IV, they must be diluted in 100–200 mL of 0.9% NS solution or D_5W solution and infused over a 20–60-minute period.

The patient should be provided with the same instructions as those given to a patient who is receiving penicillin (see "Penicillin and Patient Education" section).

Macrolide antibiotics Pregnancy Category: B		
Route	Dose	Time
Erythromycin (E-Mycin, Erythrocin, Erythrocin Lactobionate) Protein binding: 65% Half-life: PO 1–2 hours; IV 3–5 hours		
PO	250–500 mg	Every 6 hours
IV	1–4 g/day	Divided doses
Azithromyzin (Zithromax) Protein binding: 50% Half-life: 11–55 hours		
PO	500 mg	First day
	250 mg	Daily thereafter
Clarithromycin (Biaxin) Protein binding: 65–75% Half-life: 3–6 hours Pregnancy Category: C		
PO	250–500 mg	Every 12 hours

Macrolide antibiotics (*Continued*) Pregnancy Category: B		
Erythromycin, dirithromycin (Dynabac) Protein binding: UK Half-life: 20–50 hours Pregnancy Category: C		
PO	250 mg (erythromycin)	Every 6 hours
	500 mg (dirithromycin)	Once a day
IV	250–500 mg	Every 6 hours

8. Macrolides and Drug-Drug Interactions

Macrolides have various effects on other medications. Therefore, the nursing assessment should include obtaining a history of all the drugs (OTC or prescribed) or herbals that the patient may be taking. Macrolides can increase the therapeutic levels of alfentanil (Alfenta), carbamezepine (Tegretol), and cyclosporine (Sandimmune), resulting in the patient experiencing a toxic effect.

Terfenadine (Seldane) or astemizole (Hismanal) given with macrolides might cause toxicity to the heart. There is also a risk for hemorrhage if the patient takes both warfarin (Coumadin) and macrolides within the same time period. The patient may also experience increased theophylline levels, which can lead to toxicity when theophylline is given along with zanthines such as aminophylline and caffeine.

9. Macrolides, Nursing Diagnosis, and Collaborative Problems

Here are some nursing diagnoses common for patients receiving macrolides:
- Altered bowel elimination pattern
- Impaired tissue integrity related to inflammation or phlebitis at the injection site
- Fluid volume deficit related to nausea and vomiting
- Alteration in comfort related to abdominal cramping
- Sensory-perceptual disturbance related to hearing loss
- Altered protection related to loss of normal flora

Lincosamides

Lincomycin (Lincocin) has been used in the past to treat serious streptococci, pneumococci, and staphylococci infections but has generally been replaced by safer and more effective antibiotics. Clindamycin (Cleocin) is a semisynthetic derivative of lincomycin and has a similar mechanism but is more effective. It is indicated for the treatment of bone and joint infections, pelvic (female) and intraabdominal infections, bacterial septicemia, pneumonia, and skin and soft-tissue infections. In a normal dose, lincosamides prevent the growth of bacteria (bacteriostatic). In larger doses, it kills bacteria (bactericidal).

The use of lincomycin is avoided because there is a significant occurrence of pseudomembranous colitis. Clindamycin is the drug of choice because it is safer and more effective than lincomycin.

Patient assessment before lincosamide administration is the same as assessment for all antibiotics. In addition, determine whether the patient has a history of GI diseases or liver or kidney problems.

Administer lincosamides with a full glass of water or with meals to prevent esophageal ulceration. After lincosamides are administered, request for additional WBC counts to determine the effectiveness of the medication. Monitor the patient for the following conditions:

- Abdominal cramps
- Diarrhea
- Weight loss
- Weakness

The patient should be provided with the same instructions as is given to one who is receiving penicillin (see "Penicillin and Patient Education" section).

10. Clindamycins and Drug-Drug Interactions

Besides being associated with pseudomembranous colitis, clindamycin can also cause an adverse interaction with antidiarrheals, chloramphenicol (Chloromycetin), and erythromycin.

Clindamycin is known to enhance the neuromuscular blockage caused by anesthetic agents. This might result in the patient experiencing skeletal muscle weakness, respiratory depression, and even paralysis if used during or immediately after surgery.

11. Lincosamides, Nursing Diagnosis, and Collaborative Problems

Patients who receive clindamycin may also experience hypersensitivity. Therefore, you must be prepared to identify the signs and symptoms of hypersensitivity and treat them if conditions become intolerable for the patient.

Lincosamides Pregnancy Category: B		
Route	Dose	Time
Clindamycin (Cleocin, Dalacin) semisynthetic Protein binding: 94% Half-life: 2–3 hours		
PO/IM/IV	150–300 mg	Every 6 hours
Lincomycin (Lincorex) Protein binding: 70–75% Half-life: 4–6 hours		
PO	500 mg	Every 6–8 hours, maximum 8 g/day
IM	600 mg	Every day
IV	Dilute in 100 cc fluid	Every day

Here are some nursing diagnoses common for patients receiving lincosamides:

- Altered bowel elimination patterns
- Fluid volume deficits related to nausea and vomiting
- Altered protection related to neutropenia (infection), thrombocytopenia (bleeding), and loss of normal flora (superinfection)

Vancomycin

Vancomycin is a bactericidal agent used for infections of the bone and joints and bacterial septicemia caused by *Staphylococcus*. It is also used to treat *Staphylococcus*-causing endocarditis including the methicillin-resistant strains. Prescribers commonly prescribe vancomycin to patients who are susceptible to endocarditis in an effort to prevent the infection.

Vancomycin is also used for the treatment of *Clostridium difficile* and staphylococcal enterocolitis, which are treated orally or parenterally. However, parenteral vancomycin is not recommended for treating antibiotic-associated pseudomembranous colitis.

Before administering vancomycin, use the same assessment criteria as applied for all antibiotic therapy described throughout this chapter. In addition, determine whether the patient has hearing loss, kidney problems, or an inflammatory intestinal disorder. Vancomycin should be avoided or used with caution for patients who have hearing loss. Patients with kidney problems should receive lower doses of vancomycin. Carefully monitor patients who have inflammatory intestinal disorders as they are at higher risk for toxicity. Make sure that the patient has adequate renal function.

When administering vancomycin, avoid giving it as an IV bolus. Vancomycin should be infused over a 24-hour period or infused intermittently over 60 minutes. If given continuously for 24 hours, dilute 1–2 g of vancomycin in a sufficient amount of 0.09% sodium chloride (NS) or D_5W. If infused intermittently for 60 minutes, dilute the dose in 100 mL of 0.09% sodium chloride (NS) or dilute in 100 mL of 5% dextrose solution (D_5W). Rotation of the IV sites will help prevent local irritation.

After administering vancomycin, monitor the patient's renal function to ensure that there is adequate volume to excrete vancomycin. Also monitor the patient's WBC count to determine whether the drug is effective.

The patient should be provided with the same instructions as those given to a patient who is receiving penicillin (see "Penicillin and Patient Education" section).

12. Vancomycin and Drug-Drug Interactions

Vancomycin causes adverse reactions when used with some medications. You must wait for several hours before giving vancomycin to a patient who has received oral cholestyramine (Questran) or colestipol (Colestid) because these medications lower the therapeutic effect of vancomycin.

Also avoid giving vancomycin if the patient has taken any aminoglycosides because they increase the potential for ototoxicity (ear) and nephrotoxicity (kidney). If the patient receives vancomycin and aminoglycosides, then you must closely monitor vancomycin serum levels to ensure that it remains within the safe range. Drug-drug interaction may occur if vancomycin is administered with any of the following drugs:

- Amphotericin B
- Aspirin
- Bacitracin
- Parenteral bumetanide (Bumex)
- Capreomycin (Capastat)
- Cisplatin (Platinol)
- Cyclosporine (Sandimmune)
- Ethacrynate parenteral (Edecrin)
- Furosemide parenteral (Lasix)
- Paromomycin (Humatin)
- Polymyxins
- Streptozocin (Zanosar)

13. Vancomycin, Nursing Diagnosis, and Collaborative Problems

Patients who receive vancomycin may also experience nephrotoxicty (kidney). Monitor urine output for kidney function.

Here are some nursing diagnoses common for patients receiving vancomycin:

- Risk for injury related to histamine release if administered too rapidly
- Fluid volume deficit related to nausea and vomiting
- Impaired tissue integrity
- Sensory-perceptual disturbance related to ototoxicity [loss of hearing and tinnitus (ringing in the ears)]

Aminoglycosides

Aminogylcosides are potent antibiotics used to kill bacteria that cause serious or life-threatening infections. They are very effective against many bacteria (both Gram-positive and Gram-negative) but are generally used for Gram-negative infections. Safer and less toxic agents are available for treating the majority of Gram-positive infections. Since the patient is experiencing a life-threatening infection, prescribers combine animoglycosides with penicillin, cephalosporins, or ancomycin to give a one-two punch knockout to the bacteria.

Vancomycin Pregnancy Category: C		
Route	Dose	Time
Vancomycin (Vancocin) Protein binding: 10% Half-life: 5–11 hours		
IV	500 mg	Every 6 hours

There are significant side effects with aminogylcoside administration, namely, nephrotoxicity, neurotoxicity, hyersensitivity, and ototoxicity (problems with hearing and balance).

Assess the patient according to the guidelines for all antibiotics as described previously in this chapter for penicillin. Infants with botulism and patients with myasthenia gravis or Parkinsonism will experience more muscle weakness than other patients who are treated with animoglycosides. You must also ascertain whether the patient has hearing or kidney problems or allergies.

Before administering aminoglycosides, obtain a baseline assessment for the patient, including audiogram, renal function, and vestibular function studies.

When administering aminoglycosides IV, dilute the medication in solution as per the package insert and infuse it over a 30–60-minute period. Use a smaller-than-normal dose for elderly patients who are at greater risk for kidney toxicity and ototoxicity.

If aminoglycides are given IM, then give the injection deep into the upper outer quadrant of the gluteal muscle.

After administering aminoglycides, keep the patient well hydrated and monitor intake and output to determine whether there is nephrotoxicity. Monitor the patient's temperature, cultures, and WBC to determine whether the infection is working. A daily urinalysis should be obtained for signs of kidney irritation.

The patient should be provided with the same instructions as those given to one who is receiving penicillin (see "Penicillin and Patient Education" section). Advise the patient to report any hearing problem, including ringing or buzzing in the ears, as well as dizziness, numbness, tingling, twitching, or changes in urinary patterns, especially the presence of blood in the urine.

14. Aminoglycosides and Drug-Drug Interactions

Aminoglycosides can have undesirable interactions with other medications. When taken with other aminoglycosides or capremycin (Capastat), the patient has an increased potential for hearing, kidney, and neuromuscular problems. Hearing loss can lead to total deafness long after the patient stops treatment with aminoglycosides.

Neuromuscular blockage may increase when aminoglycosides are given to patients who have received anesthetics (halogenated hydrocarbon) or citrate-anticoagulated blood through massive transfusions. Methoxyflurane (Penthrane) and polymyxins, given parenterally, also increase the possibility for neuromuscular blockage as well as kidney toxicity.

In addition, patients who are treated with aminoglycides can experience interactions with the following medications:

- Amphotericin B parenteral (Fungizone)
- Aspirin
- Bacitracin parenteral
- Bumetanide parenteral aspirin
- Bacitracin
- Parenteral bumetanide (Bumex)
- Cephalothin (Keflin)

- Cisplatin (Platinol)
- Cyclosporine (Sandimmune)
- Ethacrynate parenteral (Edecrin)
- Furosemide parenteral (Lasix)
- Paromomycin (Humatin)
- Polymyxins
- Streptozocin (Zanosar)
- Vancomycin (Cancocin)

15. Aminoglycosides, Nursing Diagnosis, and Collaborative Problems

Patients who receive aminoglycosides may also experience nephrotoxicty (kidney), neurotoxicity (muscle twitching, numbness, or seizures), and hypersensitivity.

Here are some nursing diagnoses common for patients receiving aminoglycosides:

- Sensory-perceptual alterations: auditory ototoxicity (loss of hearing and tinnitus), vestibular ototoxicity (dizziness and loss of balance), and peripheral neuritis (tingling of the fingers and toes)

Aminoglycosides Pregnancy Category: C		
Route	Dose	Time
Amikacin (Amikin) Protein binding: 4–11% Half-life: 2–3 hours		
IM/IV	5 mg/kg	Every 8 hours
Gentamicin (Garamycin) Protein binding: UK Half-life: 2 hours		
IM/IV	1–1.7 mg/kg	Infusion every 8 hours
Kanamycin (Kantrex) Protein binding: 10% Half-life: 2–3 hours Pregnancy Category: D		
IM	3.75 mg/kg	Every 6 hours
Neomycin SO$_4$ (Mycifradin) Protein binding: 10% Half-life: 2–3 hours		

Aminoglycosides (*Continued*) Pregnancy Category: C		
PO (GI surgery)	1 g	Every hour for 4 doses
	1 g	Every 4 hours; thereafter for 24 hours or other regimens
(Hepatic coma)	4–12 g/day	Divided doses
IM	15 mg/kg daily	Every 6 hours for 4 doses, maximum 1 g/day
Netilmicin (Netromycin) Protein binding: 10% Half-life: 2–3 hours Pregnancy Category: D		
IM/IV	1.3–2.2 mg/kg	Every 8 hours
Streptomycin SO$_4$ Protein binding: 30% Half-life: 2–3 hours		
IM (tuberculosis)	1 g	Every day with antimycobacterials
(Endocarditis)	1 g	Every 12 hours for 1 week; dose may be decreased
Tobramycin SO$_4$ (Nebcin) Protein binding: 10% Half-life: 2–3 hours		
IM/IV	0.75 mg 1.25 mg/kg	Every 6 hours

Tetracyclines

Tetracyclines were the first broad-spectrum antibiotics used to halt the growth of many Gram-positive and Gram-negative bacteria. They are used to treat a variety of infections, including acne vulgaris, actinomycosis, anthrax, bronchitis, and other systemic bacterial infections, including bacterial urinary tract infections.

Demeclocycline, a member of the tetracycline family, is also used to treat conditions that are associated with inappropriate diuretic hormone administration since demeclocycline inhibits water-induced reabsorption in the kidneys.

Assess the patient the same way as described previously in this chapter for a patient taking penicillin. Do not use tetracyclines if the patient is pregnant or breastfeeding. Furthermore, tetracyclines should not be given to children under 8 years of age because tetracyclines can permanently mottle and discolor the teeth and decrease linear skeletal growth in both children and the fetus.

Patients who have a hypersensitivity to "-caine" medication such as lidocaine and procaine may be intolerant to tetracyclines because such medication is mixed in the tetracycline intramuscular injection.

Only doxycycline and minocycline, which are members of the tetracyclines family, can be used with patients who have renal problems. Other members of the tetracycline family should not be prescribed for those patients.

Tetracyclines should be taken with a full glass of water on an empty stomach. With the exception of doxycycline and minocycline, tetracyclines should not be administered 1 hour before or 2 hours after meals.

The patient should not be given antacids containing aluminum, calcium, or magnesium; laxatives; iron products; food; or milk or other dairy products for 1 hour before or 2 hours after tetracycline is administered.

Doxycycline and oxytetracycline can be administered IV. Doxycycline may be given in concentrations of 100 µg–1 mg/mL. Do not administer doxycycline IM or SQ. Oxytetracycline needs to be diluted in at least 100 mL of appropriate IV solution. Don't infuse rapidly.

Tetracycline may be administered IM in doses not exceeding 2 mL at each injection site. Do not administer tetracycline IV or SQ.

The patient should be provided with the same instructions as those given to one who is receiving penicillin (see "Penicillin and Patient Education" section). However, also advise the patient to avoid direct sunlight and ultraviolet light because tetracyclines might cause the patient to become sensitive to sunlight. The patient should use a sunscreen in the sun.

Advise the patient to discard unused tetracycline because tetracyline becomes toxic as it decomposes. Tetracycline should be taken on an empty stomach as food affects absorption of the drug.

16. Tetracyclines and Drug-Drug Interactions

Tetracyclines can interact with other medications. Avoid giving tetracyclines 2 hours before or after the patient receives colestipol (Colestid) or cholestyramine (Questran) because these medications decrease the absorption of tetracycline.

Give tetracycline 1–3 hours before or after giving the patient antacids, calcium supplements, choline and magnesium salicylates, iron supplements, magnesium salicylate, or magnesium laxatives, or foods containing milk and milk products. These substances lower the absorption of tetracycline.

Do not give tetracycline if the patient is taking estrogen-containing oral contraceptives since this reduces the contraceptive effectiveness and may result in breakthrough bleeding. Female patients should be advised to use alternative methods of birth control while on antibiotics.

17. Tetracyclines, Nursing Diagnosis, and Collaborative Problems

Patients who receive tetracycline may also experience nephrogenic diabetes insipidus, hepatotoxicity, pancreatitis, dizziness, or syncope, and their skin might become increasingly sensitive to sunlight.

Here are some nursing diagnoses that are common for patients receiving tetracyclines:

- Altered comfort (heartburn and abdominal cramping)
- Fluid volume deficit related to anorexia, nausea, and vomiting
- Altered bowel elimination (diarrhea)
- Altered protection related to loss of normal florae (fungal overgrowth)

Tetracyclines Pregnancy Category: D		
Route	Dose	Time
Tetracycline—short-acting Protein binding: 20–60% Half-life: 6–12 hours		
PO	250–500 mg	Every 6 hours
IM	150 mg	Every 12 hours
Oxytetracycline (Terramycin)—short-acting Protein binding: 20–40% Half-life: 6–10 hours		
PO	250–500 mg	Every 6 hours
IV	250–500 mg	Infusion every 12 hours
Democlocycline (Declomycin)—intermediate-acting Protein binding: 35–90% Half-life: 10–17 hours		
PO	150 mg	Every 6 hours
	300 mg	Every 12 hours
Doxycycline (Vibramycin)—long-acting Protein binding: 25–92% Half-life: 20 hours		
PO	100 mg	Twice the first day
	100–200 mg	Once a day thereafter

Tetracyclines (*Continued*)		
Pregnancy Category: D		
Minocycline (minocin)—long-acting		
Protein binding: 55–88%		
Half-life: 11–20 hours		
PO	200 mg	First dose
	100 mg	Every 12 hours

Chloramphenicol (Chloromycetin)

Chloramphenicol is a broad-spectrum antibiotic that slows the growth of a wide variety of Gram-positive and Gram-negative bacteria. In high doses, chloramphenicol can kill bacteria. Chloramphenicol is given for treatment of meningitis (*H. influenzae, S. pneumoniae,* and *Neisseria meningitidis*), parathyroid fever, Q fever, Rocky Mountain spotted fever, typhoid fever, typhus infections, brain abscesses, and bacterial septicemia.

Chloramphenicol should not be used for a patient who is pregnant or breastfeeding. Neonates may develop *gray syndrome*, which is blue-gray skin, hypothermia, irregular breathing, coma, and cardiovascular collapse.

Chloramphenicol is not recommended for use with a patient who is undergoing radiation therapy or who has bone marrow depression.

Monitor the chloramphenicol serum level to ensure that chloramphenicol stays within therapeutic limits. Chloramphenicol does have a seriously toxic effect on bone marrow.

Patients have infrequently reported experiencing diarrhea, nausea, or vomiting. Serious adverse effects include blood dyscrasias, optic neuritis, and possibly irreversible bone marrow depression that may lead to aplastic anemia.

18. Chloramphenicol and Drug-Drug Interactions

Chloramphenicol can have an adverse interaction with alfentanil (Alfenta) by increasing alfentanil levels in the patient. Chloramphenicol is known to increase bone marrow depression when given with anticonvulsants.

Patients who are taking antidiabetic medication may see an increase in the level of that medication when taken with chloramphenicol, resulting in hypoglycemia. Therefore, diabetics who take chloramphenicol must closely monitor their blood glucose levels.

Chloramphenicol also causes a decrease in the therapeutic effect of clindamycin, erythromycin, or lincomycin. Chloramphenicol increases the drug serum levels of phenobarbital (Luminal), phenytoin (Dilantin), or warfarin (Coumadin), which can lead to toxicity.

19. Chloramphenicol, Nursing Diagnosis, and Collaborative Problems

Patients who take chloramphenicol may also experience rash, fever, and dyspnea. Neonates experience gray syndrome.

Here are some nursing diagnoses common for patients who are taking chloramphenicol:

- Fluid volume deficit related to anorexia, nausea, and vomiting
- Altered protection resulting from dose-related bone marrow depression
- Altered bowel elimination (diarrhea)
- Altered thought processes (confusion, delirium) related to neurotoxic reactions; sensory-perceptual disturbances related to optic neuritis (blurred vision, loss of vision, eye pain); and to peripheral neuritis (tingling, numbness, and burning pain of the hands and feet)

Fluoroquinolones

Fluoroquinolones are broad-spectrum, synthetic antibiotics that stop bacterial growth in bone and joint infections, bronchitis, gastroenteritis, gonorrhea, pneumonia, urinary tract infection, and many other diseases. However, fluoroquinolones should not be prescribed for infants or children.

Chloramphenicol (Chloromycetin) Pregnancy Category: C		
Route	Dose	Time
Chloramphenicol (Chloromycetin) Protein binding: 50–60% Half-Life: 4 hours		
PO/IV	12.5 mg/kg	Every 6 hours

Make sure that the patient does not have an allergic reaction to any fluoroquinolone. If the patient is allergic to one drug within the fluoroquinolone family, then she/he is highly likely to be allergic to other fluoroquinolone medications.

Patients who take fluoroquinolones can, in rare cases, experience dizziness, drowsiness, restlessness, stomach distress, diarrhea, nausea and vomiting, psychosis, confusion, hallucinations, tremors, hypersensitivity, and interstitial nephritis (kidney).

The dose of fluoroquinolones should be lowered in patients with hepatic (liver) or renal (kidney) problems. Carefully monitor the serum level of fluoroquinolones in patients who have CNS disorders such as cerebral arteriosclerosis (hardening of the arteries in the brain), epilepsy (seizures), or alcoholism because they are at risk for CNS toxicity.

Administer fluoroquinolones with a full glass of water to minimize the possibility of crystalluria. Fluoroquinolones should be infused slowly. Ofloxacin, a member of the fluoroquinolones family, must be infused into a large vein over 60 minutes to minimize discomfort and venous irritation.

After administering fluoroquinolones, monitor the patient's urinary output. The patient should void at least 1200–1500 mL daily. Also monitor the pH of the urine; it should remain at 7.0 or less.

The patient should be provided with the same instructions as those given to a patient who is receiving penicillin (see "Penicillin and Patient Education" section). Tell the patient to report any blurred or double vision, sensitivity to light, dizziness, light-headedness, or depression. These are signs of CNS toxicity.

If fluoroquinolones are self-administered, tell the patient to avoid taking the drug within 2 hours of taking an antacid. The patient should also avoid exposure to sunlight and sunlamps. The patient must wear sunglasses and avoid bright lights.

20. Fluoroquinolones and Drug-Drug Interactions

If ciprofloxacin, a member of the fluoroquinolones family, is prescribed, then it should be given 2 hours before the patient is given antacids, ferrous sulfate, or sucralfate because these medications lower the absorption of ciprofloxacin.

Patients who are taking theophylline or other xanthines with fluoroquinolones should be aware that the theophylline plasma levels can rise, leading to toxicity.

If the patient takes fluoroquinolones concurrently with warfarin, the anticoagulant effect of warfarin increases and could result in bleeding. The prothrombin time (PT) should be monitored if both are administered together.

21. Fluoroquinolones, Nursing Diagnosis, and Collaborative Problems

Patients who receive fluoroquinolones may also experience rash, fever, dyspnea, nephritis, blood in the urine, lower-back pain, rash, edema, and photosensitivity (increased sensitivity of skin to sunlight). In addition, they might have CNS toxicity (dizziness, headache, insomnia).

Here are some nursing diagnoses that are common for patients receiving fluoroquinolones:

- Fluid volume deficit related to anorexia (nausea and vomiting)
- Altered comfort related to arthralgia (joint discomfort and stiffness)

- Impaired tissue integrity related to phlebitis (IV ciprofloxacin and ofloxacin only)

- Altered bowel elimination (diarrhea)

- Altered thought processes related to CNS stimulation (confusion, hallucinations)

Fluoroquinolones Pregnancy Category: C		
Route	Dose	Time
Ciprofloxacin (Cipro) Protein binding: 20% Half-life: 3–4 hours		
PO	250–500 mg	Every 12 hours
Fluroquinoline, severe infections	500–750 mg	Every 12 hours
IV, mild to moderate infections	400 mg	Every 12 hours
Enoxacin (Penetrex) Protein binding: 40% Half-life: 3–6 hours		
PO	200–400 mg	Every 12 hours for 1–2 weeks
Levofloxacin (Levaquin) Protein binding: 50% Half-life: 6 hours		
PO	250–750 mg	
IV	500 mg/day	7–14 days
Lomefloxacin (Maxaquin) Protein binding: UK Half-life: 6–8 hours		
PO	400 mg	10–14 days
Norfloxacin (Noroxin) Protein binding: 10–11% Half-life: 3–4 hours		
PO	400 mg	Every 12 hours for 72 hours
Ofloxacin (Floxin) Protein binding: 20% Half-life: 5–8 hours		
PO/IV	300–400 mg	Every 12 hours for 10 days

Miscellaneous Antibiotics

The following table lists other antibiotics that are likely to be prescribed to treat microbial infections.

Antibiotic	Description
Aztreonam (Azactam)	Synthetic bactericidal activity similar to that of penicillin Use: treats urinary tract, bronchitis, intraabdominal, gynecologic, and skin infections Route: IV Dose: 0.5–2 g Time: q8–12h Protein binding: 56% Half-life: 1.7–2.1 hours Pregnancy Category: B Side effects: gastric distress, diarrhea, nausea, vomiting, hypersensitivity, and thrombophlebitis at the site of injection Drug interaction: none
Imipenem-cilastatin (Primaxin IM, Primaxin IV)	Use: treats bone, joint, skin, and soft-tissue infections, bacterial endocarditis, intraabdominal bacteria infections, pneumonia, and Gram-positive/negative aerobic and anerobic organisms Route: IV/IM Dose: IV 250–500 mg q6h for mild infections to 500 mg for moderate to severe infections Maximum dose is 50 mg/kg daily IM 500–750 mg up to a maximum of 1500 mg/day Time: IV q6–8h IM q12h Protein binding: 20% Half-life: 1 hour Pregnancy Category: C Side effects: gastric distress, diarrhea, nausea, vomiting, allergic reactions, confusion, lightheadedness, convulsions, tremor Drug interaction: none Contraindication: not for use in children under 12 years old

(Continued)

Antibiotic	Description
Meropenem (Merrem IV)	Use: treats susceptible intraabdominal infections (complicated appendicitis and peritonitis) and bacterial meningitis
	Route: IV/IM
	Dose: IV 1 g over 40–60 minutes
	Time: q8h
	Protein binding: 20%
	Half-life: 1 hour
	Pregnancy Category: C
	Side effects: pseudomembranous colitis, hypersensitivity, diarrhea, nausea, vomiting, headache, and rash
	Drug interaction: none
	Contraindications: Use with caution with clients with allergy to imipenem, cilastin, or other β-lactams. Kidney problems require a reduced dosage. More than 2 g daily increases the risk for seizures.

22. Sulfonamides

Urinary tract infections (UTIs) are the most commonly reported bacterial infection in the United States. *Escherichia coli* causes 90% of them, some of which are hospital-acquired. Hospital-acquired UTIs are difficult to treat. Other UTIs are caused by *Pseudomonas aeruginosa*, *Serratia*, and *Enterobacter*.

A family of antibiotics called *sulfonamides*, which stop the growth of bacteria, are used to treat UTI. These include trimethoprim-sulfamethoxazole (TMP-SMX) and cephalasporins. Aztreonam and fluoroquinolones are used as urinary tract antiseptics. Phenazopyridine (Pyridium) is used to treat pain from a UTI.

Patients who are prescribed sulfonamides should avoid coffee, tea, and juices. These beverages are high in citric acid. They also should abstain from cola, alcohol, chocolate, and spices, which irritate the bladder.

Avoid administering sulfonamides if the patient is allergic to one member of the sulfonamide family of medication. Sulfonamides should not be administered to neonates.

Sulfonamides may adversely affect the level of some medications, causing a toxic effect. Avoid using sulfonamides with anticoagulants such as coumarin or indanedione derivatives and anticonvulsants (hydantoin) as well as oral antidiabetic agents and methotrexate.

Patients need at least 3000 mL of fluid each day in order to flush the urinary tract and follow good hygiene to reduce the likelihood of acquiring the infection again. The patient should be instructed to drink at least 3 quarts of water daily and take sulfonamides on an empty stomach. Patients should avoid the use of antacids while taking sulfonamides because antacids decrease the absorption of sulfonamides.

Sulfonamides Pregnancy Category: C		
Route	Dose	Time
Sulfadiazine Protein binding: 20–30% Half-life: 8–12 hours		
PO Drink 250 mL H_2O with each dose	2–4 mg first dose 2–4 g subsequently	7–10 days
Sulfisoxazole (Gantrisin) Protein binding: 60–70% (TMP-SMX) Half-life: 7–12 hours		
PO	2–3 g/day in 2–3 divided doses	7–10 days
Trimethoprim sulfamethoxazole Protein binding: 50–65% (TMP-SMX) Half-life: 8–12 hours Most widely used antibacterial agent in the world		
PO	160/800 mg	q12h
Sulfamethoxazole (co-trimoxazole) (TMP) Protein binding: 99% Half-life: 5.5 hours		
PO IV	160 mg TMP bid 20 mg/kg	 q6h

23. Tuberculosis

Tuberculosis is caused by acid-fast bacillus *Mycobacterium tuberculosis*. It is a major health problem and kills more people than does any other infectious disease. It is estimated that 1.5 billion people have TB. There are 8 million new cases each year. The incidence had decreased in the United States but increased again in the 1980s. This has been attributed in part to the numbers of persons with AIDS, which compromises the immune system.

The following first-line drugs are used to treat tuberculosis:

- Isoniazid (INH, Nydrazid, Laniazid) PO/IM: 5–10 mg/kg daily in a single dose; maximum 300 mg/day; prophylaxis, 300 mg/day
  - Pregnancy Category: C; protein binding (PB): 10%; $t_{1/2}$ = 104 hours

- Side effects: drowsiness, tremors, rash, blurred vision, photosensitivity
- Adverse reactions: psychotic behavior, peripheral neuropathy, vitamin B_6 deficiency
- Life-threatening: blood dyscrasias, thrombocytopenia, seizures, agranulocytosis, hepatotoxicity

Antitubular drugs				
Phase	Example 1	Example 2	Example 3	Example 4
First phase (2 months)	Isoniazid, rifampin	Isoniazid, rifampin, Pyrazinamide	Isoniazid, rifampin, streptomycin	Isoniazid, rifampin, phrazinamide, kanamycin, or ciprofloxacin
Second phase (4–7 months)	Isoniazid, rifampin	Isoniazid, rifampin, ethambutol	Isoniazid, rifampin, capreomycin, or cycloserine	Isoniazid, rifampin, ethambutol, streptomycin, kanamycin, ciprofloxacin, clarithromycin, or capreomycin

- Ethambutol HCL (Myambutol) PO: 15 mg/kg as a single dose; retreatment PO: 25 mg/kg as a single dose for 2 months; then decrease to 15 mg/kg daily
  - Pregnancy Category: C; PB: 10–20%; $t_{1/2}$ = 3–4 hours (8 hours with renal dysfunction)
- Pyrazinamide (Tebrazid): PO: 20–35 mg/kg daily in 3–4 divided doses; maximum 3 g/day
  - Pregnancy Category: C; PB: 10–20%; $t_{1/2}$ = 9.5 h—promote fluid intake
- Rifampin (Rifadin, Rimactane): PO: 600 mg/day as a single dose
  - Pregnancy Category: C; PB: 85–90%; $t_{1/2}$ = 3 hours—monitor liver enzymes
- Streptomycin SO_4: IM: 1 g daily or 7–15 mg/kg daily for 2–3 months, then 2–3 × wk
  - Pregnancy Category: C; PB: 30%; $t_{1/2}$ = 2–3 hours

Second-line drugs are as follows:

- Aminosalicylate sodium, para (aminosalicylate sodium) (PAS): PO: 14–16 g/day in 2–3 divided doses
  - Pregnancy Category: C; PB: 15%; $t_{1/2}$ = 1 hour—take after meals to reduce gastric irritation

- Capreomycin (Capastat): IM: 1 g/day for 2–4 months, then 1 g 2–3 × per week
  - Pregnancy Category: C; PB: UK; $t_{1/2}$ = 3–6 hours—hearing loss is an adverse reaction; patients should take pyridoxine (to avoid peripheral neuropathy)
- Cycloserine (Seromycin): PO: 200 mg q12h for 2 weeks; maximum 1 g/day
  - Pregnancy Category: C; PB: UK; $t_{1/2}$ = 10 h
- Ethionamide (Treacator-SC): PO: 250 mg, q8–12h
  - Pregnancy category: C; PB: UK; $t_{1/2}$ = 2–3 hours—side effects include GI discomfort; use with caution in patients with diabetes mellitus, alcoholism, and hepatic disorder
- Rifabutin (Mycobutin) PO: 300 mg/day in 1 or 2 divided doses
  - Pregnancy Category: B; PB: 85%; $t_{1/2}$ = 16–69 hours

Side effects and adverse reactions differ according to the drug prescribed. The nursing assessment should include the following information:

- History of past TB; PPD tests and reactions, chest X-ray and results, and previous allergies to any antitubercular drugs
- Medical history; usually contraindicated with severe hepatic disease (liver)
- Assessment for sign and symptoms of peripheral neuropathy

Check for hearing changes because some of the drugs are ototoxic. The following nursing diagnoses are common for TB drug therapy patients:

- Risk for infection
- Risk for impaired tissue integrity
- Risk for hearing loss

The following guidelines are nursing interventions for patients being treated for tuberculosis:

- Administer 1 hour before or 2 hours after meals.
- Administer pyridoxine as prescribed.
- Monitor serum liver enzymes.
- Collect sputum specimens in early morning (usually on three consecutive mornings).
- Arrange for eye examinations.
- Emphasize importance of complying with drug regimen.

Patient education consists of the following guidelines:

- Take before meals or 2 hours after meals for better absorption.
- Take as prescribed.

- Do not to take antacids because they decrease TB drug absorption.
- Keep medical appointments and have sputum tested.
- Check with healthcare provider before becoming pregnant.
- Report any numbness, tingling, or burning of the hands or feet.
- Avoid direct sunlight—use sunblock.
- Take rifampin (urine, feces, saliva, sputum, sweat, and tears may be a harmless red-orange color; soft contact lenses may be permanently stained).

Evaluation: Evaluate effectiveness with sputum specimens.

24. Antifungal Drugs (Antimycotic Drugs)

These drugs are used to treat two types of fungal infection:

1. Superficial fungal infections of skin or mucous membrane
2. Systemic fungal infections of the lung or CNS

The conditions may be mild, such as tinea pedis (athlete's foot), or severe, as in pulmonary conditions or meningitis.

Fungi, such as *Candida* spp. (yeast), are normal flora of mouth, skin, intestine, and vagina. Candidiasis might be an opportunistic infection when the defense mechanisms are impaired. Antibiotics, oral contraceptives, and immunosuppressives may alter the body's defense mechanisms. Infections can be mild (vaginal yeast infection) or severe (systemic fungal infection).

There are four groups of antifungal medications:

1. Polyenes, including amphotericin B and nystatin
2. Imidazoles, which include ketoconazole, miconazole, and clotrimazole
3. Antimetabolic antifungal flucytosine
4. Antiprotozoal agents

Polyenes such as amphotericin B are the drugs of choice for treating severe systemic infections. Polyenes are effective against numerous diseases, including histoplasmosis, cryptococcosis, coccidioidomycosis, aspergillosis, blastomycosis, and systemic infection; however, they are very toxic. They are not absorbed from the GI tract and thus cannot be given by mouth.

Polyenes are usually prescribed as amphotericin B (Fungizone). A test dose is given IV: 0.25–1.0 mg in 20 mL of D_5W infused over 20–30 minutes; IV: 0.25–1.0 mg/kg daily in D_5W or 1.5 mg/kg qod; maximum 1.5 mg/kg daily. Pregnancy Category: B; PB: 95%; $t_{1/2}$ = 24 hours.

Side effects and adverse reactions include flushing, fever, chills, nausea, vomiting, hypotension, paresthesias, and thrombophlebitis. Amphotericin B is *highly toxic*, causing nephrotoxicity and electrolyte imbalance, especially hypokalemia (low potassium) and hypomagnesemia (low serum magnesium). Urinary output, BUN, and serum creatinine levels should be closely monitored.

Nystatin (Mycostatin) can be given orally or topically to treat *Candida* infection. It is available in suspensions, creams, ointments, and vaginal tablets. It is poorly absorbed via the GI tract, but the oral tablet form is used for intestinal candidiasis. It is more commonly used as an oral suspension for *Candida* infection in the mouth as a "swish and swallow" rinse.

Side effects include anorexia, nausea, vomiting, diarrhea (large doses), stomach cramps, rash, and vaginal rash and/or burning sensation. There are no reported adverse reactions.

It is used topically and PO at doses of 500,000–1,000,000 U tid or q8h. Pregnancy Category: C; PB: UK; $t_{1/2}$: UK.

The imidazole group is effective against candidiasis (superficial and systemic), coccidioidomycosis, cryptococcosis, histoplasmosis, and paracoccidioidomycosis.

25. Antimalarial Drugs

Malaria is still one of the most prevalent protozoan diseases in the world. The mosquito infects the human body, and the parasite passes through two phases. The tissue phase causes no clinical symptoms in the human, and the erythrocytic phase invades red blood cells and causes chills, fever, and sweating, In the United States the 1000 cases reported annually are almost always acquired from international travel. Quinine was the only antimalarial drug from 1820 to the early 1940s when synthetic antimalarial drugs were developed. Chloroquine is commonly prescribed. If drug resistance develops, quinine is used in combination with an antibiotic such as tetracycline.

The nursing procedure related to treating malarial patients is as follows:

- Assessment:
  - Assess patient's hearing (drugs may affect the 8th cranial nerve).
  - Assess for visual changes (should undergo frequent ophthalmic examinations).
- Nursing diagnoses:
  - Risk of infection
  - Risk for impaired tissue integrity
  - Risk for sensory disturbances (auditory and visual)
- Planning:
  - Patient should be free of malarial symptoms.

- Nursing interventions:
  - Monitor urinary output (600 mL/day) and liver function (liver enzymes).
  - Report if serum liver enzymes are elevated.
- Patient education:
  - Advise patients traveling to malaria-infested countries to take prophylactic doses of antimalarial drugs before leaving, during the visit, and on return.
  - Instruct patients to take oral antimalarial drugs with food or at mealtime if GI upset occurs.
  - Monitor patients returning from international travel for malarial symptoms.
  - Instruct patients to report vision or hearing changes immediately.
  - Advise patients to avoid consuming large quantities of alcohol.
- Evaluation:
  - Evaluate the effectiveness of the drug by determining whether the patient is free of symptoms.
- Side effects and adverse reactions:
  - General side effects include GI upset, 8th cranial nerve involvement (quinine and chloroquine), renal impairment (quinine), and cardiovascular effects (quinine).

26. Anthelmintic Drugs

Helminths are large organisms (parasitic worms) that feed on host tissue. The most common site is the intestine. Other sites are the lymphatic system, blood vessels, and liver.

There are four groups of helminths:

1. Cestodes (tapeworms) [enter via contaminated food such as pork (trichinosis) and fish (dwarf)]
2. Trematodes (flukes)
3. Intestinal nematodes (roundworms)
4. Tissue-invading nematodes (tissue roundworms and filariae)

The nursing procedure related to treatment of patients who are taking antihelmiths is as follows:

- Assessment:
  - Obtain history of foods eaten, especially meat and fish and how it was prepared.

- Ascertain whether other persons in the household have been checked for worm infestations.
- Obtain baseline vital signs, and collect a stool specimen.
- Nursing diagnoses:
  - Altered comfort
  - Activity intolerance related to dizziness, headache, drowsiness
  - Altered nutrition
  - Alteration in skin integrity
- Planning:
  - Patient will be free of helminths.
  - Patient/family will understand how to prepare foods to avoid recurrence.
- Interventions:
  - Collect stool specimen.
  - Administer the prescribed anthelmintics after meals.
  - Report side effects to the healthcare provider.
- Patient education:
  - Explain the importance of hand washing.
  - Instruct the patient to take daily showers, *not* baths.
  - Instruct the patient to change sheets, bedclothes, towels, and underwear daily.
  - If the problem persists, a second course of therapy may be necessary.
  - Instruct the patient to take the prescribed drug at the designated time and keep healthcare appointments.
  - Alert the patient to the fact that drowsiness may occur and that it is dangerous to drive a car or operate other machinery if drowsiness occurs.
  - Instruct the patient to report side effects to the healthcare provider.
- Evaluation:
  - Evaluate the effects of the anthelmintics and absence of side effects.
  - Determine whether the patient is using proper hygiene, to avoid spread of parasitic worms.
- Side effects and adverse reactions:
  - Common side effects include GI upset such as anorexia, nausea, vomiting, and occasionally diarrhea and stomach cramps; neurological problems include dizziness, weakness, headache, and drowsiness; adverse reactions do not occur frequently.

Examples of anthelmiths include the following:

- Diethylcarbamzine (Hetrazan); used for nematode-filariae; PO: 2–3 mg/kg tid
- Ivermectin (Mectizan) broad-spectrum antiparasitic drug; PO: 200 µg/kg in 1 dose
- Mebandazole (Vermox); used for giant roundworm, hookworm, pinworm, whipworm. PO: 100 mg bid × 3 days; repeat in 2–3 weeks if necessary
- Niclosamide (Niclocide) used for beef and fish tapeworms: PO 2 g, single dose; treatment of dwarf tapeworms; PO: 2 g/day × 1 week
- Oxamniquine (Vansil) treatment against mature and immature worms; PO: 15 mg/kg bid for 1–2 days
- Piperazine citrate (Antepar, Vermizine); treatment of roundworms and pinworms; roundworms—PO: 3.5 g/day × 2 days; pinworms—65 mg/kg daily × 7 days, maximum 2.5 g/day
- Praziquantel (Biltricide) treatment for beef, pork, fish tapeworms; PO: 10–20 mg/kg single dose; blood flukes—PO 20 mg/kg, tid × 1 day; liver, lung, and intestinal flukes; 25 mg/kg tid for 1–2 days
- Pyrantel pamoate (Antiminth) treatment of giant roundworm, hookworm, pinworm; PO: 11 mg/kg single dose; repeat in 2 weeks if necessary
- Thiabendazole (Mintezol, Minzolum) treatment of threadworm and pork worm; PO: 25 mg/kg for 2–5 days; repeat in 2 days if necessary

Summary

When microbials invade, the body's defenses go into action to surround and kill microbials. The inflammatory response is the first line of attack, bringing white blood cells to the site of the infection in an attempt to stifle the spread of the microbial. Microbials that cause infections are called *pathogens*.

Symptoms of inflammation can disrupt the patient's normal daily activities. Anti-inflammatory medication is administered to patients to reduce the inflammatory response, enabling the patient to return to normal activities.

Sometimes the microbial attack overwhelms the body's defenses. In these cases the patient requires medication to help the body destroy the microbial. The most commonly prescribed medication to combat microbials is an antibiotic.

There are two types of antibiotics: bacteriostatic and bactericidal. *Bacteriostatic* antibiotics stop bacteria from growing inside the body. *Bactericidal* antibiotics kill the bacteria.

In this chapter, you learned about the most commonly prescribed antibiotics. You learned how they work, how to administer them, their side effects, and when they should not be administered to a patient.

In the next chapter you will learn about respiratory diseases and the medications that are prescribed to treat those diseases.

QUIZ

1. A new infection caused by a bacterium that is resistant to the present antibiotics being given is called a
   (a) communicable infection.
   (b) superinfection.
   (c) a hospital-acquired infection.
   (d) None of the above.

2. A patient should always be asked if she/he is allergic to any medications, foods, or herbals or who has a family history of allergies to antibiotics. This is because
   (a) patients who have a family member who is allergic to an antibiotic might also have an allergy to some antibiotics.
   (b) shellfish contain bacteria.
   (c) patients can contract drug-resistant bacteria from shellfish.
   (d) of all of the above.

3. Antibiotics fight off bacteria by
   (a) inhibiting the bacteria's ability to make protein called protein synthesis.
   (b) inhibiting the bacteria from growing a cell wall.
   (c) disrupting or altering the permeability of the bacteria's membrane.
   (d) all of the above.

4. All antibiotics kill bacteria.
   (a) True
   (b) False

5. Some antibiotics kill only specific bacteria.
   (a) True
   (b) False

6. What chemical mediators bring about the inflammatory reaction by vasodilatation, relaxing smooth muscles, making capillaries permeable, and sensitizing nerve cells within the affected area to pain?

    (a) Penicillin
    (b) Sulfonamides
    (c) Prostaglandin inhibitors
    (d) Prostaglandins

7. Bacteriocidal antibiotics can only stop the growth of bacteria.

    (a) True
    (b) False

8. Which of the following symptoms are possible side effects of an antibiotic?

    (a) Rash
    (b) Fever
    (c) Hives and itching
    (d) All of the above

9. The patient's white blood count should be studied after the patient is given an antibiotic.

    (a) True
    (b) False

10. Penicillin is the most effective and least toxic antibiotic.

    (a) True
    (b) False

chapter 14

Respiratory Diseases

No one looks forward to the cold season, when many of us come down with a sore throat, the sniffles, and a cough and feel utterly miserable. A lot of chicken soup and tender loving care (TLC) usually is the cure. Although chicken soup is not a drug, it does contain a mucus-thinning amino acid called *cysteine* and is considered "grandma's remedy" for the common cold. Actually, time is the best cure, and most people recover in 7–10 days with or without chicken soup.

The common cold is one of a number of respiratory diseases that can infect the human body. The common cold can be annoying. However, some respiratory diseases—such as emphysema—are debilitating and can slowly choke the life out of a person.

In this chapter, we'll explore the more common respiratory diseases and learn about the medications that are used either to destroy the disease-causing microorganism or to manage the symptoms of the disease.

1. A Brief Look at Respiration

Before learning about respiratory diseases and the medications used to treat them, let's take a few moments to briefly review the anatomy and physiology of the respiratory tract. This review will help you better understand the disease and treatment.

The respiratory tract is divided into upper and lower segments. The upper respiratory tract contains the nares, nasal cavity, pharynx, and larynx, and the lower tract consists of the trachea, bronchi, bronchioles, alveoli, and alveolar-capillary membrane.

During respiration, air is inhaled and makes its way through the upper respiratory tract and travels to the alveoli capillary membrane in the lower respiratory tract, which is the site of gas exchange. Oxygen from the air attaches to the hemoglobin of the blood while carbon dioxide leaves the blood and is expelled through the lower and upper respiratory tracts during expiration.

Respiration

There are three phases of respiration: ventilation, perfusion, and diffusion.

Ventilation

Ventilation is the process by which oxygenated air passes through the respiratory tract during inspiration.

Perfusion

Perfusion is the process in which blood from the pulmonary circulation is sufficient at the alveolar-capillary bed to conduct diffusion. In order for perfusion to occur, the alveolar pressure must be matched by adequate ventilation. The presence of mucosal edema, secretions, and bronchospasm increase resistance to the airflow, which results in decreased ventilation. Decreased ventilation causes a decrease in diffusion.

Diffusion

Diffusion is the process in which oxygen moves into the capillary bed and carbon dioxide leaves the capillary bed.

Compliance and the Lungs

There are two lungs inside the chest cavity. Each is surrounded by a membrane called the *pleura*. Each lung is divided into parts called *lobes*. The right lung has three lobes, and the left lung has two lobes.

You will frequently hear the term *lung compliance* used in reference to measuring the functionality of the lungs. This is the ability of the lungs to be distended and is expressed as a change in volume per unit change in pressure. In other words, lung compliance is a measurement of how well the lungs can stretch when filling with air.

Two factors affect compliance: (1) *connective tissue*, which consists of collagen and elastin, and (2) *surface tension* in the alveoli, which is controlled by surfactant. *Surfactant* is a surface-active agent, a substance that lowers surface tension in the alveoli, thereby preventing interstitial fluid from entering the alveoli.

Compliance is increased in patients who have chronic obstructive pulmonary disease (COPD). Compliance is decreased with patients who have restrictive pulmonary disease. A decrease in compliance results in decreased lung volume; that is, the lungs become stiff, requiring more-than-normal pressure to expand. This decrease in lung compliance is typically caused by an increase in connective tissue or an increase in surface tension in the alveoli.

Controlling Respiration

Respiration is controlled by three factors that sense the need for the body's increased or decreased requirement for oxygen: (1) oxygen (O_2) concentration, (2) carbon dioxide (CO_2) concentration, and (3) hydrogen (H^+) ion concentration in the blood.

Throughout the body, chemoreceptors sense the concentration of oxygen, carbon, and carbon dioxide and then transmit messages to the central chemoreceptors located in the medulla near the respiratory center of the brain and through cerebrospinal fluid (CSF) to respond to changes.

When an increase in carbon dioxide is detected and there is an increase in hydrogen ions, the message goes out to increase ventilation. Hydrogen ions are measured using the pH scale. The pH of normal blood is between 7.35 and 7.45. A pH lower than 7.35 indicates that the blood is acidic, and a pH higher than 7.45 indicates that pH is alkaline. The chemoreceptors respond to an increase in CO_2 and a decrease in pH by increasing ventilation. If the CO_2 level remains elevated, the stimulus to increase ventilation is lost.

There are chemoreceptors located in carotid arteries and aortic arteries that monitor changes in oxygen pressure (PO_2) levels in the arteries. These are called *peripheral chemoreceptors*. Once the oxygen pressure falls below 60 mmHg, the peripheral chemoreceptors send a message to the respiratory center in the medulla to increase the ventilation.

Tracheobronchial Tube

The *tracheobronchial tube* connects the pharynx to the bronchial tree that extends into the terminal bronchioles in the lungs, providing an unobstructed pathway for air to enter the body and for carbon dioxide to leave the body.

The tracheobronchial tube is a fibrous spiral of smooth muscles that become more closely spaced as they near the terminal bronchioles. The size of the airway can be increased or decreased by relaxing or contracting the bronchial smooth muscle. This is controlled by the parasympathetic nervous system, particularly the vagus nerve.

The vagus nerve releases acetylcholine when it is stimulated, which causes the tracheobronchial tube to contract. This is referred to as *bronchoconstriction*. The opposite effect is created when the sympathetic nervous system releases epinephrine that stimulates the β_2 receptor in the bronchial smooth muscle. This causes the tracheobronchial tube to dilate. This is called *bronchodilation*. In a healthy person the sympathetic and parasympathetic nervous systems counterbalance each other to maintain homeostasis.

2. Upper-Respiratory-Tract Disorders

Respiratory disorders are divided into two groups: upper-respiratory-tract disorders and lower-respiratory-tract disorders. Upper-respiratory-tract disorders are called *upper-respiratory infections* (URIs). These include the common cold, acute rhinitis (not the same as allergic rhinitis), sinusitis, acute tonsillitis, and acute laryngitis.

The Common Cold

The common cold is caused by the rhinovirus invading the nasopharyngeal tract. The rhinovirus is frequently accompanied by acute inflammation of the mucous membranes of the nose and increased nasal secretions. This is known as *acute rhinitis*.

Adults have between two and four colds per year. Children are more susceptible to colds. The average child has between 4 and 12 colds each year. The rhinovirus is seasonable: 50% of the infections occur in the winter and 25% during the summer. The other 25% occur anytime throughout the year. Although no one has actually died from the common cold, it does create both physical and mental discomfort for the person and leads to a loss of work and school.

The rhinovirus is contagious 1–4 days before the patient notices the symptoms of the cold. This is referred to as the *incubation period*. During this time, the rhinovirus can be transmitted by touching contaminated surfaces and from contact with droplets from an infected person who sneezes and coughs. After the incubation period, the person experiences a watery nasal discharge called *rhinorrhea*, along with nasal congestion, cough, and an increasing amount of mucosal secretions.

Many people try home remedies to battle the rhinovirus; however, these do not directly affect the virus. Instead, they may only be palliative, helping to ease the symptoms of the cold. Home remedies include rest, vitamin C, megadoses of other vitamins, and, of course, chicken soup. Vitamin C and megadoses of other vitamins have not been proven effective against the common cold.

When home remedies fail, people turn to both prescription and over-the-counter (OTC) medication. Cold medications fall into the drug groups listed in the tabular charts throughout the chapter, which provide information about specific drugs in each group.

Antihistamines (H$_1$ blocker)

Many cold symptoms are caused by the body's overproduction of histamines. *Histamines* are potent vasodilators that react to a foreign substance in the body such as the rhinovirus. They cause redness, itching, and swelling. They are part of the body's defense mechanism. *Antihistamines* are drugs that compete for the same receptor sites as histamines. Once they latch onto the site, there is no room for the histamine. Therefore, the reaction caused by the histamine does not occur. It is this reaction that produces many cold symptoms.

There are two types of histamine receptors: H_1 and H_2. H_2 *receptors* cause an increase in gastric secretions and are not involved in this response. The differences are illustrated in the charts. [See "Antihistamine" (H_1 blocker) chart and "Antihistamine Use to Treat Allergic Rhinitis" chart.]

Decongestants (Sympathomimetic Amines)

Someone who comes down with the common cold may have "runny nose." This is referred to as *nasal congestion* and is caused when the nasal mucous membranes swell in response to the rhinovirus. A *decongestant* is a drug that stimulates the α-adrenergic receptors to tell the brain to constrict the capillaries within the nasal mucosa. The result is that the nasal mucous membranes shrink, reducing the amount of fluid that is secreted from the nose. In other words, a decongestant stops a runny nose.

Decongestants are available in nasal spray, drops, tablets, capsules, or liquid form. Although decongestants address the congestion, frequent use of decongestants—especially nasal spray and drops—can lessen its effectiveness because the person becomes tolerant to the medication. In some cases, the person may even experience nasal congestion again. This is referred to as *rebound nasal congestion*. Therefore, decongestants should not be used longer than 5 days. There are three types of decongestants: (1) *nasal decongestants*, which provide quick relief; (2) *systemic decongestants*, which provide longer-lasting relief from congestion; and (3) *intranasal glucocorticoids*, which are used to treat seasonal and perennial rhinitis.

Cough Preparations

A *cough* is a common symptom of a cold brought about by the body's effort to remove nasal mucus that might drain into the respiratory tract. *Antitussives* are the ingredients used in cough medicine to suppress the cough center in the medulla. Although the cough reflex is useful for clearing the air passages, suppression of the cough reflex can provide some rest for the affected person. There are both nonnarcotic and narcotic antitussives.

Expectorants

When an individual has a cold or other respiratory infection, it is common to secrete rather thick mucus that is difficult to expectorate. *Expectorants* are medications that loosen the secretions, making it easier for the person to cough up and expel the mucus.

Expectorants work by increasing the fluid output of the respiratory tract and decreasing the adhesiveness and surface tension to promote removal of viscous mucus.

A list of drugs utilized in the treatment of upper respiratory tract disorders is provided in the Appendix. Detailed tables show doses, recommendations, expectations, side effects, and contraindications, more information is available on the book's website (see URL in Appendix).

Antihistamine Used to Treat Allergic Rhinitis	
Phenothiazines (antihistamine action); promethazine HCl (Phenergan)	PO/IM: 12.5–25 mg q4–6h PRN; maximum dose: 150 mg/day Before meals and bedtime Pregnancy Category: C Protein bound: UK (unknown) Half-life: UK
Piperazine derivative—hydroxyzine (Atarax, vistaril)	PO: 25–100 mg tid/qid Pregnancy Category: C Protein bound: UK Half-life: 3 hours
Butyrophenone derivative [terfenadine (Seldane)]	PO: 60 mg bid Pregnancy Category: C Protein bound: 97% Half-life: 20 hours
Ethanolamine derivative—carbinoxamine and pseudoephedrine (Rondec)	PO: 5 mL qid or 1 tab qid Pregnancy Category: C Protein bound: UK Half-life: UK
Clemastine fumarate (Tavist)	PO: 1.34–2.68 mg bid/tid Maximum dose: 8 mg/day Pregnancy Category: C Protein bound: UK Half-life: UK
Propylamine derivatives—brompheniramine maleate (Bromphen, Dimetane, Histaject, Hasahist B, Oraminic II)	PO: 4 mg q4 h–6h or sustained release (SR): 8 mg q8–12h Maximum dose: 24 mg/day IM/IV/SC: 10 mg q8–12h; Maximum dose: 40 mg/day Pregnancy Category: C Protein bound: UK Half-life: 25–36 hours

(Continued)

Antihistamine Used to Treat Allergic Rhinitis (*Continued*)	
Triprolidine and pseudoephedrine (Actifed)	PO: 2.5 mg q6–8h Maximum dose: 10 mg/day Pregnancy Category: B Protein bound: UK Half-life: 3 hours

Sinusitis

Sinusitis is the inflammation of the mucous membranes of the maxillary, frontal, ethmoid, or sphenoid sinuses. Patients may take systemic or nasal decongestants to reduce the congestion that frequently accompanies sinusitis. Patients are told to drink plenty of fluids, to rest, and to take acetaminophen (Tylenol) or ibuprofen for discomfort. In some cases, antibiotics are prescribed if the condition is severe or long lasting and an infection is suspected.

Acute Pharyngitis

Acute pharyngitis is inflammation of the throat. It is more commonly known as a "sore throat." The patient may have an elevated temperature, a cough, and pain when swallowing.

Pharyngitis is caused by a virus (viral pharyngitis) or by bacteria (bacteria pharyngitis) such as the β-hemolytic streptococci. Patients know this as "strep throat." A throat culture is taken to rule out β-hemolytic streptococcal infection. Sometimes patients experience acute pharyngitis along with other upper-respiratory-tract disease such as a cold, rhinitis, or acute sinusitis.

Patients who have viral pharyngitis are given medications that treat the symptoms rather than attack the underlying virus. Acetaminophen or ibuprofen is given to reduce the patient's temperature and discomfort. Saline gargles, lozenges, and increased fluid intake are usually helpful to soothe the sore throat.

Patients who have bacterial pharyngitis are given antibiotics to destroy the β-hemolytic streptococci bacteria. However, antibiotics are prescribed only if the result of the throat culture is positive for bacteria. Patients are also given the same treatments for viral pharyngitis to address the symptoms of pharyngitis.

Acute Tonsillitis

Acute tonsillitis is inflammation of the tonsils, which can be caused by a streptococcus microorganism. Patients who acquire acute tonsillitis experience a sore throat, chills, fever, aching muscles, and pain when they swallow.

A throat culture is taken to determine the cause of the infection before an appropriate antibiotic is prescribed to the patient. The patient is also given acetaminophen or ibuprofen to reduce the fever and the aches and pains associated with acute tonsillitis. The patient is also encouraged to use saline gargles, lozenges, and increased fluid to soothe the soreness brought on by infected tonsils. Antibiotics are used only if a bacterial infection is suspected.

Acute Laryngitis

Acute laryngitis is an infection that causes swelling (edema) of the vocal cords. This results in the patient developing a weak or hoarse voice. Acute laryngitis can be caused by a viral infection. Sometimes it is caused by stress or overuse of the vocal cords—a common occurrence for fans whose team wins the Super Bowl.

Refraining from speaking and avoiding exposure to substances that can irritate the vocal cords, such as smoking, is the preferred treatment for acute laryngitis.

3. Lower-Respiratory-Tract Disorders

Lower-respiratory-tract disorders are conditions that obstruct or restrict tracheobronchial tubes and prevent the exchange of gas within the lungs. These conditions are referred to collectively as *chronic obstructive pulmonary disease* (COPD) and include chronic bronchitis, bronchiectasis, emphysema, and asthma.

Chronic obstructive pulmonary disease obstructs the patient's airway by increasing resistance of the airflow during inspiration and expiration. The result is an impairment of oxygen reaching lung tissues that can in some cases irreversibly damage those tissues.

The airway obstruction occurs when the bronchioles constrict (bronchospasm) and mucous secretions increase, causing the patient to experience difficulty breathing (dyspnea).

Pneumonia

Pneumonia is an infection in the lungs that can be caused by various microorganisms, including viruses, bacteria, or fungi. It often starts following a URI. Symptoms can occur 2–3 days after onset of a cold or sore throat. Symptoms include fever, chills, cough, rapid breathing, wheezing, and/or grunting respirations, labored breathing, vomiting, chest pain, abdominal pain, loss of appetite, decreased activity, and, in extreme cases, signs of hypoxia (low oxygen levels) or cyanosis such as a bluish tint around the mouth or fingernails. Vaccines are available on the market to prevent certain types of pneumonia. Pneumonia treatment is based on the underlying cause. Viral pneumonia is usually treated symptomatically; specifically, bronchodilators, antipyretics (fever-reducing agents), analgesics such as ibuprofen, cough medications that include expectorants, mucolytics, and suppressants to help the patient sleep. Bacterial and fungal pneumonia are treated with antimicrobials as well as the abovementioned treatment for viral pneumonia. Choice of the antimicrobial is based on the specific microorganism causing the pneumonia. Antimicrobials are discussed in Chapter 13. Antipyretics such as ibuprofen are discussed in Chapter 12. Pneumonia is contagious and is spread from person to person via droplets in the air from coughing and sneezing.

Tuberculosis

Tuberculosis (TB) is caused by the acid-fast bacillus *Mycobacterium tuberculosis.* The pathogen is frequently referred to as the *tubercle bacillus.* It is a major health problem in the world and kills more persons than any other infectious disease. More than 1.5 billion people in the world may have TB, and many do not know it. Each year there are more than 8 million new cases of TB. Many of these new cases can be attributed, in part, to the increased number of persons with acquired immunodeficiency syndrome (AIDS). Active TB develops in these people because of their compromised immune systems. It can also be attributed to the increasingly crowded living conditions in urban areas. Individuals susceptible to TB are those with alcohol addiction and AIDS, and those in a debilitated condition.

Tuberculosis is transmitted from one person to another by droplets dispersed in the air through coughing and sneezing. The organisms are inhaled into the alveoli (air sacs) of the lung. The tubercle bacilli can spread from the lungs to other organs of the body via the blood and lymphatic system. If the body's immune system is strong or intact, the phagocytes stop the multiplication of the tubercle bacilli. When the immune system is compromised, the tubercle bacilli spread within the lungs and to other organs. Dissemination of tuberculosis bacilli can be found in the liver, kidneys, spleen, and other organs. Symptoms of TB include anorexia, cough, sputum production, increased fever, night sweats, weight loss, and positive acid-fast bacilli (AFB) in the sputum. Medications used to treat and prevent TB are discussed in Chapter 13.

Chronic Bronchitis

Chronic bronchitis is an inflammation of the bronchi that persists for a long period of time or occurs repeatedly. It is a form of COPD. Smoking is the main cause for bronchitis. Second-hand smoke may also cause chronic bronchitis. Air pollution, infection, and allergies make it worse. Patients who develop chronic bronchitis have excess mucus production that irritates the bronchial tubes, causing the patient to develop a persistent productive cough.

Patients exhibit a gurgling lung sound (*rhonchi*) on both inspiration and expiration. The excess mucus blocks the airway, causing a buildup of carbon dioxide in the blood (hypercapnia) and a decrease in oxygen (hypoxemia), which leads to respiratory acidosis.

Bronchiectasis

Bronchiectasis is the enlargement and distension of the airways so that pockets are formed where infection can develop. This condition alters the lining of the airways and damages the lung's ability to filter air. Dust, mucus, and bacteria accumulate in the lungs, causing infection.

Emphysema

Emphysema is a progressive form of COPD. The alveoli become enlarged and damaged, trapping air in the overexpanded alveoli, preventing an adequate exchange of oxygen and carbon dioxide.

Emphysema is caused by smoking cigarettes, inhaling contaminants from the environment, or the lack of the α_1-antitrypsin protein. The lung contains bacteria that release proteolytic enzymes that destroy alveoli. The α_1-antitrypsin protein inhibits proteolytic enzymes and protects the alveoli.

Excess mucus as well as the residue from cigarette smoking and airborne pollutants find their way down the airways and plug the terminal bronchioles. The network of alveoli then loses their fiber and become inelastic and unable to spring back to size after expanding during inspiration. Alveoli enlarge as many of the alveolar walls are destroyed. Air becomes trapped in the overexpanded alveoli, leading to inadequate gas exchange (O_2 and CO_2).

Asthma

Acute asthma is a *reactive airway disease* (RAD) that occurs when lung tissue is exposed to extrinsic (environmental) or intrinsic (internal) factors that stimulate the bronchoconstrictive response. This causes bronchospasms that result in the patient wheezing and having difficulty breathing. More than 500,000 patients are hospitalized, and 5000 die from asthma each year, making acute asthma the third leading cause of preventable hospitalizations in the United States.

Various allergens (an *allergen* is an agent that causes an allergic reaction) can trigger an asthma attack. These include humidity, air pressure changes, temperature changes, smoke, fumes (exhaust, perfume), stress, emotional upset, and allergies to animal dander, dust mites, and drugs such as aspirin, indomethacin, and ibuprofen.

Allergens attach to mast cells and basophils in connective tissues, causing an antigen-antibody reaction to occur. Mast cells stimulate release of chemical mediators. These chemicals constrict the bronchi, increase mucus secretions, stimulate the inflammatory response, and cause pulmonary congestion. Asthma medications are administered to dilate the bronchi and reduce the congestion.

Chemical mediators include histamines (proteins that are potent vasodilators), cytokines [small proteins that mediate and regulate the immune system, inflammatory response, and hematopoiesis (red blood cell production)], serotonin (CNS neurotransmitter), eosinophil chemotatic factor of anaphylaxis (ECF-A), and leukotriene. Histamine and ECF-A are strong bronchoconstrictors that stimulate the contraction of bronchial smooth muscles. Cyclic adenosine monophosphate (cyclic AMP or cAMP) maintains bronchodilation. Histamines, ECF-A, and leukotrienes inhibit the action of Camp, resulting in bronchoconstriction. An increase in the serum level of eosinophils indicates that the inflammatory response has occurred.

The first line of treatment for an acute asthma attack is administration of sympathomimetics (β-adrenergic agonists), which promote the production of cAMP and thereby cause bronchodilation.

Long-term management includes controlling extrinsic factors that caused the attack, educating the patient and the patient's family, school officials, and employers about how to reduce exposure to those factors; and using various combinations of medications according to the severity of the disease. Many asthmatics take two types of medications to address the bronchial constriction and to reduce the congestion. They also take medications that treat the disease every day and additional medications that are called *rescue medications* for use when their respiratory symptoms become acute.

Medications Used to Treat COPD

Four types of medication are used to treat this disease.

Bronchodilator   Bronchodilators relax smooth muscles around the bronchioles, restoring airflow to the lungs. *Sympathomimetics* are bronchodilators that increase the production of cyclic AMP, causing dilation of the bronchioles by acting as adrenergic agonistic.

Some sympathomimetics are selective to particular adrenergic receptors, which are referred to as α_1-, β_2-, and β_2-adrenergic. Other sympathomimetics are nonselective sympathomimetics that affect all types of adrenergic receptor sites.

Epinephrine (adrenalin) is a nonselective sympathomimetic that is given subcutaneously, IV, or via an endotracheal tube in emergency situations to restore circulation and increase airway patency.

Selective β_2-adrenergic agonists have fewer side effects than epinephrine and are given by aerosol or as a tablet. These include albuterol (Proventil, Ventolin), isoetharine HCl (Bronkosol), metaproterenol sulfate (Alupent), samleterol (Serevent), and terbutaline SO_4 (Brethine).

Ipratropium bromide (Atrovent) is an anticholinergic drug that inhibits vagus-mediated response by reversing the action of acetylcholine, producing smooth-muscle relaxation. It is a newer medication that dilates bronchioles with few systemic effects. Ipratropium bromide (Atrovent) is used 5 minutes before glucocorticoid (steroid) or cromolyn is inhaled to allow the bronchioles to dilate, enabling the steroids to be deposited in the bronchioles. Sometimes ipratropium bromide is combined with albuterol sulfate (Combivent) to treat chronic bronchitis for more effective and longer duration than if each is used alone.

Methylxanthine (xanthine) derivatives are a second group of bronchodilators used to treat asthma. They include aminophylline, theophylline, and caffeine, which stimulate the central nervous system (CNS) to increase respirations, dilate coronary and pulmonary vessels, and increase urination (diuresis).

Leukotriene Modifiers

Bronchoconstrictors cause the contraction of smooth muscle around the bronchi, restricting airflow to the lungs. Leukotriene (LK) is the primary bronchoconstrictor that increases migration of eosinophils, increases mucus production, and increases edema in the bronchi, resulting in bronchoconstriction.

There are two types of LK modifers: lymphotoxin (LT) receptor antagonists and LT synthesis inhibitors. These agents are effective in reducing the inflammatory symptoms of asthma triggered by allergic and environmental stimuli.

Leukotriene modifiers include zafirlukast (Accolate), zileuton (Zyflo), and nontelukast sodium (Singulair).

Anti-inflammatory Medications

Chronic obstructive pulmonary disease causes inflammation in the respiratory tract that results in respiratory distress for the patient. Glucocorticoids (steroids) are the primary medication given to reduce the inflammation. Glucocorticoids (steroids) are discussed in further detail in Chapter 12.

Glucocorticoids (steroids) can be administered orally, via aerosol inhalation, intramuscularly, and intravenously. Glucocorticoids employed for aerosol inhalation use beclomethasone (Beconase, Vanceril), dexamethasone (decadron), flunisolide (Aerobid, Nasalid), or triamcinolone (Azmacort, Kenalog, Nasacort).

Glucocorticoids used for other routes include betamethasones (Celestone), cortisone acetate (Cortone acetate, Cortistan), dexamethasone (Decadron), hydrocortisone (Cortef, Hydrocortone), methylprednisolone (Medrol, Solu-Medtol, Depo-Medrol), and prednisolone, prednisone, and triamcinolone (Aristocort, Kenacort, Azmacort).

Expectorants   As you learned previously in this chapter, an expectorant—referred to as a *mucolytic* drug—liquefies and loosens thick mucous secretions so that they can be removed through coughing. A commonly prescribed expectorant for chronic obstructive pulmonary disease is acetylcysteine (Mucomyst), which is administered by nebulizor 5 minutes after the patient receives a bronchodilator.

Acetylcysteine should not be mixed with other medications and can cause nausea, vomiting, oral ulcers (stomatitis), and a runny nose. Acetylcysteine is also an antidote for acetaminophen overdose if given within 12–24 hours after the overdose.

Mast Stabilizer Drugs   Mast cells release histamines, leukotrienes, and other mediators of the inflammatory process. Mast cell stabilizer drugs inhibit the early asthmatic response and the late asthmatic response. They have no bronchodilator effect, nor do they have any effect on inflammatory mediators already released in the body. They are indicated for the prevention of bronchospasms and bronchial asthma attacks. They are administered by aerosol inhalation. The exact action of the drugs have not been determined. However, they are believed to have a modest effect in lowering the required dose of corticosteroids. The most common mast stabilizer drugs are cromolyn (Intal) and nedocromil (Tilade).

A list of drugs utilized in the treatment of lower-respiratory-tract disorders is provided in the Appendix. Detailed tables show doses, recommendations, expectations, side effects, and contraindications; more information is available on the book's website (see URL listed in the Appendix).

Summary

Respiratory diseases interfere with air passages or gas exchanges of the respiratory system. They are grouped together according to the portion of the respiratory tract that they affect. These are the upper respiratory tract and the lower respiratory tract.

Diseases that affect the upper respiratory tract are called *upper respiratory infections* (URIs). These include the common cold, acute rhinitis (not the same as allergic rhinitis), sinusitis, acute tonsillitis, and acute laryngitis.

Diseases that affect the lower respiratory tract are called *lower respiratory infections* (LRIs). Lower respiratory infections include pneumonia and tuberculosis.

Some conditions obstruct or restrict tracheobronchial tubes and prevent the exchange of gas within the lungs. These conditions are referred to collectively as *chronic obstructive pulmonary disease* (COPD). These conditions include bronchitis, bronchiectasis, emphysema, and asthma.

Some patients treat URIs with home remedies to treat the infection; however, these remedies do not kill the bacteria or the virus that causes the infection. Home remedies at times do help to ease the symptoms of the disease.

When home remedies do not work, patients often use OTC or prescription drugs. The most commonly used are antihistamines (which block the histamines produced by the body), decongestant (reduces swollen nasal mucous membranes), antitussives (suppress the coughing reflex), and expectorants (loosen mucus).

Patients suffering from COPD take prescription medication to ease their symptoms. These include bronchodilators (dilate bronchial tubes), steroids (reduce inflammation), and leukotriene modifiers (reduce inflammation and decrease bronchoconstriction).

QUIZ

1. Compliance is
   (a) the ability of the lungs to be contracted.
   (b) the ability of the lungs to be distended.
   (c) the ability of the lungs to exchange gases.
   (d) none of the above.

2. All cases of pharyngitis are caused by bacteria.
   (a) True
   (b) False

3. The common cold is referred to as
   (a) rhinovirusites.
   (b) nasoitis.
   (c) rhinitis.
   (d) all of the above.

4. A runny nose is caused by nasal congestion
   (a) True
   (b) False

5. Acute laryngitis is an infection that causes swelling (edema) of the vocal cords.
   (a) True
   (b) False

6. Bronchiectasis is a form of
   (a) URI.
   (b) acute pulmonary disease.
   (c) chronic obstructive pulmonary disease.
   (d) none of the above.

7. Constriction of the bronchioles is called *bronchospasm*.

    (a) True
    (b) False

8. The lack of the α_1-antitrypsin protein causes

    (a) bronchiectasis.
    (b) bronchitis.
    (c) emphysema.
    (d) asthma.

9. The lung contains bacteria that release proteolytic enzymes that destroy alveoli.

    (a) True
    (b) False

10. The vagus nerve releases acetylcholine when stimulated, which causes the tracheobronchial tube to contract.

    (a) True
    (b) False

chapter **15**

Nervous System Drugs

The human nervous system is our Internet over which sensory impulses travel the neural pathways to the brain. There they are interpreted and analyzed for an appropriate response. Another impulse is then generated by the brain and transmitted along the same pathway to tell appropriate parts of the body to respond.

Sometimes those responses are voluntary, such as using your hand to swat a bug from your nose. Involuntary responses include your heartbeat. Some responses can be a combination, such as breathing. You can hold your breath, and you can make yourself breathe faster, but your involuntary nervous system will take over and slow down your breathing or make you take a breath. Medication is available to interrupt impulses that flow along the neural pathway and prevent the body from responding normally to a stimulant. Likewise, there are medications that cause an impulse to stimulate parts of the body. These include drugs that increase the heart rate.

In this chapter, you'll learn about medications that affect the central nervous system (CNS) and the peripheral nervous system (PNS).

1. A Brief Look at the Nervous System

In order to understand the therapeutic effects of medication used to treat the nervous system, you'll need some knowledge of the anatomy and physiology of the system. The nervous system is composed of the brain, the spinal cord, nerves, and ganglia. Collectively, they receive stimuli and transmit information.

There are two nervous systems. These are the CNS and the PNS. The CNS consists of the brain and spinal cord, which are responsible for regulating body function. The CNS receives information from the PNS, which is interpreted, and then the CNS sends an appropriate signal to the PNS to stimulate cellular activity. Depending on the signal, the stimulation either increases or blocks nerve cells, which are called *neurons*.

The PNS is organized into two divisions. These are the somatic nervous system (SNS) and the autonomic nervous system (ANS). The SNS acts on skeletal muscles to produce voluntary movement. The ANS, also known as the *visceral system*, is responsible for involuntary movement and controls the heart, respiratory system, gastrointestinal (GI) system, and the endocrine system (glands).

The ANS is further divided into the sympathetic and parasympathetic nervous systems (see Section 4, "Autonomic Nervous System" in this chapter).

The SNS is also called the *adrenergic system* and uses the norephinephrine neurotransmitter to send information. The parasympathetic system, called the *cholinergic system*, uses the acetylcholine neurotransmitter to transmit information.

Both the sympathetic and parasympathetic nervous systems innervate organs within the body. The sympathetic system excites the organ, while the parasympathetic system inhibits the organ. For example, the sympathetic system increases the heart rate whereas the parasympathetic system decreases it.

Neurological Pathways

Neurological pathways extend from locations in the spinal cord to various areas of the body. These pathways contain two types of nerve fibers. These preganglionic and postganglionic fibers are connected together by a ganglion. The preganglionic nerve fiber carries messages from the CNS to the ganglion. The postganglionic nerve fiber transmits that message to specific tissues and organs from the ganglion.

Neurological pathways in the sympathetic nervous system originate from the thoracic (T1–T12) and the upper lumbar segments (L1 and L2) of the spinal cord. This is why the sympathetic nervous system is also referred to as the *thoracolumbar division* of the ANS.

The preganglionic fibers of the sympathetic nervous system extend from the spinal cord to the ganglionic fiber. These are relatively short. However, sympathetic postganglionic fibers are long from the ganglion to the body cells.

Neurological pathways in the parasympathetic nervous system originate from cranial nerves III, VII, IX, and X from the brain stem and the sacral segments S2, S3, and S4 from the spinal cord. This is why the parasympathetic nervous system is also known as the *craniosacral division* of the ANS.

Preganglionic fibers are long from the spinal cord to the ganglion, and the postganglionic fibers are short from the ganglion to the body cells.

2. CNS Stimulants

Medication is given to stimulate the CNS in order to induce a therapeutic response. These include medications that treat narcolepsy, attention-deficit disorder (ADD), and obesity, and for reversal of respiratory distress.

There are four major groups of medications that stimulate the CNS: (1) *amphetamines*, which stimulate the cerebral cortex of the brain; (2) *caffeine*, which also stimulates the cerebral cortex and stimulates respiration by acting on the brain stem and medulla; (3) *analeptics*, which affect the brain stem and medulla in the same way as caffeine does; and (4) *anorexiants*, which inhibit appetite by stimulating the cerebral cortex and the hypothalamus.

Amphetamines, analeptics, and anorexiants are commonly referred to as "uppers" when used to prevent sleep. Anorexiants and amphetamines can produce psychological dependence, and the body can become tolerant to its effect if abused. Abrupt discontinuation of these medications may result in withdrawal symptoms, including depression. Amphetamines are also taken to decrease weight and increase energy, enabling the patient to perform work quickly without rest.

Analeptics are substances that stimulate breathing and heart activity. Methylphenidate (Ritalin) is an analeptic often prescribed for children with attention-deficit hyperactivity disorder (ADHD).

Amphetamines, analeptics, and anorexiants stimulate release of the neurotransmitters norepinephrine and dopamine from the brain and from the peripheral nerve terminals of the sympathetic nervous system. The result is euphoria and increased alertness. The patient can also experience sleeplessness, restlessness, tremors, and irritability; and cardiovascular problems (increased heart rate, palpitations, dysrhythmias, and hypertension). Some examples of anorexiants and analeptics are benzphetamine (Didrex), diethylpropion (Tenuate), fenfluramine (Pondimin), and phentermine (Phentride). Caffeine is also a stimulant found in many beverages, foods, OTC drugs, and prescription drugs. Caffeine is found in many drugs, including Anacin, Excedrin, Cafergot, Fiorinal, and Midol.

See amphetamine-like drugs provided in the Appendix. Detailed tables show doses, recommendations, expectations, side effects, and contraindications; further information is available on the book's website (see URL in Appendix).

Migraine Headaches

Migraines are a debilitating neurovascular disorder that affect 28 million people over the age of 11. The cause of migraines is not clearly understood, although research indicates that the expansion of blood vessels and the release of certain chemicals—such as dopamine and serotonin—cause inflammation and pain. Dopamine and serotonin are found normally in the brain. A migraine can occur if an abnormal amount of these chemicals is present or if the blood vessels are unusually sensitive to them.

Patients who have migraines experience intense, throbbing, headache pain, which is often accompanied by nausea, photophobia (sensitivity to light), phonophobia (sensitivity to sound), and temporary disability. Migraines are sometimes preceded by an aura such as a breeze, odor, a beam of light, or a spectrum of colors. Migraines can occur on one side of the head (unilateral), and the pain is frequently reported as pulsating or throbbing.

Treatment of migraine is divided into prevention and symptomatic relief. There are six categories of medication used to prevent migraines. These are blood vessel constrictors and dilators (see Chapter 26), antiseizure drugs (discussed later in this chapter), antidepressants (discussed later in this chapter), β blockers (see Chapter 26), and analgesics (see Chapter 16). Patients are given a selected combination of these medications to prevent migraines. The prescriber determines the most effective combination for each patient according to the patient's response to these medications.

Commonly prescribed medications to prevent migraines are amitriptyline, divalproex sodium, propranolol, timolol, topiramate, bupropion, cyproheptadine, diltiazem, doxepin, fluvoxamine, ibuprofen, imipramine, and methysergide. Methysergide is particularly effective. However, there are side effects that might make this drug less tolerable.

Bringing about symptomatic relief from the pain associated with migraines and other migraine symptoms is achieved by prescribing antiemetics (antinausea drugs; see Chapter 18), ergot alkaloids and related compounds, NSAIDs (see Chapter 12), and other analgesics (nonopioids); opioids; and triptans (see chart).

Other Triptans	
Almotriptan	6.25–12.5 mg and repeat one dose if necessary; use with greater caution in patients with liver and kidney impairment; less side effects reported
Eletriptan	20–40-mg tablets repeated in 2 hours; high drug-drug interaction
Frovatriptan	2.5 mg at onset and may repeat after 2 hours; has longest half-life with a slow onset of action
Naratriptan	1–2.5-mg tablets and repeat after 4 hours; onset of action is slower but has the second longest half-life; has fewer side effects
Rizatriptan	5–10 mg repeated in 2 hours; fast-acting
Zolmitriptan	2.5–5-mg dose with 2-hour repeats available PO and nasal spray; increased risk of drug-drug interaction

A list of drugs utilized in the treatment of migrane headaches is provided in the Appendix. Detailed tables show doses, recommendations, expectations, side effects, and contraindications; more information is available on the book's website (see URL in Appendix).

3. CNS Depressants

Central nervous system depressants are medications that suppress the transmission of information throughout the CNS. There are seven broad classifications of CNS depressants. These are sedative-hypnotics, general and local anesthetics (discussed later in this chapter), analgesics, narcotic analgesics (Chapter 16), anticonvulsants, antipsychotics, and antidepressants (discussed later in this chapter).

Sedative-Hypnotics

Sedative-hypnotics are commonly referred to as *sedatives* and are the mildest form of CNS depressant. Sedative-hypnotics are given in low doses to diminish the patient's physical and mental responses without affecting the patient's consciousness.

With increased doses, the patient experiences a hypnotic effect that induces sleep. Even higher doses of sedative-hypnotics anesthetize the patient. Such is the case of the ultra-short-acting barbiturate thiopental sodium (Pentothal) that produces anesthesia.

Sedative-hypnotics and barbituates were first used to reduce tension and anxiety. However, other medications have been developed for this use. Chronic use of any sedative-hypnotic should be avoided.

It is important to understand that sedative-hypnotics are not the same as sleep medications purchased OTC, such as Nytol, Sominex, Sleep-eze, and Tylenol PM. Over-the-counter sleep medications such as diphenhydramine contain an antihistamine, not barbiturates, to achieve sedation.

Short-acting sedative-hypnotics are ideal for patients who need assistance falling asleep but who must awaken early without experiencing a lingering aftereffect from the medication. Intermediate-acting sedative-hypnotics are useful to sustain sleep. Patients may experience a residual drowsiness (hangover) after awakening.

The use of sedative-hypnotics for sleep (hypnotic) should be short term; otherwise there is a chance that the patient could become dependent on the medication or develop a tolerance. Patients who take high doses of sedative-hypnotics over long time periods must gradually discontinue the medication rather than abruptly stopping the drug, which can cause withdrawal symptoms. Sedative-hypnotics should not be administered to patients who have severe respiratory disorders or who are pregnant.

Before being prescribed a sedative-hypnotic to aid with sleep, the patient should try nonpharmacological methods that promote sleep, such as the following guidelines:

- Arise at a specific hour in the morning.
- Take few or no daytime naps.
- Avoid heavy meals or strenuous exercise before bedtime.
- Take a warm bath, read, or listen to music before bedtime.
- Decrease exposure to loud noises.
- Avoid watching disturbing television programs or news before sleep.
- Avoid drinking a large amount of fluids before sleep.
- Drink warm milk before sleep.

See sedative-hypnotic–benzodiazepine provided in the Appendix. Detailed tables show doses, recommendations, expectations, side effects, and contraindications; more information is available on the book's website (see URL in Appendix).

Barbiturates

Barbiturates are a type of sedative-hypnotic that is used to induce sleep, as an anesthetic, and in high doses to control epileptic seizures. Barbiturates are classified by duration of action, referred to as ultra-short-acting, short-acting, intermediate-acting, and long-acting.

Ultra-short-acting barbiturates such as thiopental sodium (Pentothal) was a commonly used anesthetic but has been largely replaced by propofol. Secobarbital (Seconal) and pentobarbital (Nembutal) are short-acting barbiturates that induce sleep. For longer periods of sleep, patients are prescribed intermediate-acting barbiturates such as amobarbital (Amytal), aprobarbital (Alurate), and butabarbital (Butisol). Phenobarbital and mephobarbital are long-acting barbiturates used for controlling epileptic seizures.

Barbiturates are Class II controlled substances, because of their addiction potential—both physical and psychological—should be prescribed for no more than 2 weeks because of the adverse side effect potential. Barbiturates increase CNS depression in the elderly and should not be used for sleep. Because of the potential for addiction, they have been replaced by benzodiazepines.

See "Sedative-Hypnotic—Barbituates and Others" provided in the Appendix. Detailed tables show doses, recommendations, expectations, side effects, and contraindications; more information is available on the book's website (see URL in Appendix).

Other Barbiturates			
Short-acting:	Secobarbital sodium (seconal sodium) Class II	Preoperative sedation; used to induce sleep	PO 100–200 mg before surgery; hypnotic: PO/IM 100–200 mg hs (hora somni; at bedtime); status epilepticus: IV; 5.5 mg/kg; repeat in 3–4 hours; with spinal anesthesia IV; 50–100 mg; infused over 30 seconds; maximum dose of 250 mg
Intermediate-acting	Amobarbital sodium (amytal sodium)	Sleep sustainers	PB 50–60%; half-life 20–40 hours; sedative: PO 30–50 mg bid/tid; hypnotic: PO/IM 65–200 mg hs, IV: 65–200 mg
Other	Chloral hydrate Class IV	No hangover and less respiratory depression; give with meals or fluids to prevent gastric irritation	Pregnancy Category C; PB 70–80%; half-life 8–10 hours; PO 250 mg tid before meals; hypnotic: PO 500 mg–1 g hs
Other	Paraldehyde Class IV	Exhaled via the lungs; strong odor and disagreeable taste; seldom used; has been used to control delirium tremens (DTS) in alcoholics; can be used for drug poisoning	Status epilepticus and tetanus to control convulsions; Pregnancy Category C, PB UK; half-life 7.5 hours; sedative PO 5–10 mL q4–6h PRN in water or juice; maximum dose 30 mL; hypnotic: PO 10–30 mL hs

Anesthetic Agents

Anesthetic agents depress the CNS, causing a loss of consciousness. They are classified as general and local.

Anesthetic agents were introduced in surgery in the early 1800s in the form of nitrous oxide (laughing gas), which is still used today for dental procedures. Other anesthetic agents were widely used by the mid-1800s. These included ether and chloroform. Ether is a highly flammable liquid with a pungent odor that causes nausea and vomiting and is seldom used today. Chloroform is toxic to the liver and is no longer used.

General anesthetics are used for general surgery, cardiac surgery, neurosurgery, and pediatric surgery. They are administered by an anesthesiologist or a nurse anesthetist. They are inhaled through a mask or breathing tube.

A general anesthetic can consist of one medication or a combination of medications—called *balanced anesthesia*—depending on the patient's age, weight, medical history, general health, and allergies and the type of procedure to be performed.

This balanced approach is used when administering general anesthetics to patients in phases to minimize cardiovascular problems, decrease the amount of general anesthetic needed, reduce possible postanesthetic nausea and vomiting, minimize the disturbance of organ function, and increase recovery from anesthesia with fewer adverse reactions.

The night before the surgery, the patient may be given a hypnotic to assist with a good night's sleep. On the day of surgery, premedication may be given to the patient about 1 hour before surgery. Premedication typically consists of two medications. One is a benzodiazepine, such as lorazepam (Ativan). This medication sedates and decreases anxiety. The other is an anticholinergic such as atropine to decrease secretions. A short-acting barbiturate such as thiopental sodium (Pentothal) is then administered in the operating room to induce anesthesia. The patient is then given inhaled gas and oxygen to maintain anesthesia. Sometimes the anesthetic is administered IV. Depending on the nature of the operation, the patient may also receive a muscle relaxant.

The patient experiences four stages of anesthesia, some of which are not observable because they occur rapidly. These stages are described in the following paragraphs.

Stage 1: Analgesia

The patient experiences analgesia (a loss of pain sensation) but remains conscious and can carry on a conversation.

Stage 2: Excitement

The patient may experience delirium or become violent. Blood pressure rises and becomes irregular, and breathing rate increases. This stage is typically bypassed by administering a barbiturate such as sodium pentothal before the anesthesia.

Stage 3: Surgical Anesthesia

Skeletal muscles relax. Breathing becomes regular. Eye movement slows and then stops. It is at this point when surgery begins.

Stage 4: Medullary Paralysis

Breathing and other vital functions cease to function because the respiratory center (medulla oblongata) is paralyzed. Death results if the patient is not revived quickly. Careful administration of the anesthesia prevents the patient from reaching this stage.

A list of anesthetic drugs is provided in the Appendix. Detailed tables show doses, recommendations, expectations, side effects, and contraindications; more information is available on the book's website (see URL in Appendix).

Commonly Administered IV Anesthetic Agents	
Ketamine (Ketalar)	Affects the senses, and produces a dissociative anesthesia (catatonia, amnesia, analgesia) in which the patient may appear awake and reactive; but cannot respond to sensory stimuli. These properties make it especially useful in developing countries and during warfare medical treatment. Ketamine is frequently used in pediatric patients because anesthesia and analgesia can be achieved with an intramuscular injection. It is also used in high-risk geriatric patients and in shock cases, because it also provides cardiac stimulation.
Thiopental (Pentothal)	A barbiturate that induces a rapid hypnotic state of short duration. Because thiopental is slowly metabolized by the liver, toxic accumulation can occur; therefore, it should not be continuously infused. Side effects include nausea and vomiting on awakening.
Opioids	Fentanyl, sufentanil, and alfentanil are frequently used prior to anesthesia and surgery as a sedative and analgesic, as well as a continuous infusion for primary anesthesia. Because opioids rarely affect the cardiovascular system, they are particularly useful for cardiac surgery and other high-risk cases. Opioids act directly on spinal cord receptors, and are frequently used in epidurals for spinal anesthesia. Side effects may include nausea and vomiting, itching, and respiratory depression.
Propofol (Diprivan)	Nonbarbiturate hypnotic agent and the most recently developed IV anesthetic. Its rapid induction and short duration of action are identical to those of thiopental, but recovery occurs more quickly and with much less nausea and vomiting. Also, propofol is rapidly metabolized in the liver and excreted in the urine, so it can be used for long durations of anesthesia, unlike thiopental. Hence, propofol is rapidly replacing thiopental as an anesthetic agent.

Topical Anesthetic Agents

Topical anesthetic agents (see chart) are solutions, liquid sprays, ointments, creams, and gels that are applied to mucous membranes, broken or unbroken skin surfaces, and burns to decrease the sensitivity of nerve endings in the affected area.

The first topical anesthetic agent was TAC, which is a combination of tetracaine, adrenaline (epinephrine), and cocaine, and was used for face and scalp lacerations. A version of TAC called *LET* is used today. LET is a combination of lidocaine, epinephrine, and tetracaine. Lidocaine has replaced cocaine. LET gel is generally preferred over TAC as analgesia for skin that is not intact because LET has a superior safety record and is more cost-effective than TAC.

Perhaps the best known topical anesthetic for intact skin is a eutectic mixture of local anesthetics (EMLA). EMLA is commonly used to anesthetize skin before IM injections, venipuncture, and simple skin procedures such as curettage or biopsy. EMLA is most effective if administered 90 minutes before the procedure.

ELA-Max (4% liposomal lidocaine) is another topical anesthetic used for intact skin that works more rapidly than EMLA. ELA-Max is an OTC medication that uses the liposomal delivery system. *Liposomes* are tiny lipid (fat) balls that deliver moisture to the skin. Because of their small molecular size, they are able to penetrate the cell wall reasonably well and can be used to deliver medications.

Other topical anesthetics can be delivered using *iontophoresis*—a type of therapy that uses a local electric current to introduce the ions of a medicine into the tissues—and anesthetic patch.

Topical Anesthetic Agents	
TAC (0.5% tetracaine, 1:2000 epinephrine, and 11.8% cocaine)	2–5 mL (1 mL/cm of laceration) applied to the wound with cotton or gauze for 10–30 minutes; onset effective 10–30 minutes after application; duration not established; may be as effective as lidocaine for lacerations on face and scalp; rare severe toxicity, including seizures and sudden cardiac death
LET (4% lidocaine, 1:2000 epinephrine, and 0.5% tetracaine)	1–3 mL applied directly to wound for 15–30 minutes; onset 20–30 minutes; duration not established; similar to TAC for face and scalp lacerations; less effective on extremities; no severe adverse effects reported
EMLA (2.5% lidocaine and 2.5% prilocaine)	Thick layer (1–2 g/10 cm^2) applied to intact skin with covering patch of Tegaderm; onset—must be left on for 1–2 hours; duration: 0.5–2 hours; variable, depending on duration of application; contact dermatitis, methemoglobinemia (very rare)
Iontophoresis	Small current applied to lidocaine-soaked sponges on intact skin; onset 10 minutes; duration 10–20 minutes; good for small procedures, depth of anesthesia greater than EMLA; stinging sensation; may burn skin if high current

Other Local Anesthetic Agents	
Procaine (Novocaine)	Short-acting (0.5–1 hour)—ester, first synthetic local anesthetic, relatively safe, due to rapid metabolism in the plasma, rapid onset, short duration, not good for topical anesthesia
Cocaine	Ester, only local anesthetic that is a vasoconstrictor, only local anesthetic that produces euphoria, used by ear-nose-throat specialists (ENTs) for surgical procedures because it reduces pain and controls bleeding
Tetracaine (Pontocaine)	Long-acting—ester—used for spinal anesthesia and topical applications
Bupivicaine	Long-acting—amide—can be cardiotoxic at high concentrations, used for infiltration, epidural, and nerve blocks

Local Anesthesia

A *local anesthetic* (see chart) blocks pain at the site where the medication is administered without affecting the patient's consciousness. It is commonly used for dental procedures, suturing of skin lacerations, short-term surgery at a localized area, spinal anesthesia by blocking nerve impulses (nerve block) below the insertion of the anesthetic, and diagnostic procedures such as lumbar puncture.

Local anesthetics are divided into two groups according to their basic chemical structure: (1) *esters*, which are chemical compounds formed from acid–alcohol reactions; and (2) *amides*, which are organic chemical compounds formed by reactions between acid chlorides, acid anhydrides, or esters and amines. Amides have a lower incidence of causing allergic reactions than do esters.

See "Local Anesthetics" listing provided in the Appendix. Detailed tables show doses, recommendations, expectations, side effects, and contraindications; more information is available on the book's website (see URL in Appendix).

Spinal Anesthesia

Spinal anesthesia is a local anesthetic injected into the spinal column in the third or fourth lumbar space to produce a regional neural block. If it is given too high, the respiratory muscles could be affected and respiratory distress or failure could result. There are four types of spinal anesthesia: subarachnoid block, epidural block, saddle block, and a caudal block.

A *subarachnoid block* is the injection into the subarachnoid space in the third or fourth lumbar space to produce anesthesia.

The *epidural block* occurs when the anesthetic is injected into the outer covering (dura mater) of the spinal cord near the sacrum.

The *saddle block* is given at the lower end of the spinal column to block the perineal area for procedures such as childbirth.

The *caudal block* is placed near the sacrum.

The patient may experience headaches and hypotension as a result of these procedures because of a change in cerebrospinal fluid pressure when the needle is inserted into the spine. The patient should remain in the supine position following the procedure and increase fluid intake.

4. Autonomic Nervous System

The autonomic nervous system—also known as the *visceral system*—involuntarily regulates smooth muscles and glands, including the heart, respiratory system, GI tract, peristalsis (digestion), bladder, and eyes.

The autonomic nervous system (ANS) has two sets of nerves: the sensory neurons (afferent) and the motor neurons (efferent). *Sensory neurons* send impulses to the CNS; these impulse are transmitted to the brain, where they are interpreted. The brain then sends a response to the motor neuron's brain through the spinal cord that directs specific organ cells to respond to the sensory neuron's impulse.

Previously in this chapter you learned that the ANS has two branches: the sympathetic branch and the parasympathetic branch. Both branches act on the same organ cells but in opposite ways. The *sympathetic branch* stimulates a response, and the *parasympathetic branch* depresses a response by the organ cell. Together, they keep the organ in balance (homeostasis).

The sympathetic branch stimulates a response using norepinephrine, a neurotransmitter. Medications that mimic the effect of norepinephrine are called *adrenergic drugs* or *sympathomimetics* (agents that mimic sympathetic nervous system actions) (see chart). These drugs are also known as *adrenergic agonists* because they initiate a response at the adrenergic receptor sites. There are four types of adrenergic receptors: α_1, α_2, β_1, β_2 (see chart).

The parasympathetic branch depresses a response using adrenergic blockers—also known as *sympatholytics*. *Lytic* means to stop or halt an effect. Adrenergic blockers prevent the norepinephrine response at the adrenergic receptor sites.

The parasympathetic branch is sometimes referred to as the *cholinergic system* because an acetylcholine neurotransmitter is used to innervate muscle cells at the end of the neuron. Acetylcholine stimulates receptor cells to produce a response. However, the enzyme acetylcholinesterase can inactivate the acetylcholine before it reaches the receptor cell.

Receptor	Physiologic Responses
α_1	Increases force of contraction of heart. Vasoconstriction: increases blood pressure. Mydriasis: dilates pupils of the eyes. Glandular (salivary): decreases secretions. Bladder and prostate: capsule increases contraction and ejaculation.
α_2	Inhibits the release of norepinephrine, dilates blood vessels, and produces hypotension; decreases gastrointestinal motility and tone.
β_1	Increases heart rate and force of contraction; increases rennin secretion, which increases blood pressure.
β_2	Dilates bronchioles; promotes GI and uterine relaxation; promotes increase in blood sugar through glycogenolysis in the liver; increases blood flow in the skeletal muscles.

Drugs that mimic acetylcholine are cholinergic agonists because they initiate a response. These are also known as *cholinergic drugs* or *parasympathomimetics* (see chart).

Drugs that block the effect of acetylcholine are called *anticholinergic*, or *parasympatholytics*. They are also known as *cholinergic antagonists* because they inhibit the effect of acetylcholine on the organ.

There are two types of cholinergic receptors: (1) *nicotinic* receptors, which are stimulated by the alkaloid nicotine; and (2) *muscarinic* receptors, which are stimulated by muscarine.

Sympathetic Stimulants	Parasympathetic Stimulants

Sympathomimetics (adrenergics, adrenomimetics, or adrenergic agonists)
  Increase blood pressure
  Increase pulse rate
  Relax bronchioles
  Dilate pupils of eyes
  Relax uterine muscles
  Increase blood sugar
	Direct-acting
	Parasympathomimetics (cholinergics, or cholinergic agonists)
	  Decrease blood pressure
	  Decrease pulse rate
	  Constrict bronchioles
	  Constrict pupils of eyes
	  Increase urinary contraction
	  Increase peristalsis
	Indirect-acting
	Cholinesterase Inhibitors (anticholinesterase)
	Increase muscle tone

Sympathetic Depressants	Parasympathetic Depressants

Sympatholytics (adrenergic blockers, adrenolytics, or adrenergic antagonists)
  Decrease blood pressure
  Decrease pulse rate
  Constrict bronchioles
	Parasympatholytics (anticholinergics, cholinergic antagonists, or antispasmodics)
	  Increase pulse rate
	  Decrease mucous secretions
	  Decrease gastrointestinal motility
	  Increase urinary retention
	  Dilate pupils of eyes

The Fight-or-Flight Response

Norepinephrine and acetylcholine neurotransmitters produce a fight-or-flight response (see chart). In a *fight response*, the pupils of the eyes dilate, enabling the person to see better and causing the lungs to inspire more oxygen while increasing the heart rate. Blood vessels constrict, increasing blood pressure. Smooth muscles along the bladder and the GI tract relax, so that energy is not expended on digestion. Salivary glands reduce the secretion of saliva, giving the person the dry mouth feeling in an emergency.

The *flight response* is really a misnomer because it does not help the person run away. Instead, the flight response is really the opposite of fight and allows the individual to relax and function normally. In the flight response or the nonfight mode, pupils constrict, the heart rate slows, the GI tract reduces function, and breathing slows down.

Body Tissue/Organ	Sympathetic (Fight) Response	Parasympathetic (Flight) Response
Eye	Dilates pupils	Constricts pupils
Lungs	Dilates bronchioles	Constricts bronchioles and increases secretions
Heart	Increases heart rate	Decreases heart rate
Blood vessels	Constricts	Dilates
Gastrointestinal	Relaxes smooth muscles	Increases peristalsis
Bladder	Relaxes bladder muscle	Constricts bladder
Uterus	Relaxes uterine muscle	
Salivary gland		Increases salivation

Adrenergics and Adrenergic Blockers

Andrenergics are medications that stimulate α_1 receptors and β_2-adrenergic receptors. The α_1 receptors are located in the smooth muscle of vascular (vessels) tissues. β_2-Adrenergic receptors are in the smooth muscle of the lungs, arterioles of skeletal muscles, and the uterine muscles. Adrenergics also stimulate the dopaminergic receptor located in the renal, mesenteric, coronary, and cerebral arteries to dilate and increase blood flow. Dopamine is the only adrenergic that can activate this receptor.

Adrenergic blockers inactivate these receptors in three ways:

1. They promote reuptake of the transmitter back into the neuron (nerve cell terminal).
2. Transmitters are transformed or degraded by enzymes, making them unable to attach to a receptor. Two enzymes that inactive norepinephrine are monoamine oxidase (MAO) and catechol-*o*-methyltransferase (COMT). MAO is inside the neuron, and COMT is outside the neuron.
3. Transmitters are diffused away from receptors.

Sympathomimetic drugs stimulate adrenergic receptors and are classified into three groups according to their effects on organ cells:

1. *Direct-acting sympathomimetics*—directly stimulate receptors.

2. *Indirect-acting sympathomimetics*—stimulate the release of norepinephrine from terminal nerve endings.

3. *Mixed-action sympathomimetics*—have the effect of both direct-acting sympathomimetics and indirect-acting sympathomimetics. They simulate the adrenergic receptor sites and stimulate the release of norepinephrine from terminal nerve endings. Ephedrine is an example of a mixed-action sympathomimetic and is used to treat idiopathic orthostatic hypotension and hypotension resulting from spinal anesthesia. Ephedrine also stimulates β_2 receptors to dilate bronchial tubes and is used treat mild forms of bronchial asthma.

Many adrenergic medications stimulate more than one adrenergic receptor site. For example, epinephrine (Adrenalin) acts on α_1-, β_1-, β_2-receptor sites. These receptor sites include an increase in blood pressure, pupil dilation, increase in heart rate (tachycardia), and bronchodilation.

Epinephrine (Adrenalin) is used to treat cardiogenic and anaphylactic shock because it increases blood pressure, heart rate, and airflow through the lungs by means of bronchodilation. Because it affects three different receptors, it lacks selectivity.

α-Adrenergic blockers inhibit the response at the α-adrenergic receptor sites. There are two types of α-adrenergic blockers: selective and nonselective blockers. Both types decrease symptoms of benign prostatic hypertrophy (BPH) (enlarged prostate) and promote vasodilation and treat peripheral vascular disease such as Raynaud's disease.

Doxazosin (Cardura) is a selective α_1 blocker, and phentolamine (Regitine) is a nonselective α-adrenergic blocker. Both can be used to treat hypertension.

However, α-adrenergic blockers can cause orthostatic hypotension (drop in blood pressure when an individual stands up), dizziness, and reflex tachycardia. They are not as frequently prescribed as β blockers.

β-Adrenergic blockers (see chart)—also known as *β blockers*—decrease heart rate and decrease blood pressure, resulting in bronchoconstriction. Therefore, β-adrenergic blockers should be used with caution for patients who have COPD or asthma.

Other Adrenergics	
Ephedrine HCl (α_1, β_1, β_2)	PO 25–50 mg tid/qid; SC/IM: 25–50 mg; IV: 10–25 mg PRN; maximum dose 150 mg/24 hr; effective for relief of hay fever, sinusitis, and allergic rhinitis; may be used for treating mild cases of asthma; Pregnancy Category C; PB UK; half-life 3–6 hours

(Continued)

Other Adrenergics (Continued)	
Norepinephrine bitartrate (Levophed) (α_1, β_1)	Potent vasoconstrictor; IV: 4 mg in 250–500 mL of D_5W or NSS infused initially 8–12 µg/min; then 4 µg/min; titrated according to blood pressure; Pregnancy Categories C, D; PB: UK; half-life UK
Metaraminol bitartrate (Aramine) (α_1, β_1)	V/Inf: 15–100 mg in 500 mg D_5W at a rate adjusted according to blood pressure; Pregnancy Category C; PBL UK; half-life UK
Dobutamine HCl (Dobutrex) (β_1)	To treat cardiac decompensation due to depressed myocardial contractility that may result from organic heart disease, cardiac surgery; IV 2.5–20 µg/kg · min initially; increase dose gradually; maximum dose of 40 µg/kg · min; Pregnancy Category C; PB: UK; half-life 2 minutes
Dopamine HCl (Intropin) (α_1, β_1) IV/Inf	1–5 µg/kg · min initially; gradually increase to 5–10 µg/kg · min to a maximum of 50 µg/kg · min; it does not decrease renal function in doses <5 µg/kg · min; Pregnancy Category C; PB: UK; half-life 2 minutes

There are also two types of β-adrenergic blockers: selective and nonselective. For example, metoprolol tartrate (Lopressor) is a selective α-adrenergic blocker that blocks β_1 receptors to decrease pulse rate and decrease blood pressure. Propranolol hydrochloride (Inderal) is a nonselective α-adrenergic blocker that blocks both β_1 and β_2 receptors, resulting in a slower heart rate, decreased cardiac output, and lower blood pressure.

Other β Blockers	
Doxazosin mesylate (Cardura) α_1	Mild to moderate hypertension; PO: 1 mg/day; titrate dose up to maximum of 16 mg/day; maintenance 4–8 mg/day; Pregnancy Category C; PB: 95%; half-life 3 hours
Carvedilol (Coreg) α_1, β_1, β_2	Use for hypertension and mild to moderate heart failure; can be used with a thiazide diuretic; PO: 6.25 mg bid; may increase to 12.5 mg bid to maximum 50 mg/day; Pregnancy Category C; PB: UK; half-life 7–10 hours
Labetalol (Normodyne) α_1, β_1, β_2	Mild to severe hypertension; angina pectoris; PO: 100 mg bid; dose may be increased to a maximum of 2.4 g/day; IV: 20 mg or 102 mg/kg; repeat 20–80 mg at 10-minute interval to maximum dose of 300 mg/day; Pregnancy Category C; PB: 50%; half-life 6–8 hours
Nadolol (Corgard) β_1, β_2	Management of hypotension and angina pectoris; contraindicated in bronchial asthma and severe COPD; PO: 40–80 mg/day, maximum 320 mg/day; Pregnancy Category C; PB: 30%; half-life 10–24 hours

Selective β-Adrenergics	
Metoprolol tartrate (Lopressor)—β₁	Management of hypertension, angina pectoris, post–myocardial infarction; hypertension; PO: 50–100 mg/day in 102 divided doses; maintenance 100–450 mg/day in divided doses to maximum of 450 mg/day in divided doses; for management of myocardial infarction: IV 5 mg q2m × 3 doses, then PO: 100 mg bid; Pregnancy Category C; PB: 12%; half-life 3–4 hours
Atenolol (Tenormin)—β₁	Mild to moderate hypertension and angina pectoris; may be used in combination with antihypertensive drugs; PO: 25–100 mg/day; Pregnancy Category C; PB: 6–16%; half-life 6–7 hours; esmolol HCl (Brevibloc)—β₁; supraventricular tachycardia, atrial fibrillation/flutter, and hypertension; contraindications—heart block, bradycardia, cardiogenic shock, uncompensated CHF; IV: loading dose 500 μ/kg · min for 1 minute; then 50 μg/kg · min for 4 minutes; Pregnancy Category C; PB: UK; half-life 9 minutes

5. Cholinergics

Cholinergics mimic the parasympathetic neurotransmitter acetylcholine. Acetylcholine (Ach) is a neurotransmitter located in the ganglions and terminal nerve endings of parasympathetic nerves that connect to receptors in organs, tissues, and glands.

There are two types of cholinergic receptors: (1) *muscarinic* receptors, which stimulate smooth muscles and slow the heart rate; and (2) *nicotinic* receptors, which affect skeletal muscles. Some cholinergic medications are selective and affect either muscarinic receptors or nicotinic receptors, while other cholinergic medications are nonspecific and affect both types of receptors.

Direct-acting cholinergics act on the receptors to activate a tissue response. Indirect-acting cholinergic drugs inhibit the action of cholineresterase (acetylcholinesterase) by forming a chemical complex that permits acetylcholine to persist and attach to the receptor. These drugs are called *cholinesterase inhibitors* or *anticholinesterase drugs.*

Pilocarpine is a commonly used direct-acting cholinergic that is administered to treat glaucoma. Pilocarpine reduces intraocular pressure by constricting pupils and opening the canal of Schlemm, enabling drainage of aqueous humor (fluid).

There are two types of cholinesterase inhibitors: (1) *reversible* inhibitors, which bind to the cholinesterase enzyme for a period of time and then unbind, enabling the cholinesterase enzyme to function properly; and (2) *irreversible* inhibitors, which permanently bind to the cholinesterase enzyme.

Cholinergics stimulate (see chart) the bladder, constrict pupils (miosis), increase neuromuscular transmission, and provide muscle tone to the GI tract. Other effects include a decreased heart rate and blood pressure while increasing secretion of the salivary glands.

A direct-acting cholinergic list is provided in the Appendix. Detailed tables show doses, recommendations, expectations, side effects, and contraindications; more information is available on the book's website (see URL in Appendix).

6. Anticholinergics

Anticholinergic drugs (see chart) inhibit acetylcholine by occupying the acetylcholine receptors. Anticholinergics are also called *parasympatholytics, cholinergic blocking agents, cholinergic* or *muscarinic antagonists, antiparasympathetic agents, antimuscarinic agents,* or *antispasmodics.*

Anticholinergic drugs block parasympathetic nerves, thereby enabling impulses from sympathetic nerves to take control. Anticholinergic and adrenergic drugs produce many of the same responses.

A list of anticholinergic drugs is provided in the Appendix. Detailed tables show doses, recommendations, expectations, side effects, and contraindications; more information is available on the book's website (see URL in Appendix).

7. Anti-Parkinsonism-Anticholinergic Drugs

Anti-Parkinsonism-anticholinergic drugs are used to treat the early stages of Parkinson's disease. These are typically combined with levodopa to control Parkinsonism or alone to treat pseudo-Parkinsonism. These are the Parkinson-like side effects of phenothiazines, which is an antipsychotic medication.

Drugs for Parkinsonism

Parkinsonism, better known as *Parkinson's disease,* is a chronic neurological disorder that affects balance and locomotion at the extrapyramidal motor tract. It is considered a syndrome because it has a combination of symptoms. Parkinsonism has three major features: rigidity, bradykinesia (slow movements), and tremors.

Rigidity is the abnormal increase in muscle tone that causes the patient to make postural changes such as shuffling gate, with chest and head thrust forward, and knees and hips flexed. The patient walks without swinging her/his arms. These movements are slow (bradykinesia), and the patient exhibits involuntary tremors of the head and neck, which may be more prevalent at rest and pill-rolling movements of the hands. Another characteristic symptoms is the masked facies (no facial expression) common in patients with Parkinson's disease.

TABLE 15−1 Foods That Can Cause a Hypertensive Crisis If Taken with MAO Inhibitors	
Foods	Effects
Cheese (cheddar, Swiss, bleu)	Sweating, tremors
Bananas, raisins	Bounding heart rate
Pickled foods	Increased blood pressure
Red wine, beer	Increased temperature
Cream, yogurts	
Chocolate, coffee	
Italian green beans	
Liver	
Yeast	
Soy sauce	

Note: The patient should avoid taking barbiturates, tricyclic antidepressants, and OTC medications with MAO inhibitors.

There are four types of drugs used to treat Parkinson's disease: dopaminergics, dopamine agonists, MAO-B inhibitors, and anticholinergics, which were discussed earlier in this chapter.

Dopaminergics decrease the symptoms of Parkinson's disease by permitting more levodopa to reach the nerve terminal where levodopa is transformed into dopamine and the tremors are reduced.

Dopamine agonists stimulate the dopamine receptors and reduce the symptoms of Parkinson's disease. MAO-B inhibitors inhibit the catabolic enzymes that break down dopamine, thereby extending the effects of dopamine. However, they can cause a hypertensive crisis if taken with certain foods (see Table 15–1).

A list of drugs utilized in the treatment of Parkinson's disease is provided in the Appendix. Detailed tables show doses, recommendations, expectations, side effects, and contraindications, and more information is available on the book's website (see URL in Appendix).

Muscle Spasms and Pain

Muscle spasms and pain are associated with traumatic injuries and many chronic debilitating disorders such as multiple sclerosis. Spasms are caused by hyperexcitable neurons stimulated by cerebral neurons or from lack of inhibition of the stimulus in the spinal cord or at the skeletal muscles.

Muscle relaxants are used to treat muscle spasms. There are two groups of muscle relaxants: (1) *centrally acting* relaxants, which depress neuron activity in the spinal cord or the brain, and are used to treat acute spasms from muscle trauma, but are less effective for treating spasms caused by chronic neurological disorders; and (2) *peripherally acting* relaxants, which depress neuron activity in the skeletal muscles.

Centrally Acting Muscle Relaxants

Carisoprodol (Soma), Cyclobenzaprine (Flexeril), and Methocarbamol (Robaxin) These drugs decrease pain, increase range of motion, and exert a sedative effect on the patient. Centrally acting muscle relaxants should not be taken concurrently with CNS depressants such as barbiturates, narcotics, and alcohol.

Diazepam (Valium) and Baclofen (Lioresal) These drugs are used to treat acute spasms from muscle trauma and for treating spasms caused by chronic neurologic disorders.

Peripherally Acting Muscle Relaxants

Dantrolene Sodium (Dantrium) This is a peripherally acting muscle relaxant. Peripherally acting muscle relaxants depress neuron activity at the skeletal muscles and have a minimal effect on the CNS. They are most effective for spasticity or muscle contractions caused by chronic neurologic disorders. They are also used to treat malignant hypertension, which is an allergic reaction to anesthesia.

Myasthenia Gravis

Myasthenia gravis is a disease characterized by failure of the nerve impulses to reach the nerves in muscle endings (myoneural junctions), which, in turn, is a result of an inadequate secretion or loss of acetylcholine due to action of acetylcholinesterase, an enzyme that destroys acetylcholine at the myoneural junction.

Patients experience fatigue and muscle weakness, particularly in respiratory muscles, facial muscles, and muscles in the extremities. They have drooping eyelids (ptosis) and difficulty in chewing and swallowing, and their respiratory muscles become paralyzed; this condition ultimately leads to respiratory arrest. Acetylcholinesterase (ACE inhibitors) are used to treat the symptoms of this disease. They include ambenonium (Mytelase), edrophonium Cl (Tensilon), neostigmine bromide (Prostigmin), and pyridostigmine bromide (Mestinon).

Multiple Sclerosis

Multiple sclerosis (MS) is an autoimmune disease affecting the CNS. Multiple lesions of the myelin sheath that surround the nerve fibers occur; these lesions are collectively called *plaque*. Myelin enables nerves to conduct impulses. Because some axons are spared, symptoms are different in each patient. The absence of the myelin causes impulses to jump or not transmit at all. MS patients can live a normal lifespan. At times patients are asymptomatic, and at other times symptoms can become severe and debilitating. These patients are said to have *relapsing-remitting MS*. Other patients have no periods of remission.

There is no cure for MS. However, the disease is treated palliatively and symptomatically using several medications.

Corticosteroids

These are used for treating periods when the patient experiences symptoms of MS (exacerbations). These are also known as "attacks," "relapses," and "flare-ups."

Interferon β-1B (Betaseron) and Interferon β-1a (Avonex)

These drugs are used to reduce the frequency and severity of relapses.

Copolymer 1

This drug is effective for treatment of relapsing-remitting MS.

Copaxone (Glatiramer Acetate Injection)

This drug reduces new brain lesions and the frequency of relapses in people with relapsing-remitting multiple sclerosis.

Alzheimer's Disease

Alzheimer's disease is a form of dementia common in older people that affects the patient's ability to carry out daily activities. Part of the patient's brain that controls thought, memory, and language becomes impaired.

It is estimated that 4.5 million Americans are afflicted with Alzheimer's disease. Alzheimer's disease affects 5% of people between 65 and 74 years of age, and 50% of those older than 85 years. Alzheimer's disease is not a normal part of the aging process.

Although the cause of Alzheimer's disease remains unknown, investigators have discovered that Alzheimer's patients have abnormal clumps of amyloid plaques and tangled bundles of fibers called *neurofibrillary tangles* in areas of their brains. There are also low levels of chemicals that carry messages between nerve cells in the brain. Amyloid plaques, neurofibrillary tangles, and decreased chemical levels impair thinking and memory by disrupting the transmission of these messages and cause nerve cells to die. The course of the disease varies from person to person. Eventually, the patient loses mental capacity and the ability to perform daily activities. This can range from mild memory problems to severe brain damage.

Although there is no curative treatment for Alzheimer's disease at this time, certain medications provide some relief to patients who are in the early and middle stages of the disease.

Razadyne (Galantamine), Exelon (Rivastigmine), and Aricept (Donepezil) These drugs prevent some symptoms from becoming worse for a limited time.

Memantine (Namenda) This medication is used to treat moderate to severe cases. The FDA has approved Aricept and NAMZARIC, a combination of Namenda and donepezil for the treatment of moderate to severe disease.

Tranquilizers, Mood Elevators, and Sedatives These can help control behavioral symptoms such as sleeplessness, agitation, wandering, anxiety, and depression.

A list of anticholinergic drugs is provided in the Appendix. Detailed tables show doses, recommendations, expectations, side effects, and contraindications; more information is available on the book's website (see URL in Appendix).

Effects of Cholinergic and Anticholinergic Drugs		
Body Tissue	**Cholinergic Response**	**Anticholinergic Response**
Cardiovascular*	Decreases heart rate, lowers blood pressure due to vasodilation, and slows conduction of atrioventricular node.	Increases heart rate with large doses. Small doses can decrease heart rate.
Gastrointestinal†	Increases the tone and motility of the smooth muscles of the stomach and intestine. Peristalsis is increased and the sphincter muscles are relaxed.	Relaxes smooth-muscle tone of GI tract, decreasing GI motility and peristalsis. Decreases gastric and intestinal secretions.
Genitourinary	Contracts the muscles of the urinary bladder, increases tone of the ureters, and relaxes the bladder's sphincter muscles. Stimulates urination.	Relaxes the bladder detrusor muscle and increases constriction of the internal sphincter. Urinary retention can result.
Eye†	Increases papillary constriction, or miosis (pupil becomes smaller), and increases accommodation (flattening or thickening of eye lens for distant or near vision).	Dilates pupils of the eye (mydriasis) and paralyzes ciliary muscle (cycloplegia), causing a decrease in accommodation.
Glandular* Bronchi (lung)*	Increases salivation, perspiration, and tears Stimulates bronchial smooth-muscle contraction and increases bronchial secretions.	Decreases salivation, sweating, and bronchial secretions. Dilates the bronchi and decreases bronchial secretions.

(Continued)

Effects of Cholinergic and Anticholinergic Drugs (Continued)		
Body Tissue	Cholinergic Response	Anticholinergic Response
Striated muscle†	Increases neuromuscular transmission and maintains muscle strength and tone.	Decreases tremors and rigidity of muscles.
Central nervous system		Drowsiness, disorientation, and hallucination can result from large doses.

*Tissue responses to large doses of cholinergic drugs.
†Major tissue responses to normal doses of cholinergic drugs.

Epilepsy

Epilepsy is a seizure disorder where there is an abnormal electric discharge from the cerebral neurons resulting in loss or disturbance of consciousness and convulsion (abnormal motor reaction). Epilepsy affects 1% of people in the United States.

Half the epilepsy cases are secondary to trauma, brain anoxia, infection, lesions, or cerebrovascular disorder (CVA) (commonly referred to as a "stroke"). Cause of the other half is unknown (idiophatic). Seventy-five percent of persons with seizures had their first seizure before 18 years of age. There are various types of seizures defined by the international classification of seizures. These include grand mal (tonic-clonic), petit mal (absence), and psychomotor seizures.

Epilepsy is treated by using anticonvulsant medication.

Hydantoins (Phenytoin, Mephenytoin, Ethotoin) These drugs treat grand mal (tonic-clonic) seizures and psychomotor seizures.

Barbiturates (Phenobarbital, Mephobarbital, Primidone) These drugs are used for treating grand mal and acute episodes or status epilepticus; meningitis, toxic reactions, and eclampsia

Succinimides (Ethosuximide) These agents are used to treat absence seizures and may be used in combination with other anticonvulsants.

Oxazolidones (Trimethadione) Oxazolidones are used to treat petit mal seizures and may be used in combination with other drugs or singly for treating refractory petit mal seizures.

Benzodiazepines (Diazepam, Clonazepam) These agents are effective in controlling petit mal seizures.

Carbamazepine This drug is effective in treating refractory seizure disorders that have not responded to other anticonvulsant therapies. It is also used to control grand mal and partial seizures and a combination of these seizures.

Valproate (Valproic Acid) This drug is used to treat petit mal, grand mal, and mixed types of seizures.

Keppra (levetiracetam) is used for partial onset, myoclonic, or tonic-clonic seizures. Anticonvulsant medication works in one of three ways:

1. It can suppress the sodium influx by binding to the sodium channel, prolonging the channel's inactivation and preventing neurons from firing.

2. It suppresses the calcium influx, preventing stimulation of the T calcium channel.

3. It increases the action of the γ-aminobutyric acid (GABA) by inhibiting neurotransmitters throughout the brain and thereby suppressing seizure activity.

A list of drugs utilized in the treatment of epilepsy is provided in the Appendix. Detailed tables show doses, recommendations, expectations, side effects, and contraindications; and more information is available on the book's website (see URL in Appendix).

8. Antipsychotics

Psychosis is a disorder that is characterized by a number of symptoms. These include difficulty processing information and reaching a conclusion, experiencing delusions or hallucinations, being incoherent or in a catatonic state, or demonstrating aggressive violent behavior.

Psychosis is divided into major categories, one of which is schizophrenia. *Schizophrenia* is a chronic psychotic disorder where patients exhibit either positive or negative symptoms. *Positive symptoms* are exaggerations of normal functions such as agitation, incoherent speech, hallucination, delusion, and paranoia. *Negative symptoms* are characterized by a decrease in or loss of motivation or function such as social withdrawal, poor self-care, and a decrease in the content of speech. Negative symptoms are more chronic and persistent than positive symptoms.

Psychosis is caused by an imbalance in the neurotransmitter dopamine in the brain. Antipsychotic medication, also known as *dopamine antagonists*, block the D_2-dopamine receptors in the brain, thereby reducing the psychotic symptoms.

A number of antipsychotic medications block the chemoreceptor trigger zone and vomiting (emetic) center of the brain. When this occurs, an antiemetic effect is produced. Although blocking dopamine improves the patient's thought processes and behavior, it can cause side effects.

These side effects include symptoms of Parkinsonism (see discussion of Parkinsonism earlier in this chapter). Patients who undergo long-term treatment for psychosis using antipsychotic medications also might be prescribed drugs to treat the symptoms of Parkinsonism.

Antipsychotic medications are divided into two categories. These are sometimes called *traditional* and *atypical*. The atypical category of antipsychotic medication is further subdivided into phenothiazines and nonphenothiazines.

Phenothiazines block norepinephrine causing sedative and hypotensive effects early in treatment.

Nonphenothiazines include butyrophenone haloperidol (Haldol), whose pharmacologics are similar to those of phenothiazines as it alters the effects of dopamine by blocking the dopamine receptor sites.

Atypical antipsychotic drugs are used to treat schizophrenia and other psychotic disorders for patients who do not respond to the typical antipsychotic medication.

A list of antipsychotic drugs is provided in the Appendix. Detailed tables show doses, recommendations, expectations, side effects, and contraindications; more information is available on the book's website (see URL in Appendix).

9. Phenothiazines

Phenothiazines are divided into three groups. These are aliphatic, piperazine, and piperidine. Each category has different side effects (see Table 15–2). The aliphatic group produces a strong sedative effect, decreases blood pressure, and may moderate extrapyramidal symptoms (EPSs). Chlorpromazine is a member of this group.

TABLE 15–2 Effects of Antipsychotic Drug Categories				
Group	Sedation	Hypotension	EPS	Antiemetic
Aliphatic (Chlorpromazine and triflupromazine)	+++	+++	++	++ +++
Piperazine	++	+	+++	+++
Piperidine	+++	+++	+	–
Nonphenothiazines				
Haloperidol	+	+	+++	++
Loxapine	++	++	+++	–
Molindone	+/++	+	+++	–
Thiothixene	+	+	+++	–
Atypical antipsychotics				
Risperidone	+	+	+/0	–

Key: – no effect; + mild effect; ++ moderate effect; +++ severe effect.

The piperazine group produces a low sedative effect and a strong antiemetic effect, more EPS, and little effect on blood pressure. Included in this group are prochlorperazine (Compazine), fluphenazine (Prolixin), perphenazine (Trilafon), and trifluoperazine (Stelazine).

The piperidine group includes mesoridazine besylate (Serentil) and thioridazine HCl (Mellaril). These produce few EPS or antiemetic effects and can cause hypotension.

Anxiolytics

Anxiolytics are medications used to treat anxiety and insomnia. These have replaced sedatives that were traditionally used because they have fewer and less potent side effects, especially if an overdose of the medication is given to the patient. Benzodiazepine is the major group of anxiolytics.

Anxiolytics are prescribed when the patient's anxiety reaches a level where she/he becomes disabled and is unable to perform normal activities. Anxiolytics have a sedative-hypnotic effect on the patient, but not an antipsychotic effect.

There are two types of anxiety: primary anxiety and secondary anxiety. *Primary anxiety* is not caused by a medical condition or drug use but may be situational. *Secondary anxiety* is caused by a medical condition or by drug use. Anxiolytics are seldom administered for secondary anxiety unless the secondary cause is severe or untreatable. Instead, the secondary cause is treated.

Benzodiazepines are prescribed to treat severe or prolonged anxiety, but are also used to treat convulsions and hypertension, and as a sedative-hypnotic and preoperative medication. Benzodizepines include chlordiazepoxide (Librium), diazepam (Valium), clorazepate dipotassium (Tranxene), oxazepam (Serax), lorazepam (Ativan), and alprazolam (Xanax).

10. Depression

About 20% of Americans are depressed; however, one-third receives medical or psychiatric help for their depression. Depression is characterized by mood changes and loss of interest in normal activities. Patients who are depressed might have insomnia, fatigue, a feeling of despair, and an inability to concentrate. Some may have suicidal thoughts. Depression is associated with two-thirds of all suicides.

Causes and Types of Depression

Depression is caused by a number of factors, including genetic predisposition, social and environmental factors, and biologic conditions such as insufficient monoamine neurotransmitter (norepinephrine and serotonin).

There are three types of depression: reactive, major (unipolar), and bipolar affective.

Reactive (Exogenous) Depression

Reactive depression has a sudden onset and lasts for months and is usually caused by an event such as the loss of a loved one. Benzodiazepine is used to treat reactive depression.

Major (Unipolar) Depression

Major depression is characterized by losing interest in work and home. The patient is unable to complete tasks and falls into a deep depression. Causes of major depression can include genetic predisposition, social and environmental factors, and biologic conditions. Benzodiazepines are the drugs of choice to treat major depressions.

Bipolar Affective (Manic-Depressive) Depression

Bipolar affective depression is characterized by mood swings, with the patient exhibiting behavior ranging from manic (euphoric) to depressive (dysphoric). Lithium is prescribed for bipolar affective disorders.

Antidepressants

Antidepressants are used to treat depression; however, they also can mask suicidal tendencies (Table 15–3). There are four groups of antidepressants: tricyclics, second-generation antidepressants [serotonin reuptake inhibitors (SSRIs)], atypical antidepressants, and monoamine oxidase (MAO) inhibitors.

Tricyclics are the most commonly prescribed drug to treat major depression. Tricyclics include clomipramine HCl (Anafranil), desipramine HCl (Norpramin, Pertofrane), doxepin HCl (Sinequan), imipramine HCl (Tofranil), Nortriptyline HCl (Aventyl), Protriptyline HCl (Vivactil), and trimipramine maleate (Surmontil).

Second-generation antidepressants have fewer side effects than tricyclics. They do not cause hypotension, sedation, anticholinergic effects, or cardiotoxicity. Second-generation antidepressants include

- SSRI: fluoxetine HCl (Prozac), paroxetine HCl (Paxil), sertraline HCl (Zoloft), fluvoxamine (Luvox)

- Atypical: amoxapine (Asendin), bupropion HCl (Wellbutrin), maprotiline HCl (Ludiomil), nefazodone HCl (Serzone), trazodone HCl (Desyrel)

Monamine Oxidase Inhibitors (MAOIs)

The enzyme monoamine oxidase inactivates norepinephrine, dopamine, epinephrine, and serotonin. With the inhibition of monoamine oxidase, the levels of these

TABLE 15–3 Side Effects of Antidepressants

Category	Anticholinergic Effect	Sedation	Hypotension	GI Distress	Cardiotoxicity	Seizures	Insomnia/Agitation
Tricyclic Antidepressants							
Amitriptyline (Elavil)	+++	++++	+++	−	++++	+++	−
Clomipramine (Anafranil)	++++	++++	++	−	++++	++	−
Desipramine (Norpramin)	+	++	++	−	++	++	+
Doxepin (Sinequan)	+++	++++	++	−	++	++	−
Imipramine (Tofranil)	+++	+++	+++	+	++++	++	+
Nortriptyline (Aventyl)	+	+++	+	−	+++	++	−
Protriptyline (Vivactil)	+++	+	++	−	+++	+	+
Trimipramine (Surmontil)	+++	++++	+++	−	++++	++	−
Selective Serotonin Reuptake Inhibitors							
Fluoxetine (Prozac)	−	+	−	+++	−	0/+	++
Fluvoxamine (Luvox)	−	++	−	++	−	−	++
Paroxetine (Paxil)	−	+	−	+++	−	−	++
Sertraline (Zoloft)	−	+	−	+++	−	−	++
Atypical (Heterocyclic) Antidepressants							
Amoxapine (Asendin)	+++	++	+	−	+	+++	++
Bupropion (Wellbutrin)	++	−	0/+	+	+	++++	++
Nefazodone (Serzone)	+	++	+	+	0/+	−	−
Trazodone (Desyrel)	−	+++	++	+	+	+	−
Maprotiline (Ludiomil)	+++	+++	+	−	++	++	−
Monoamine oxidase inhibitors	+	+	++	+	−	−	++

neurotransmitters rise. Examples of these drugs include isocarboxazid (Marplan), phenelzine sulfate (Nardil), and tranylcypromine sulfate (Parnate).

A list of drugs utilized in the treatment of depression is provided in the Appendix. Detailed tables show doses, recommendations, expectations, side effects, and contra-indications; more information is available on the book's website (see URL in Appendix).

Summary

There are many medications that either interfere with impulses transmitted over the neural pathways or stimulate those impulses. Medications that interfere with impulses are called *inhibitors* and usually compete with neurotransmitters for receptor sites. In other words, the medication reaches the receptor site before the neurotransmitters, blocking the neurotransmitters from delivering the impulse to the receptor site. Medications that cause an impulse to be generated are called *stimulants*.

There are four major groups of medications that stimulate the CNS: amphetamines, caffeine, analeptics, and anorexiants. *Amphetamines* stimulate the cerebral cortex of the brain. *Caffeine* also stimulates the cerebral cortex and stimulates respiration by acting on the brain stem and medulla. *Analeptics* have a similar effect on the brain stem and medulla as caffeine. *Anorexiants* inhibit appetite by stimulating the cerebral cortex and the hypothalamus.

There are seven broad classifications of medications that depress the CNS: sedative-hypnotics, general and local anesthetics, analgesics, narcotic analgesics, anticonvul-sants, antipsychotics, and antidepressants.

Sedative-hypnotics diminish the patient's physical and mental responses without affecting consciousness. *General anesthetics* cause a loss of consciousness and relieve pain. *Local anesthetics* block pain at the site where the medication is administered without affecting the patient's consciousness.

Analgesics are drugs that reduce pain and include aspirin, acetaminophen, and ibu-profen. *Narcotic analgesics* are drugs that reduce pain and produce a state of stupor or drowsiness by blocking the transmission of pain signals in the brain.

Anticonvulsants are medications that prevent or lessen the likelihood that a patient will experience convulsions, which are abnormal motor reactions such as those found in epilepsy. *Antipsychotics* are drugs used to minimize symptoms of psychosis. *Psychosis* is a disorder that is characterized by one of a number of symptoms such as difficulty processing information and reaching a conclusion. *Antidepressants* are med-ications used to treat depressions.

The next chapter continues our exploration of drugs that affect the CNS by examin-ing narcotic agonists. A *narcotic agonist* is a medication that relieves pain—called an *analgesic*.

QUIZ

1. **Amphetamines**
   (a) inhibit the release of neurotransmitters.
   (b) stimulate the release of neurotransmitters.
   (c) lower the heart rate.
   (d) do none of the above.

2. **Patients who experience migraines**
   (a) can be treated with a combination of migraine medications.
   (b) should not be treated with a combination of migraine medications.
   (c) should be treated with amphetamines.
   (d) should be treated with Prozac.

3. **Muscarinic receptors**
   (a) stimulate smooth muscles.
   (b) stimulate skeletal muscles.
   (c) increase the heart rate.
   (d) do all of the above.

4. **Tricyclic medications are used to treat depression.**
   (a) True
   (b) False

5. **Anticholinergics drugs inhibit acetylcholine.**
   (a) True
   (b) False

6. **β-Adrenergic blockers**
   (a) decrease blood pressure.
   (b) decrease the heart rate.
   (c) cause bronchoconstriction.
   (d) do all of the above.

7. **Selective blockers affect specific receptors, while nonselective blockers affect multiple receptors.**
   (a) True
   (b) False

8. Indirect-acting sympathomimetics

   (a) stimulate receptors.
   (b) stimulate the release of norepinephrine from terminal nerve endings.
   (c) stimulate both receptors and the release of norepinephrine from terminal nerve endings.
   (d) do none of the above.

9. The saddle block can be used during childbirth.

   (a) True
   (b) False

10. A local anesthetic blocks pain at the site where the medication is administered without affecting the patient's consciousness.

   (a) True
   (b) False

chapter **16**

Narcotic Agonists

Pain is something that all of us feel, yet it is difficult for healthcare providers to accurately assess because pain is whatever you say it is. You know that it hurts when you twist an ankle or have a pounding headache. All you want is fast relief. You want a magic pill to make the pain go away. The pill may be a narcotic agonist that blocks transmission of impulses from the site of the injury to the area of the brain that interprets pain.

This chapter explores pain and how healthcare providers assess and manage pain. You'll also learn about narcotic and nonnarcotic analgesics and how they are used to treat pain.

1. A Close Look at Pain

Narcotic agonists are medications that relieve pain. These are safe and effective when properly administered. These medications are opioid-based and are used to treat acute or chronic pain from trauma, tumor growth, and surgical procedures. They are also used to treat pain caused by the progression of diseases or complications from other conditions.

For example, pain from a sickle cell crisis can be debilitating and require the patient to receive a narcotic analgesic such as morphine. This medication blocks the pain and creates a euphoric effect, giving the patient relief from the pain of the disease.

However, fear of inducing addiction or respiratory depression interferes with pain management. Addiction has become a concern in clinical practice. Studies have revealed that 50% of patients who receive an opioid analgesic for an acute injury are still using that medication or have progressed to intravenous (IV) heroin use 3 months later. Some patients who are treated with opioid analgesics can develop a tolerance to the medication, requiring an increased dose to maintain pain relief. However, the need to increase the dose of the medication can be related to an increase in pain due to disease progression or complications. Physical dependence on a medication occurs when the physiological condition of the patient is altered.

Increased doses of opioid analgesics also expose the patient to adverse side effects such as respiratory depression. However, this effect seldom occurs with long-term use in patients with chronic conditions such as cancer. Prescribers can avoid this side effect by titrating doses over time to deliver pain relief without adversely affecting the respiratory system.

2. Influences on Administrating Pain Medication

The concerns about addiction and the potential for adverse side effects of opioid analgesics influence how the medication is administered. Patients may avoid or postpone taking pain medication until the pain is unbearable for fear of becoming addicted or developing a tolerance for the medication. This is especially true with patients who suffer chronic debilitating diseases. They realize that pain increases as the disease progresses, and they are fearful that the medication will lose its effectiveness.

Some healthcare providers are also hesitant to administer pain medication for some of the same reasons that patients refuse to take the drug. Furthermore, healthcare providers might be skeptical that the patient is actually in pain since pain is subjective and difficult to measure in the clinical setting.

Many studies have demonstrated that women, the elderly, children, and those addicted to illegal drugs are at greater risk for being undertreated for acute pain. These studies indicate that some healthcare providers believe females react emotionally and pain is not as severe as reported. Others believe the elderly and children do not feel pain as acutely as other patients. Also, many healthcare providers believe that addicts are simply seeking drugs to forego withdrawal symptoms, even when it is clear that the addict is suffering pain from an acute injury or illness.

3. Components of Pain

There are two components of pain: the physical sensation and the psychological component. The *physical* sensation of pain occurs when nerve endings are stimulated, causing the nerve to send an impulse along the nerve pathways to the brain, which transmits a pain response.

The *psychological* component is a person's emotional response to pain based on the person's pain threshold. The *pain threshold* is the level of nerve-ending stimulation that causes the person to have the feeling of unbearable pain.

For example, applying heat to the skin will cause the sensation of pain. However, the point beyond which pain becomes unbearable (pain tolerance) varies widely among individuals. Pain tolerance is also different for the same person depending on the circumstance in which sensation is detected. For example, a toothache might hurt more when you're at home than at work, where you have a lot of distractions from the pain.

4. The Gate Control Theory

The *gate control theory* is an attempt to describe the mechanism of pain transmission. The dorsal horn of the spinal cord contains a gate mechanism that alters the transmission of painful sensations from peripheral nerve fiber to the thalamus and cortex of the brain. The thalamus and the cortex are where the painful sensations are recognized as pain.

The transmission flows through the gate mechanism. The gate is closed by large-diameter, low-threshold afferent fibers and is opened by small-diameter, high-threshold afferent fibers. In addition to these two sets of fibers, the gate is also influenced by descending control inhibition from the brain to close the gate.

When the patient experiences slower-acting painful stimuli, the large-diameter fibers are stimulated. This causes the gate to close, stopping transmission of the painful stimuli.

Nonpharmacological pain relief treatments, such as a massage, are based on the gate control theory to ease the patient's pain.

5. Defining Pain

Pain is whatever the patient who is experiencing pain says it is. Healthcare providers describe pain in terms of intensity, duration, frequency, and type of pain. However, these terms are subjective and characterized by the patient.

Pain is classified in six different ways:

1. **Acute Pain:** *Acute pain* is the presence of severe discomfort or an uncomfortable sensation that has a sudden onset and subsides with treatment. For example, a fractured bone causes acute pain since the uncomfortable sensation occurs suddenly when the bone is broken and subsides when the bone is immobilized in a cast. Pain associated with myocardial infarction (heart attack), appendicitis, and kidney stones are also examples of acute pain. Acute pain can be treated with NSAIDs or opioid analgesics.

2. **Chronic Pain:** *Chronic pain* is a persistent or recurring pain that continues for 6 months or more. This is the type of pain caused by cancer, rheumatoid arthritis, and other chronic conditions. Chronic pain is treated with combinations of NSAIDs and opioid analgesics as well as medications to reduce swelling and anxiety.

3. **Visceral Pain:** *Visceral pain* is the dull, aching pain caused by stimulating nerve endings in smooth muscle or sympathetically innervated organs. Visceral pain is *referred pain*. This makes it difficult to localize the source of the pain. Pain of a myocardial infarction (MI) is an example of visceral pain. MI can be described as crushing chest pain and also described as pain in the left arm or hand and even the shoulder, left back, or the left ear. Visceral pain is best treated with opioid analgesics.

4. **Somatic Pain:** *Somatic pain* is pain that occurs from skeletal muscles, fascia, ligaments, vessels, and joints. Somatic pain is an aching, throbbing pain over the affected area. Somatic pain is best treated with nonsteroidal anti-inflammatory agents.

5. **Neuropathic Pain:** *Neuropathic pain* is a burning, shooting, and sometimes tingling pain that is caused by peripheral nerve injury. This type of pain is often caused by the invasion of a cancerous tumor or nerve damage. Neuropathic pain is treated with a combination of medications such as anticonvulsants, tricyclic antidepressants, and opioid analgesics.

6. **Psychogenic Pain:** *Psychogenic pain* is pain caused by psychiatric illness or psychosocial stimuli such as anxiety, depression, and fear. Drug therapy alone may bring brief relief. Psychotherapy may bring long-lasting relief from psychogenic pain.

6. Pain Assessment

The most common method used to assess pain is the *pain scale*. One of the pain scales ranges from 0 to 10, 0 is freedom from pain and 10 is the most severe pain. There are a number of variations of this pain scale, including the face-rating scale and the color scale. The *face-rating scale* uses expressions of cartoon faces to assess pain, while the *color scale* uses colors ranging from blue to red, where blue is freedom from pain and red is the most severe pain.

In addition to rating the intensity of the patient's pain, you also must assess other characteristics of pain. These are onset, duration, frequency, what started the pain (precipitating factors or cause), and what relieves the pain.

Patients who have chronic pain should keep a pain diary. A pain diary helps the healthcare professional develop a pain management plan. The patient is asked to keep a timed record of the pain experience to include when the pain starts, what starts it, how severe it is, what relieves the pain, and any other factors that may explain how the patient is responding to the pain. This record can help the healthcare provider and the patient plan effective pain management.

The *pain management plan* contains both pharmacological and nonpharmacological strategies for managing the patient's pain. *Pharmacological strategies* involve using pain medication. *Nonpharmacological strategies* involve treatments other than medication. These include massage, imagery, music, distraction, humor, acupuncture, chiropractic interventions, hypnosis, herbal therapies, therapeutic touch, and transcutaneous electronerve stimulation. Surgical interventions are also sometimes performed to relieve pain.

7. Pharmacologic Management of Pain

Pharmacologic management of pain involves administering pain medication to relieve the patient's pain. These include nonnarcotic analgesics, nonsteroidal anti-inflammatory drugs (NSAIDs), narcotic analgesics, and salicylates.

Nonnarcotic analgesics (see chart) are used to treat mild to moderate pain. Many of these medications are not addictive and are available over the counter. Nonnarcotic analgesics are used to treat headaches, menstrual pain (dysmenorrhea), pain from inflammation, minor abrasions, muscular aches and pain, and mild-to-moderate arthritis. Nonnarcotic analgesics also lower elevated body temperature (antipyretic). Nonnarcotic analgesics include acetaminophen and NSAIDs (aspirin, ibuprofen, and COX-2 inhibitors), which were discussed in Chapter 12.

See "Non-narcotic Analgesic" in the Appendix. Detailed tables show doses, recommendations, expectations, side effects, and contraindications; more information is available on the book's website (see URL in Appendix).

Narcotic Analgesics

Narcotic analgesics are known as *narcotic agonists*, and act on the CNS to provide relief from moderate and severe pain. Narcotic analgesics are also used to suppress coughing by acting on the respiratory and cough centers in the medulla of the brain stem.

Opioids are a category of narcotic analgesics. All relieve pain, and all, except meperidine (Demerol), have an antitussive (cough suppression) and antidiarrheal effects.

See "Narcotic Agonist-Opiate Analgesic" and "Opioid Agonist" listed in the Appendix. Detailed tables show doses, recommendations, expectations, side effects, and contraindications; more information is available on the book's website (see URL in Appendix).

Narcotic Agonist-Antagonists

A *narcotic agonist-antagonist* (agonist) is an opioid narcotic mixed with naloxone (antagonist) to try to curb a form of drug misuse. Although the exact mechanism of action is unknown, these agents exert both agonist and antagonist effects on the opioid receptors. Generally, these drugs are less potent and have a lower dependence potential than opioids, and withdrawal symptoms are not as severe. Commonly used narcotic agonist-antagonists are pentazocine (Talwin), butorphanol tartrate (Stadol), duprenorphine (Buprenex), and nalbuphine hydrochloride (Nubain). Their pharmacokinetics, adverse, and side effects are similar to those of morphine.

Other Narcotic Analgesics of the Opium and Synthetic Group	
Drug	Purpose
Codeine (sulfate, phosphate), CSS II	For mild to moderate pain
Hydromorphone HCl (Dilaudid) CSS II	For severe pain
Levorphanol tartrate (Levo-Dromoran) CSS II	For moderate to severe pain
Meperidine (Demerol) synthetic narcotic CSS II	For moderate pain
Fentanyl (Duragesic, Sublimaze) CSS II	Short-acting potent—used with short-term surgery; patches for controlling chronic pain
Sufentanil (Duragesic, Sublimaze) CSS II	Short-acting potent—used as part of balanced anesthesia
Methadone (Dolophine)	Similar to morphine but longer duration of action; used in drug abuse programs

See "Narcotic Agonist-Antagonist" listed in the Appendix. Detailed tables show doses, recommendations, expectations, side effects, and contraindications; more information is available on the book's website (see URL in Appendix).

Narcotic Antagonists

Narcotic antagonists (see chart) are antidotes for overdoses of narcotic analgesics. They have a higher affinity to the opiate receptor site than the narcotic analgesic and block the narcotic analgesic from binding to the opiate receptor site. They also reverse the respiratory and CNS depression caused by the narcotics.

Naloxone (Narcan) is a narcotic antagonist and can be used to determine whether an unconscious patient has used an opioid narcotic drug. If the patient wakes up after Narcan is administered IV, she/he is likely to have ingested or injected an opioid narcotic.

Summary

Pain is sensed when a nerve ending is stimulated, sending an impulse along the neural pathway to the brain that interprets the impulse as pain. Pain is assessed in a patient by asking her/him to describe the intensity of the pain on a pain scale—the higher the value, the more severe the pain. Besides intensity, pain is assessed according to onset, duration, frequency, what started the pain (precipitating cause), and what relieves the pain.

There are six classifications of pain: acute pain, chronic pain, visceral pain, somatic pain, neuropathic pain, and psychogenic pain. Pain can be treated either nonpharmacologically or pharmacologically.

Nonpharmacological pain treatment includes massage, imagery, music, distraction, humor, acupuncture, chiropractic interventions, hypnosis, herbal therapies, therapeutic touch, and transcutaneous electronerve stimulation. Surgical interventions are also sometimes performed to relieve pain.

Pharmacological pain treatment involves administering medication that relieves the patient of pain. There are four categories of pain medication: nonnarcotic analgesics, nonsteroidal anti-inflammatory drugs (NSAIDs), narcotic analgesics, and salicylates (discussed in Chapter 12).

Narcotic analgesics are opioid narcotics that can induce respiratory depression. The effects of a narcotic analgesic can be reversed by administering a narcotic antagonist.

Many patients and healthcare providers are concerned that a patient will become addicted to narcotic analgesics or develop a tolerance for these drugs. Both can occur. However, proper pain management can alleviate these potential problems.

This chapter concludes the look at pain medications. In the next chapter, we'll take a look at medications that are used to control the immune system.

QUIZ

1. **Physical sensation of pain**
   - (a) occurs when nerve endings are stimulated, causing it to send an impulse along the nerve pathways to the brain.
   - (b) is a person's emotional response to pain, based on a person's pain threshold.
   - (c) occurs when the brain stimulates nerve endings at the site of the injury.
   - (d) none of the above.

2. **Nonpharmacological pain relief treatments apply the**
   - (a) pain oppression theory.
   - (b) pain suppression theory.
   - (c) brain suppression theory.
   - (d) gate control theory.

3. The presence of severe discomfort or an uncomfortable sensation that has a sudden onset and subsides with treatment is

   (a) neuropathic pain.

   (b) visceral pain.

   (c) chronic pain.

   (d) acute pain.

4. The color scale uses colors ranging from blue to red, where blue is freedom from pain and red is the most severe pain.

   (a) True

   (b) False

5. Naloxone (Narcan) is the antidote to an opioid narcotic.

   (a) True

   (b) False

6. Pain occurring from skeletal muscles, fascia, ligaments, vessels, and joints is called

   (a) neuropathic pain.

   (b) visceral pain.

   (c) chronic pain.

   (d) none of the above.

7. Surgical interventions are sometimes performed to relieve pain.

   (a) True

   (b) False

8. Patients who are in chronic pain should

   (a) stay in bed.

   (b) keep a pain diary.

   (c) avoid vacations.

   (d) do none of the above.

9. Most opioids suppress coughs.

   (a) True

   (b) False

10. Music can help relieve pain.

   (a) True

   (b) False

chapter **17**

Immunologic Agents

The body's immune system is its natural defense against microorganisms that cause diseases (pathogens) and against cells that are not the body's own cells, such as transplanted organs. The immune system also treats its own abnormal cells, such as cancer cells, as foreign and attacks them with the same energy as it attacks microorganisms.

However, when the immune system is compromised through diseases, including HIV, the body loses its ability to fight off microorganisms and to destroy its own abnormal cells. The patient encounters more episodes of infection that can ultimately lead to death.

In this chapter, you'll learn about the therapies used to help the immune system combat preventable diseases and you'll also learn about medications that inhibit the growth of HIV.

1. A Brief Look at Immunity

The *immune system* is the body's way of combating the invasion of microscopic organisms such as bacteria, viruses, molds, spores, pollens, protozoa, and cells from transplant donors (human or animal). The immune system prevents an invasion from attacking internal organs, and, if that fails, the immune system neutralizes, destroys, and eliminates any nonself proteins and cells (ie, proteins and cells that are foreign to the body), including microorganisms.

Nonself proteins and cells also include self-cells (the body's own cells) that have become infected or debilitated. One example is malignant transformation that changes healthy cells into cancer cells. The ability of the immune system to differentiate between the body's own cells and non-self-cells is called *self-tolerance*.

The immune system is able to recognize self-cells by using unique proteins that are on the surfaces of all self-cells. Think of these proteins as an identification code. Foreign cells have a different identification code. These are called *antigens* and stimulate the immune response of the host.

When bacteria invade your body, your immune system detects the bacteria's surface protein as not being a self-cell. This triggers your immune system to launch an attack against the bacteria.

The immune system originates in the bone marrow. Mature immune system cells are released from the bone marrow into the bloodstream, where they circulate throughout the body searching for invaders.

Three processes are necessary for immunity: inflammation, antibody-mediated immunity (humoral immunity), and cell-mediated immunity (CMI).

Inflammation

This is discussed in detail in Chapter 12.

Antibody-Mediated Immunity

Antibody-mediated immunity occurs when the immune system produces antibodies that neutralize, eliminate, or destroy an antigen (foreign protein). Antibodies are produced by B lymphocytes. The body must be exposed to sufficient amounts of an antigen before the immune system produces an antibody to combat the antigen. Patients can be given vaccinations that stimulate the immune system to generate antibodies before the microorganism actually invades the body. In this way, the antibodies already exist and can attack at the first sign of the microorganism.

Cell-Mediated Immunity

Cell-mediated immunity, also known as *cellular immunity*, uses T leukocytes [referred to as *natural killer cells* or (NK) cells] to attack non-self-cells. Cell-mediated immunity also causes the body to release cytokines, which regulate the activities of antibody-mediated immunity and inflammation.

Cell-mediated immunity is especially useful in identifying and ridding the body of self-cells that are infected by organisms that live within host cells and of self-cells that mutate at the DNA level, transforming them into abnormal and potentially harmful cells. Cell-mediated immunity is critically important in preventing development of cancer and metastasis after exposure to carcinogens.

HIV and the Immune System

Human immunodeficiency virus (HIV) is a retrovirus that gradually destroys the immune system's function if left untreated. When a person becomes infected with HIV, the virus infects the CD4$^+$ T cells and uses them to replicate at a rapid pace. In the process, the CD4$^+$ T cells are destroyed and the person's CD4$^+$ T-cell count decreases as the HIV viral load increases. Eventually, the immune system responds to the HIV infection, causing the viral load to decrease and stabilize at a viral setpoint. Once this happens, the CD4$^+$ T-cell count begins to increase, but seldom returns to preinfection levels. An acutely infected person may display symptoms of viral infection such as fever, swollen glands, sore throat, rash, muscle and joint pains, and headache. These symptoms usually appear within 2–4 weeks of the initial infection and resolve on their own. Many acutely infected people experience mild or no symptoms, so the initial infection may be missed unless the clinician takes a through history. This initial stage is referred to as primary *HIV infection* or *acute retroviral syndrome* (ARS). HIV can be transmitted during any stage of infection, but the risk is greatest during acute HIV infection.

Without diagnosis and treatment, the HIV-infected person progresses to the clinical latency stage, often referred to as *asymptomatic HIV infection* or *chronic HIV infection*. The infected person can transmit the HIV virus during this period of clinical latency. HIV continues to replicate throughout the body, but the person may be asymptomatic. Clinical latency may last for up to 10 years. Without antiretroviral treatment (ART) to suppress HIV, the CD4 count will continue to drop and the HIV viral load will continue to rise. If the infected person starts taking HIV medications (ART), the viral load becomes undetectable; HIV infection will remain a chronic disease. If left untreated, however, HIV infection will progress to acquired immunodeficiency syndrome, commonly known as "AIDS."

AIDS is the final stage of HIV infection. At this stage, the immune system is so badly damaged that the person becomes susceptible to opportunistic infections. AIDS is defined as a CD4 cell count below 200 cells/mm (ie, 200 cells mm^{-1}) and/or one or more opportunistic infection(s). Common symptoms of AIDS include chills, fever, sweats, swollen lymph glands, weakness, and weight loss. Without treatment, people who have progressed to AIDS typically survive about 3 years. Once a person with AIDS develops a dangerous opportunistic infection, malignancy, or secondary infection, without treatment, life expectancy decreases to about 1 year. With treatment, CD4 immune function can recover and CD4 cells can increase to >200 cells/mm. However, once people have a diagnosis of AIDS, it remains regardless of CD4 count. People with AIDS whose viral load is not suppressed with ART can have a high viral load and can transmit the virus.

CD4 measurements are used to determine the health of the immune system in a person with HIV infection. The *viral load* (VL) is another test used to evaluate the effectiveness of the medication in preventing viral replication and the person's adherence to HIV medication. When a person takes ART, it stops the virus from replicating and the viral load decreases to undetectable, or less than 200 copies/mL. ART must be taken every day for the rest of the person's life in order for the HIV viral load to remain undetectable. If the person is not taking HIV medications consistently, stops taking the medication, or develops resistance to the HIV medication, HIV begins to replicate and the viral load will become detectable once again. Eventually, CD4 levels will decrease, placing the person at risk of developing AIDS.

HIV drug resistance testing or genotype is recommended when an HIV viral load becomes detectable, HIV viral suppression is not achieved and there is a viral load of >1000 copies/mL, when an HIV-positive person has been on many different ART medications intermittently over time and may have developed resistance, and at entry into HIV care to guide selection of the initial ART regimen.

Three types of tests are used to screen for HIV: antibody tests, combination or fourth-generation tests, and nucleic acid tests (NATs). Antibody tests use either blood or saliva for testing. It can take 3–12 weeks for an acutely infected person's body to produce enough antibodies to enable detection of HIV infection. Negative HIV antibody test results within 3 weeks of a possible HIV exposure require a retest in 3 months. A positive HIV antibody test requires a follow-up confirmatory test.

Combination or fourth-generation screening tests look for both HIV antibodies and antigens. In HIV infection, an antigen called *p24* is produced before antibodies develop. It can take 2–6 weeks (13–42 days) for a person's body to produce enough antigens and antibodies for a combination, or fourth-generation, test to detect HIV. Negative combination test result during the 2–6-week period after a possible exposure should be retested after 3 months. Combination screening tests are recommended for testing performed in laboratories. There is now a rapid combination test available.

NATs look for HIV in the blood and can detect HIV infection about 7–28 days after a person has been infected with HIV. NATs are expensive and not routinely used for HIV screening unless the person had a high-risk exposure or a possible exposure with early symptoms of HIV infection.

HIV is transmitted through direct contact with certain body fluids—blood, semen, pre-seminal fluid, rectal fluids, vaginal fluids, and breast milk—from a person who has HIV. Body fluids must come in contact with a mucous membrane or damaged tissue or be directly injected into the bloodstream for transmission to occur. In the United States, HIV transmission occurs mainly in one of two ways. Transmission can occur through unprotected anal or vaginal sexual contact with an HIV-positive person and when needles and other equipment used to prepare drugs for injection are shared with someone who is HIV-infected. Less common modes of transmission in the United States include vertical transmission during pregnancy, birth, or breastfeeding if a woman is living with HIV. Recommendations to test all pregnant women for HIV and start HIV treatment immediately have lowered the incidence of HIV-infected newborns. Occupational HIV exposure (usually from a needlestick) accounts for a small number of transmissions in the United States.

The HIV virus can replicate only inside cells. HIV uses three enzymes to genetically encode, replicate, and assemble a new HIV virion within a host cell. These enzymes are integrase, reverse transcriptase, and protease. There are seven stages to HIV replication: binding, fusion, reverse transcription, integration, replication, assembly, and budding.

The HIV virus enters the cell by binding or attaching to receptors on the surface of the CD4 molecule. The HIV envelope and the CD4 cell membrane fuse together, allowing HIV to enter the cell. Once inside the cell, the virus is uncoated with the help of the reverse transcriptase enzyme, enabling conversion of the virus' single-stranded RNA to DNA. The viral DNA migrates to the nucleus of the cell, where it is spliced into the host DNA with the help of the integrase enzyme. Once integrated into the cell's DNA, HIV uses the CD4 cell to make HIV proteins. The HIV proteins and RNA move to the surface of the cell and assemble into immature HIV cells. The immature HIV proteins bud out of the CD4 cell, and the protease enzyme assists in the assembly of a new HIV virion.

Combinations of ART medications stop the HIV replication process at different points, thereby decreasing the viral load to undetectable levels. Once the viral load is undetectable, CD4 cells do not become infected during the replication process. CD4 levels increase, and the immune system begins to recover, preventing opportunistic infections and keeping the person in good clinical condition. ART is recommended for all HIV-infected patients who have detectable HIV RNA in their plasma, regardless of their CD4 level or clinical stage of HIV.

Potential Benefits of ART

- Control of viral replication and mutation
- Reduction of viral burden
- Prevention of progressive immunodeficiency
- Maintenance of the normal immune system
- Reconstruction of the normal immune system
- Delay in the progression to AIDS and prolongation of life
- Decreased risk of resistant virus
- Decreased risk of viral transmission

Potential Risks

- Inconvenience of adhering to the medication regimen
- Unknown long-term toxicity of antiretroviral drugs

HIV Medication

Medications that are highlighted in bold type are no longer used or recommended in the guidelines; however, some patients may still be taking them if they come from another country. The Centers for Disease Control (CDC) publishes up-to-date recommendations for the pharmacological treatment of HIV patients, including adults, women, adolescents, children, and neonates. ART is recommended for everyone living with HIV. ART is a combination of HIV medicines that generally includes three HIV medicines from at least two different drug classes. Currently, six classes of antiretroviral agents exist:

Nonnucleoside Reverse Transcriptase Inhibitors (NNRTIs) NNRTIs bind to *reverse transcriptase*, a protein that HIV needs to make more copies of itself. In doing so, reverse transcriptase becomes disabled. Drugs within this category include Delavirdine (**Rescriptor, DLV**), Efavirenz (Sustiva, EFV), Etravirine (Intelence, ETR), Rilpivirine (Endurant, RPV), and **Neviapine (Viramune, NVP)**.

Nucleoside Reverse Transcriptase Inhibitors (NRTIs) NRTIs are faulty version reverse transcriptase. Reproduction of HIV is stalled when HIV uses NRTI instead of the normal reverse transcriptase. Drugs within this category include Abacavir (Ziagen, ABC), **Didanosine (Videx, ddI, Videx EC)**, Emtricitabine (Emtriva, FTC, Coviracil), Lamivudine (Epivir, 3TC), **Stavudine (Zerit, d4T)**, Tenofovir DF (Viread, TDF), **Zalcitabine (Hivid, ddC)**, and Zidovudine (Retrovir, AZT, AZV).

Protease Inhibitors (PIs) Protease inhibitors disable protease, a protein that HIV needs to make more copies of itself. Drugs within this category include **Amprenavir (Agenerase, APV)**, Atazanavir (Reyataz, ATV), Darunavir (DRV), Fosamprenavir (Lexiva, FPV), **Indinavir (Crixivan, IDV)**, Lopinavir (Kaletra, LPV/r), **Nelvinavir (Viracept, NFV)**, Ritonavir (Norvir, RTV), **Saquinavir (Fortovase, SQV; Invirase)**, and **Tipranavir (Aptivus, TPV)**.

Integrase Strand Transfer inhibitors (INSTIs) *Integrase strand transfer inhibitors* (INSTIs) block integrase (an HIV enzyme). HIV uses integrase to insert (integrate) its viral DNA into the DNA of the host CD4 cell. Blocking integrase prevents HIV from replicating. Drugs in this class include Dolutegravir (Tivicay, DTG), Elvitegravir (Vitekta, EVG), and Raltegravir (Isentress, RAL).

Fusion Inhibitors Fusion Inhibitors prevent HIV from entry into cells. They include Enfuviritide (Fuzeon, T-20). This medication is rarely used because of the side effect of pain at the injection site and the availability of other more easily tolerated medications.

Chemokine Coreceptor Antagonists (CCR5 Antagonists) CCR5 antagonists block the CCR5 co-receptor on the surface of certain CD4 T lymphocytes (CD4 cells). This prevents HIV from entering the cell. There is only one drug in this class, Maraviroc (Selzentry, MVC).

harmacokinetic Enhancers Pharmacokinetic enhancers are used in HIV treatment to increase the effectiveness of protease inhibitor (PI) medications when they are used in an ART regimen. There are two drugs in this class: Cobicistat (tybost, COBI) and Ritonavir (Norvir, RTV). Although ritonavir is a weak PI, it is used as a pharmacokinetic enhancer with other PI medications.

Combination HIV Medicines Generally, an HIV regimen includes two NRTIs plus an INSTI, an NNRTI, or a PI boosted with cobicistat (Tybost, COBI) or ritonavir (Norvir, RTV). In order to facilitate dosing and adherence, 14 combination HIV medications are available in addition to the individual medications in the six classes of ART. Combination HIV medicines contain two or more HIV medicines from one or more drug classes. Combination medications include Abacavir/Lamivudine (ABC/3TC, Epzicom), Abacavir/Dolutegravir/Lamivudine (ABC/DTG/3TC, Triumeq), **Abacavir/ Lamivudine/Zidovudine (ABC/3TC/ZDV, Trizivir)**, Atazanavir/ cobicistat (ATV/ COBI, Evotaz), Dauravir/Cobicistat (DRV/COBI, Prezcobix), Efavirenz/Emtricitabine/ Tenofovir (EFV/FTC/TDF), Elvitegravir/Cobicistat/Emtricitibine/Tenofovir (EVG/ COBI/FTC/TDF, Stribild), Emtricitibine/Rilpivirine/Tenofovir (FTC/RPV/TDF, Complera), Emtricitabine/Tenofovir (FTC/TAF, Discovy), Emtricitabine/Tenofovir (FTC/TDF, Truvada), Lamivudine/Zidovudine (3TC/ZDV, Combivir), and Lopinivir/ Ritonavir (LPVr, LPV/RTV, Kaletra).

Aggressive prophylaxis and treatment of opportunistic infections is recommended for people who have progressed to full-blown AIDS in addition to an ART regimen. Nutritional therapy, complementary therapy, and supportive care are also necessary. A list of drugs used in the treatment of HIV is provided in the Appendix. Detailed tables show doses, recommendations, expectations, side effects, and contraindications; more information is available on the book's website (see URL in Appendix).

HIV Therapy and Pregnancy

Special care must be taken when an HIV patient is pregnant. The objective is to reduce the risk of transmission of HIV to the fetus. Pregnant women should take ART during pregnancy; they can continue on the same medications they are already taking. If they are not taking medications, they should start as soon as possible. Most HIV medications do not cause birth defects. A cesarean section is recommended for pregnant women who have high or unknown viral loads. The patient is given ZDV (zidovudine) intravenously in a 10-hour loading dose of 2 mg/kg of body weight, followed by a continuous infusion of 1 mg/kg of body weight per hour at beginning of labor and until delivery. ZDV passes across the placenta and protects the baby from any HIV that passed from mother to child during childbirth.

The newborn is then given PO ZDV at 2 mg/kg body weight per dose every 6 hours for the first 6 weeks of life, beginning 6–12 hours after birth. A 4-week neonatal AZT prophylaxis regimen can be used for full-term infants if the mother received ART during pregnancy with sustained viral suppression and if there are no concerns related to maternal adherence. Otherwise, a 6-week course as part of a combination infant prophylaxis regimen is recommended. The National Perinatal HIV Hotline (1-888-448-8765) provides free clinical consultation on all aspects of perinatal HIV, including infant care.

Occupational Postexposure Prophylaxis (PEP)

Postexposure prophylaxis is administered to all healthcare workers who experience an occupational exposure to HIV according to the Public Health Service Statement on the Management of Occupational Exposures to HIV and Recommendations. The policy for PEP is institution-specific and should be available to all employees. Clinicians caring for healthcare workers who might have been exposed can call the PEPline (1-888-448-4911), which offers around-the-clock advice on managing occupational exposures to HIV.

Nonoccupational Postexposure Prophylaxis (nPEP)

Nonoccupational postexposure prophylaxis (nPEP) should be taken within 72 hours of a recent possible exposure to HIV. nPEP is not a substitute for other proven methods of preventing HIV transmission, such as using condoms or using new sterile needles when injecting drugs. The CDC publishes guidelines for nonoccupational exposure, and clinicians can call the PEPline for guidance.

Preexposure Prophylaxis (PrEP)

Preexposure prophylaxis (or PrEP) is for people who have a high risk for HIV infection. PrEP reduces the risk of contracting HIV from sex by >90%. This risk can be even lower if PrEP is used in conjunction with condoms. Among people who inject drugs, PrEP reduces the risk of HIV infection by 70%. A combination of two HIV medicines, tenofovir and emtricitabine (TDF/FTC, Truvada), in one pill is approved for daily use as PrEP.

2. Vaccines

The immune system develops antibodies to attack a pathogen using one of two methods: active immunity and passive immunity.

Active immunity occurs when the immune system generates antibodies on the first exposure to the pathogen. This immune response is relatively slow, resulting in the patient showing the signs and symptoms of the disease.

However, the immune system remembers the pathogen and is quick to dispatch antibodies should the pathogen attack a subsequent time. This happens more rapidly than the initial response and can generally eliminate the pathogen before the patient experiences the signs and symptoms of the disease. The patient may have a lifelong immunity to the pathogen owing to the body's active natural immunity.

Active natural immunity can also occur through immunization when the patient receives a vaccination against the pathogen. The vaccination contains a small amount of the pathogen to stimulate the production of antibodies, but insufficient in strength to develop the signs and symptoms of the disease.

There are five ways in which the pathogen in vaccines is produced:

1. Whole microorganism or components of an inactivated (dead) microorganism.

2. Live, but weakened microorganisms.

3. Toxoids, which are inactivated toxins produced by some microorganisms.

4. Conjugates, which are vaccines that link a protein (toxoid) from an unrelated organism to the outer coat of the disease-causing microorganism. The result is a substance that is recognized by the immature immune system of young infants. *Haemophilus influenzae* type b is an example.

5. Recombinant subunit vaccine is where DNA of a pathogen is inserted into a cell or organism. The cell or organism then produces massive quantities of the pathogen that are used in place of the whole pathogen. Examples are hepatitis B and LYMErix for Lyme disease.

A booster dose of a vaccine is sometimes required to maintain sufficient immunity. The immune system has a memory, and when the vaccinated individual is later exposed to the actual pathogen, the body can mount a rapid immune response and prevent the disease. This is called *artificially acquired immunity*.

Passive immunity occurs when the patient receives antibodies from another source rather than generating her/his own antibodies. Newborns have natural passive immunity to protect them from pathogens. The newborn receives natural passive immunity from antibodies that cross the placenta. Antibodies may also be acquired from a pool of antibodies from human or animal sources. This is *acquired passive immunity*.

Passive immunity is transient—lasting no more than several weeks to a few months. The individual does not mount her/his own immune response to antigens. Acquired passive immunity is important when time does not permit active vaccination alone, when the exposed individual is at high risk for complications of the disease, or when the person suffers from an immune system deficiency that renders her/him unable to produce an effective immune response.

3. Preventing Diseases

More than 20 infectious diseases in the United States can be prevented by vaccination. Some vaccines are routinely administered to both children and adults. Other vaccines are given under special circumstances to military personnel, travelers whose destinations are certain foreign countries, and the chronically ill.

These preventable diseases include adenovirus, cholera, diphtheria, *H. influenzae* type b (Hib), hepatitis A, hepatitis B, influenza, Japanese encephalitis, Lyme disease, measles, meningococcal disease, poliomyelitis, rabies, rotavirus, rubella, tetanus, tuberculosis, typhoid, varicella, and yellow fever.

The Centers for Disease Control (CDC) recommends a vaccination schedule for children, available on their website (http://www.cdc.gov/mmwr/preview/mmwrhtml/mm5351-Immunizationa1.htm).

Adult Immunizations

Adults are frequently overlooked when it comes to vaccination because emphasis is placed on preventing children from developing preventable diseases. However, the CDC suggests that adults review their immunizations on decade birthdays (20, 30, 40, 50, and 60).

Adults should also review their immunizations every time they travel to a foreign country, regardless of their age. The CDC provides information regarding appropriate immunizations on their website (http://www.cdc.gov/).

Adverse Events of Vaccine

Biologic products such as vaccines do not undergo the pharmacokinetic process that is associated with other drug therapies. Vaccines are generally safe. Some common mild reactions include swelling at the injection site and fever. Absolute contraindications for the use of vaccines include anaphylactic reaction to a specific vaccine or component of another vaccine or moderate or severe illness.

Healthcare providers are expected to report vaccine adverse events to public health officials, who, in turn, report these to the CDC every week using the Vaccine Adverse

Events Reporting System (VAERS), which is used to provide compensation for injury and death caused by vaccination.

Determining Whether Someone Is Vaccinated

Patients may not know if they've been vaccinated. Therefore, healthcare professionals perform a blood test to determine detectable levels of antibodies in the bloodstream for preventable diseases such as rubella.

If antibodies are detected in sufficient quantity, then the patient is immune to the disease. If the antibodies are not detected, then the patient needs to be revaccinated. Healthcare professionals are required to be vaccinated for many common communicable diseases in order to prevent them from acquiring the disease and passing it along to their patients.

Nursing Actions for Vaccinations

Here are the steps that should be followed when vaccinating a patient:

- Obtain immunization history.
- Obtain medical history of immune deficiency diseases such as malignancy (cancer) or HIV.
- Obtain pregnancy history and pregnancy test.
- Obtain drug history including high-dose immunosuppressants, blood transfusions, and immune globulin.
- Obtain a complete allergy history, including drugs, foods, and environmental allergies.
- Do not administer vaccines to a pregnant patient.
- Ascertain whether anyone in the patient's household is not vaccinated or is immunodeficient.
- Assess for symptoms of moderate to severe acute illness with or without fever.
- Adhere to storage requirements for the vaccine to ensure its potency.
- Administer vaccine within stated time limit after preparation.
- If two or more vaccines are being administered at the same time, use different injection sites.
- Do not mix vaccines in the same syringe.
- Observe the patient for signs and symptoms of adverse reactions to vaccines.
- Keep epinephrine available in the case of anaphylactic reaction.
- Document that a Vaccine Information Statement (VIS) is available from the CDC for each vaccine administered and is provided to the patient/family. Be sure

to include the date of vaccination, route and site, vaccine type, manufacturer, lot number, and expiration date, name, address, and title of individual administering vaccine.

- Provide the patient with a record of immunizations.

Patient Education for Vaccinations

Here are facts that patients should know about vaccinations:

- Explain risk of contracting vaccine-preventable diseases.

- Female patients of childbearing age must avoid becoming pregnant within a month of receiving the vaccine.

- Provide the patient or family with current VIS forms, available from CDC for each vaccine administered. Be sure to include the date of vaccination, route and site, vaccine type, manufacturer, lot number, and expiration date, name, address, and title of individual administering vaccine.

- Remind the patient or family to bring the VIS record to all visits.

- Provide the patient or family with date for return for next vaccination.

- Discuss common side effects of receiving the vaccine.

- Tell patient or family to contact healthcare provider if they observe signs of a serious reaction to the vaccine.

Immunosuppressants

The development of organ transplants—which include kidneys, liver, heart, lungs, and pancreas—has led to the development of immunosuppressant drugs. These drugs are meant to suppress the body's natural reaction to reject the foreign protein to ensure that the patient will not reject the transplanted organ. Some of these drugs include azathioprine (Imuran), cyclosporine (Sandimmune), muromonab-DC3 (Orthoclone OKT3), mycophenolate mofetil (Cell Cept), and tacrolimus (FK506 Prograf).

Some of the side effects of these drugs include nausea and vomiting and an increased risk of tumor growth. Significant leukopenia and thrombocytopenia may occur. These drugs are expensive and must be continued for the life of the patient.

Summary

The immune system provides a natural defense against pathogens and against abnormal cells that might lead to cancer. This system differentiates between self-cells and non-self-cells by proteins on the cell surfaces. Abnormal self-cells are considered non-self-cells. Microorganisms are antigens and considered non-self-cells and cause the immune system to generate antibodies that neutralize and destroy the antigen.

There are three processes in immunity: inflammation, antibody-mediated immunity (humoral immunity), and cell-mediated immunity (CMI).

Human immunodeficiency (HIV) is a retrovirus that destroys the immune system. When the retrovirus becomes active, the patient exhibits acquired immunodeficiency syndrome (AIDS).

Highly active antiretroviral therapy (HAART) is the use of antiretroviral medications designed to slow or inhibit reverse transcriptase and protease enzymes that replicate HIV. The patient must adhere to HAART therapy; otherwise the virus will become resistant and the antiretroviral agents will lose their therapeutic effects. Four classes of medication are approved by the FDA for treatment of HIV: NNRTI, NRTI, PI, and fusion inhibitors.

A vaccine contains a small amount of a pathogen that is sufficient to stimulate the production of antibodies, but not sufficient for the patient to acquire the disease. Once antibodies for a specific pathogen are generated, the immune system can quickly regenerate the antibodies when the pathogen invades the body again.

In the next chapter we look at medications that are used to treat gastrointestinal and digestive diseases.

QUIZ

1. **The immune system is able to recognize self-cells by**
   - (a) using unique RNA molecules that are on the surface of all self-cells.
   - (b) using unique lipids that are on the surface of all self-cells.
   - (c) using unique proteins that are on the surface of all self-cells.
   - (d) none of the above.

2. **Antibody-mediate immunity occurs when the immune system produces**
   - (a) antibodies that neutralize, eliminate, or destroy an antigen (foreign protein).
   - (b) antigens that neutralize, eliminate, or destroy an antibody (foreign protein).
   - (c) antibodies that generate an antigen (foreign protein).
   - (d) antigens that generate antibodies (foreign protein).

3. **HIV is transmitted via**
   - (a) injection of infected blood or blood products.
   - (b) sexual contact.
   - (c) maternal-fetal transmission.
   - (d) all of the above.

4. Cell-mediated immunity, also known as *cellular immunity*, uses T leukocytes referred to as natural-killer cells (NK cells) to attack non-self-cells.

   (a) True
   (b) False

5. Cell-mediated immunity is especially useful in identifying and ridding the body of self-cells that are infected by organisms that live within host cells.

   (a) True
   (b) False

6. NNRTI inhibits HIV by

   (a) binding to ART.
   (b) binding to protease.
   (c) binding to reverse transcriptase.
   (d) none of the above.

7. A newborn whose mother is HIV positive should not be treated for HIV unless the newborn shows signs and symptoms of HIV.

   (a) True
   (b) False

8. When administering a vaccination, which of the following should you have on hand?

   (a) Immune globulin
   (b) Whole blood
   (c) Plasma
   (d) Epinephrine

9. Passive immunity can also occur through immunization by giving the patient a vaccination against the pathogen.

   (a) True
   (b) False

10. The HIV virus enters the cell through the CD4 molecule on the cell surface.

    (a) True
    (b) False

chapter 18

Gastrointestinal System

At some point, all of us have had a bellyache—especially right before an exam—that suddenly disappeared once the exam was over. However, a stomachache and other aliments of the gastrointestinal system are not as easily cured by removing stress. Some require more sophisticated treatment with medication.

Problems with the gastrointestinal system can include vomiting, ingesting toxins, diarrhea, constipation, peptic ulcers, and gastroesophageal reflux disease. Each is treatable with the proper medication.

In this chapter, you'll learn about common gastrointestinal disorders and about the medications that are frequently prescribed to treat these conditions.

1. A Brief Look at the Gastrointestinal System

The gastrointestinal (GI) system consists of the alimentary canal and the digestive tract that begins with the oral cavity and extends to the anus. The major structures of the GI system are the oral cavity (mouth, tongue, and pharynx), the esophagus, the stomach, the small intestine (duodenum, jejunum, and ileum), the large intestine (cecum, colon, rectum), and the anus.

In addition to these major structures, the GI system has several accessory organs and glands that include the salivary glands, the pancreas, the gallbladder, and the liver.

Food that enters the oral cavity is broken down into small pieces in the mouth. Starches are then digested by amylase found in saliva. Small pieces of food are voluntarily moved to the back of the mouth and moved down to the esophagus in a process

315

commonly referred to as *swallowing*. When the food reaches the esophagus, it is moved to the stomach and intestines with an involuntary movement called *peristalsis*.

The *esophagus* is a tube connecting the oral cavity to the stomach and is lined with mucous membranes that secrete mucus. The esophagus has two sphincters. These are the superior (hyperpharyngeal) sphincter and the lower sphincter, which prevents gastric juices from entering the esophagus (gastric reflux).

The *stomach* is a hollow organ that holds between 1000 and 2000 mL of contents that takes about 2–3 hours to empty. It, too, has two sphincters. These are the cardiac sphincter (located at the opening of the esophagus) and the pyloric sphincter (that connects the stomach to the head of the duodenum).

The stomach has mucosal folds containing glands that secrete gastric juices used to break down food (digest) into its chemical elements. Lipid-soluble drugs and alcohol are absorbed in the stomach. There are four types of cells in the stomach: (1) *chief cells*, which secrete proenzyme pepsinogen (pepsin); (2) *parietal cells*, which secrete hydrochloric acid (HCl); (3) *gastrin-producing cells*, which secrete *gastrin*—a hormone that regulates the release of enzymes during digestion; and (4) *mucus-producing cells*, which release mucus, which protects the stomach lining from the gastric juices.

The small intestine extends from the ileocecal valve at the stomach to the duodenum. The cecum is attached to the duodenum, which is the site where most medication is absorbed. Most foods are also absorbed in the small intestine.

The duodenum releases secretin, which is a hormone that suppresses gastric acid secretion. This results in the intestinal juices having a higher pH than the gastric juices in the stomach. The hormone cholecystokinin is also released. It simulates the flow of bile into the duodenum. Hormones, bile, and the pancreatic enzymes trypsin, chymotrypsin, lipase, and amylase digest carbohydrates, protein, and fat in preparation for absorption in the small intestine.

The small intestine leads into the large intestine, where undigested material from the small intestine are collected. The large intestine also absorbs water and secretes mucus while moving the undigested material—using peristaltic contractions—to the rectum, where it is eliminated through defecation.

2. Gastrointestinal Diseases and Disorders and Methods

Vomiting

Vomiting (emesis) is the expulsion of gastric contents of the stomach through the esophagus and out the oral cavity. It is a protective mechanism that serves to eliminate harmful substances from the stomach and duodenum. Vomiting is sometimes preceded by nausea, which is a queasy sensation, although vomiting can occur without nausea. Vomiting can occur for a number of reasons. These include motion sickness, viral and bacterial infections, food intolerance, surgery, pregnancy, pain, shock, effects of selected drugs, radiation, and disturbances of the middle ear affecting equilibrium.

Vomiting occurs when two major centers in the cerebrum are stimulated. These are the *chemoreceptor trigger zone* (CTZ), which lies near the medulla, and the *vomiting center* in the medulla. The CTZ receives impulses from drugs, toxins, and the vestibular center in the ear. These impulses are transmitted by the neurotransmitter dopamine to the vomiting center. The neurotransmitter acetylcholine is also a vomiting stimulant. Sensory impulses such as odor, smell, taste, and gastric mucosal irritation are transmitted directly to the vomiting center.

When the vomiting center is stimulated, motor neurons respond, causing contraction of the diaphragm, the anterior abdominal muscles, and the stomach. The glottis closes, the abdominal wall moves upward, and the stomach contents are forced up the esophagus.

When vomiting occurs, try to identify the cause before treating the patient. Begin treatment with nonpharmacological measures such as having the patient drink weak tea, flattened carbonated beverages, gelatin, Gatorade, and for children, Pedialyte. Crackers and dry toast may also be helpful.

Nausea and vomiting that occur during the first trimester of pregnancy should be treated with nonpharmacologic remedies since antiemetics can cause possible harm to the fetus.

If dehydration occurs because vomiting is severe, intravenous fluids may be needed to restore body fluid balance.

If nonpharmacological measures fail, then administer antiemetic medication. There are two groups of antiemetics: nonprescription and prescription. Nonprescription antiemetics are purchased over-the-counter (OTC) and are used to prevent motion sickness. They have little effect in controlling severe vomiting. They must be taken 30 minutes before traveling and are not effective once vomiting occurs.

Antihistamine antiemetics such as diphenhydramine (Dramamine), meclizine hydrochloride (Antivert), and diphenhydramine hydrochloride (Benadryl) are OTC medications that prevent nausea, vomiting, and dizziness (vertigo) caused by motion by inhibiting stimulation in the middle ear. They also cause drowsiness, dryness of the mouth, and constipation.

Several OTC drugs—such as bismuth subsalicylate (Pepto-Bismol)—act directly on the gastric mucosa to suppress vomiting. Such drugs can be taken for gastric discomfort or diarrhea. Do not give Pepto-Bismol to children who are vomiting and who might be at risk for Reyes syndrome as it contains salicylates.

Phosphorated carbohydrate solution (Emetrol), a hyperosmolar carbohydrate, is also available OTC. It decreases nausea and vomiting by changing the gastric pH or by decreasing smooth-muscle contractions of the stomach. This drug has a high sugar content and should not be used by diabetics.

Prescription antiemetics act as antagonists to dopamine, histamine, serotonin, and acetylcholine. Antihistamines and anticholinergics act on the vomiting center and decrease stimulation of the CTZ and vestibular pathways.

Antiemetics

There are eight classifications of prescription antiemetics.

Antihistamines

Antihistamines are used to decrease nausea and vomiting that occur after surgery. They are also used for the management of motion sickness and to treat allergic symptoms. Examples are Vistaril (hydroxyzine), Atarax (hydroxyzine), and Phenergan (promethazine).

See antihistamines in the Appendix. Detailed tables show doses, recommendations, expectations, side effects, contraindications, and more; available on the book's website (see URL in Appendix).

Anticholinergics

Anticholinergics are used to prevent and treat nausea, vomiting, and motion sickness. They are also used to treat vertigo that is associated with vestibular system disease. Scopolamine is an example of an anticholinergic agent.

See anticholinergics in the Appendix. Detailed tables show doses, recommendations, expectations, side effects, contraindications, and more and are available on the book's website (see URL in Appendix).

Dopamine Antagonists

Dopamine antagonists suppress emesis by blocking dopamine receptors in the CTZ. These include phenothiazines, butyrophenones, and metoclopramide. Common side effects are extrapyramidal symptoms (EPSs), which are caused by blocking the dopamine receptors—and hypotension. Phenothiazines are the largest group of antiemetics. They are also used for anxiety (see Chapter 15). Dopamine antagonists suppress emesis by blocking dopamine receptors. They act by inhibiting the CTZ. Not all phenothiazines are effective antiemetics. The dose is generally smaller when phenothiazines are used as an antiemetic. Promethazine (Phenergan) is a phenothiazine. It was introduced as an antihistamine with sedative side effects and can be used for motion sickness.

Phenothiazines and the miscellaneous antiemetics such as benzquinamide, diphenidol, metoclopramide, and trimethobenzamide act on the CTZ center.

Chlorpromazine (Thorazine) and prochlorperazine edisylate (Compazine) are tranquilizers used for both psychosis and vomiting.

Butyrophenones include haloperidol (Haldol) and droperidol (Inapsine). They block dopamine receptors in the CTZ. Extrapyramidal side effects (EPSs) are likely to occur if these drugs are used over an extended period of time. Hypotension can also occur.

Metoclopramide (Reglan) suppresses emesis by blocking the dopamine and serotonin receptors in the CTZ. High doses can cause sedation and diarrhea. The occurrence of EPS is more prevalent in children than adults.

Benzodiazepines

Benzodiazepines indirectly control nausea and vomiting. Lorazepam (Ativan) is the choice drug in this category and may be given with metoclopramide.

Serotonin Antagonists

Serotonin antagonists suppress nausea and vomiting by blocking the serotonin receptors in the CTZ and the afferent vagal nerve terminals in the upper GI tract. Two serotonin antagonists—ondansetron (Zofran) and granisetron (Kytril)—are effective in suppressing chemotherapy-induced emesis. They do not block the dopamine receptors. Therefore, they do not cause EPS. Zofran is commonly used to prevent and treat postoperative nausea and vomiting.

Glucocorticoids

Glucocorticoids (corticosteroids) include dexamethasone (Decadron) and methyl-prednisolone (Solu-Medrol). They are administered intravenously for short-term use. This reduces the side effects caused by using glucocorticoids. (See Chapter 12 for a discussion on the use of steroids.)

Cannabinoids (for Cancer Patients)

The cannabinoids act on the cerebral cortex and have the same side effects and adverse reactions as the antihistamines and anticholinergics. These include drowsiness, dry mouth, blurred vision, tachycardia, and constipation. Cannabinoids include dronabinol and nabilone. These drugs should not be administered to glaucoma patients because they dilate the pupils (ie, cause mydriasis). They are contraindicated for use in patients with psychiatric disorders and are also used as an appetite stimulant for patients with AIDS. Side effects include mood changes, euphoria, drowsiness, dizziness, headaches, depersonalization, nightmares, confusion, incoordination, memory lapse, dry mouth, orthostatic hypotension, hypertension, and tachycardia. Less common symptoms include depression, anxiety, and manic psychosis.

Miscellaneous

Miscellaneous antiemetics include benzquinamide hydrochloride (Emete-Con), diphenidol (Vontrol), and trimethobenzamide (Tigan). They do not act strictly as antihistamines, anticholinergics, or phenothiazines. They suppress the impulses to the CTZ. Diphenidol also prevents vertigo by inhibiting impulses to the vestibular area. Benzquinamide appears to have antiemetic, antihistaminic, and anticholinergic effects. It inhibits stimulation to the CTZ center and decreases activity in the vomiting center. It can also increase cardiac output and elevate blood pressure. Side effects and adverse reactions of the miscellaneous antiemetics include drowsiness and anticholinergic symptoms such as dry mouth, increased heart rate, urine retention, constipation, and blurred vision. Benzquinamide should be used cautiously in clients with cardiac problems such as dysrhythmias. It can cause CNS stimulation, including nervousness, excitement, and insomnia. Trimethobenzamide can cause hypotension, diarrhea, and EPS.

A list of antiemetic drugs appears in the Appendix. Detailed tables show doses, recommendations, expectations, side effects, contraindications, and more and are available on the book's website (see URL in Appendix).

Emetics—Inducing Vomiting

When a patient ingests a toxic substance, it may be critical that the toxin be expelled or neutralized before the body can absorb it. Although the use of emetics is no longer the standard of care when a patient ingests a toxic substance, it is important to understand the action of emetic medication. They are classified according to the site of action. Centrally acting emetics include apomorphine and morphine; peripherally acting emetics include mustard, potassium tartrate, and hypertonic sodium chloride. Vomiting should not be induced if the toxin is a caustic substance such as ammonia, chlorine bleach, lye, toilet cleaners, or battery acid. Regurgitating these substances can cause additional injury to the esophagus. Vomiting should also be avoided if petroleum distillates are ingested. These include gasoline, kerosene, paint thinners, and lighter fluid. Vomiting should never be induced in an unconscious patient.

In cases where vomiting is contraindicated, the patient should be administered activated charcoal, which is available in tablets, capsules, or suspension. Charcoal absorbs (detoxifies) ingested toxic substances, irritants, and intestinal gas. Activated charcoal can be given as a slurry (30 g in ≥8 oz of water) or 12.5–50 g in aqueous or sorbitol suspension. It is usually given as a single dose.

In cases where vomiting is desired, use one of the following two ways to expel a toxin:

The nonpharmacological treatment is to induce vomiting by stimulating the gag reflex by placing a finger or a toothbrush in the back of the patient's throat.

Pharmacological treatment involves administering an emetic to induce vomiting. Ipecac is the most commonly used emetic. Ipecac, available OTC, should be purchased as a syrup—not a fluid extract. The syrup induces vomiting by stimulating the CTZ in the medulla and acts directly on the gastric mucosa.

Ipecac should be taken with ≥8 oz of water or juice (do not use milk or carbonated beverages). If vomiting does not occur within 20 minutes, then the dose should be repeated. If vomiting cannot be induced, then administer activated charcoal. The absorption of ipecac is minimal. Protein binding is unknown, and the half-life is short. Duration of action is only 20–25 minutes. Do not attempt to induce vomiting if the patient is not fully awake and alert.

Antidiarrhea Medication

Diarrhea is defined as frequent liquid stools that can be caused by foods, fecal impaction, bacteria (*Escherichia coli*, *Salmonella*), virus (*parvovirus, rotavirus*), toxins, drug reaction, laxative abuse, malabsorption syndrome caused by lack of digestive enzymes, stress and anxiety, bowel tumor, and inflammatory bowel disease such as ulcerative colitis or Crohn's disease.

Diarrhea can be mild (lasting one bowel movement) or severe (lasting several bowel movements). Intestinal fluids are rich in water, sodium, potassium, and bicarbonate, and diarrhea can cause minor or severe dehydration and electrolyte imbalance. The loss of bicarbonate places the patient at risk for developing metabolic acidosis. Severe diarrhea can be life-threatening in young, elderly, and debilitated patients. However, one bowel movement does not need medication. Patients should be advised to stay hydrated and maintain a normal diet.

Children who are not dehydrated should continue to maintain a regular diet, and infants who are breastfeeding should continue to do so unless at least one of the parents is told otherwise by the clinician. Dehydrated children require rehydration (replacement of lost fluid), and suitable oral rehydration solutions are the most physiologic. After being rehydrated, severely affected children will be able to resume a normal diet.

Diarrhea is a symptom of an underlying cause. Therefore, you should treat the underlying cause while treating the diarrhea. Diarrhea can be treated with a combination of medications and nonpharmacological measures such as clear liquids and oral solutions—Gatorade, Pedialyte, or Ricolyte—and intravenous electrolyte solutions.

For example, traveler's diarrhea, also known as "Montezuma's revenge," is an acute condition usually caused by *E. coli* that lasts less than 2 days, but it can become severe. A patient experiencing traveler's diarrhea may be given fluoroquinolone antibiotics and loperamide (Imodium) to slow peristalsis and decrease the frequency of the stools. Fluoroquinolone treats the underlying cause of diarrhea, and loperamide treats the diarrhea itself.

Antidiarrhea medications decrease the hypermotility (increased peristalsis) that stimulates frequent bowel movements. Antidiarrheals should not be used for longer than 2 days and should not be used if a fever is present. Antidiarrhea medication is available in four classifications.

See antidiarrheals listed in the Appendix. Detailed tables show doses, recommendations, expectations, side effects, contraindications, and more and are available on the book's website (see URL in Appendix).

Opiates

Opiates decrease intestinal motility, thereby decreasing persistalsis. Constipation is a common side effect. Examples are tincture of opium, paregoric (camphorated opium tincture), and codeine. Opiates are frequently combined with other antidiarrheal agents and can cause central nervous system (CNS) depression when taken with alcohol, sedatives, or tranquillizers. Duration of action is about 2 hours.

Opiate-Related Agents

Opiate-related agents are drugs that are synthetic compounds similar to opiates. These drugs include diphenoxylate (Lomotil) (50% atropine to discourage abuse; amount of atropine is subtherapeutic) and loperamide. Both are synthetic drugs that are chemically related to meperidine (Demerol). Loperamide causes less CNS depression than diphenoxylate and can be purchased OTC. It protects against diarrhea longer than a similar dose of Lomotil, reduces fecal volume, and decreases intestinal fluid and electrolyte losses. These drugs can cause nausea, vomiting, drowsiness, and abdominal distention. Tachycardia, paralytic ileus, urinary retention, decreased secretions, and physical dependence can occur with prolonged use.

Absorbents

Adsorbents coat the wall of the GI tract and adsorb bacteria or toxins that are causing the diarrhea. Adsorbents include kaolin and pectin, which are combined in the OTC drug Kaopectate, and other antidiarrheals. Pepto-Bismol is considered an adsorbent because it adsorbs bacterial toxins. Bismuth salts can also be used for gastric discomfort. Colestipol and cholestyramine (Questran) are prescription drugs that have been used to treat diarrhea.

Antidiarrhea Combinations

Antidiarrhea combinations are miscellaneous antidiarrheals that include colistin sulfate, furazolidone, loperamide, lactobacillus, and octreotide acetate. You may know these brand-name drugs to alleviate diarrhea: Lomotil (diphenoxylate HCl with atropine sulfate) and parepectolin (paregoric, kaolin, pectin, alcohol). Most contain a synthetic narcotic ingredient.

Constipation

Constipation is the accumulation of hard fecal material in the large intestine. It is a common occurrence for the elderly as a result of insufficient water intake and poor dietary habits. Other factors that cause constipation are fecal impaction, bowel obstruction, chronic laxative use, neurologic disorders such as paraplegia, a lack of exercise, and ignoring the urge to have a bowel movement. Drugs such as anticholinergics, narcotics, and certain antacids can also cause constipation.

Constipation can be treated nonpharmacologically and pharmacologically. The nonpharmacological approach is to include bulk (fiber) and water in the patient's diet and have the patient exercise and develop routine bowel habits. The normal number of bowel movements is 1–3 per day to 1–3 per week. Normal bowel movements vary from person to person.

The pharmacological approach is to administer laxatives and cathartics to eliminate fecal matter. Laxatives promote a soft stool, and cathartics promote a soft-to-watery stool with some cramping. Harsh cathartics that cause a watery stool with abdominal cramping are called *purgatives*. Frequency of the dose determines whether the drug acts as a laxative or a cathartic.

Laxatives should be avoided if there is any question as to whether the patient has an intestinal obstruction, severe abdominal pain, or symptoms of appendicitis, ulcerative colitis, or diverticulitis. Most laxatives stimulate peristalsis. Laxative abuse from chronic use of laxatives is a common problem, especially with the elderly. Dependence can become a problem.

There are four types of laxatives, described in the following paragraphs.

Osmotics (Saline)

Osmotic laxatives (hyperosmolar) are salts or saline products, lactulose, and glycerin. The saline products are composed of sodium or magnesium, and a small amount is systemically absorbed. They pull water into the colon and increase water in the feces to increase bulk, which stimulates peristalsis. Saline cathartics cause a semiformed-to-watery stool depending on dose. However, they are contraindicated for patients who have congestive heart failure.

Osmotic laxatives contain three types of electrolyte salts: sodium salts (sodium phosphate or phosphosoda, sodium biphosphate), magnesium salts [magnesium hydroxide (milk of magnesia), magnesium citrate, magnesium sulfate (Epsom salts)], and potassium salts (potassium bitartrate, potassium phosphate). Serum electrolytes should be monitored to avoid electrolyte imbalance. Good renal function is needed to excrete any excess salts.

High doses of salt laxatives are used for bowel preparation for diagnostic and surgical procedures. Also used for bowel preparation is poly(ethylene glycol) (PEG) with electrolytes, commonly referred to as *Colyte* or *GoLYTELY*. PEG is administered in amounts of 3–4 L over 3 hours. Patients may be advised to keep GoLYTELY refrigerated to make it more palatable. PEG is an isotonic, nonabsorbable osmotic substance that contains sodium salts. Therefore, patients with renal impairment or cardiac disorder can be administered potassium chloride.

Lactulose, another saline laxative, is not absorbed and draws water into the intestines and promotes water and electrolyte retention. Lactulose decreases the serum ammonia level and is useful in liver diseases such as cirrhosis. Glycerin acts like lactulose by increasing water in the feces in the large intestine. The bulk that results from the increased water in the feces stimulates peristalsis and defecation. Patients who have diabetes mellitus should avoid lactulose because it contains glucose and fructose.

Adequate renal function is needed to excrete excess magnesium. Patients who have renal insufficiency should avoid magnesium salts. Hypermagnesemia can result from continuous use of magnesium salts, causing symptoms such as drowsiness, weakness, paralysis, complete heart block, hypotension, flushing, and respiratory depression. Side effects from excess use are flatulence, diarrhea, abdominal cramps, nausea, and vomiting.

Stimulants (Contact or Irritants)

Stimulant laxatives increase peristalsis by irritating sensory nerve endings in the intestinal mucosa. Stimulant laxatives include those containing phenolphthalein (Ex-Lax, Feen-A-Mint, Correctol), bisacodyl (Dulcolax), cascara sagrada, senna (Senokot), and castor oil (purgative). Bisacodyl and phenolphthalein are two of the most frequently used and abused laxatives.

Results occur in 6–12 hours. Stimulant laxatives such as bisacodyl (Dulcolax) are used to empty the bowel before diagnostic tests (eg, barium enema) because they are minimally absorbed from the GI tract. Most are excreted in feces. However, a small amount of bisacodyl absorption excreted in the urine changes the color to reddish-brown. With excessive use, fluid and electrolyte imbalances can occur (especially potassium and calcium). Mild cramping and diarrhea are side effects.

Castor oil is a harsh laxative (purgative) that acts on the small bowel and produces a watery stool within 2–6 hours. Therefore, this should not be taken at bedtime. Castor oil is used mainly for bowel preparation and is seldom used to correct constipation. Castor oil should not be used in early pregnancy because it stimulates uterine contractions, and spontaneous abortion can occur. Prolonged use of castor oil can damage nerves, resulting in loss of intestinal muscular tone.

Bulk-Forming Laxatives

Bulk-forming laxatives are natural fibrous substances that promote large, soft stools by absorbing water into the intestines and increasing fecal bulk and peristalsis. Bulk-forming laxatives are nonabsorbable. Defecation usually occurs within 8–24 hours but can take up to 3 days after the start of therapy for the stool to become soft and formed.

Powdered bulk-forming laxatives are available in flavored and sugar-free preparations and should be mixed and stirred in a glass of water or juice. The patient should drink it immediately, followed by a half to a full glass of water. Insufficient fluid intake can cause the drug to solidify in the GI tract, resulting in intestinal obstruction. Bulk-forming laxatives do not cause dependence and may be used by patients with diverticulosis, irritable bowel syndrome, ileostomy, and colostomy.

Calcium polycarbophil (FiberCon), methylcellulose (Citrucel), fiber granules (Perdiem), and psyllium hydrophilic mucilloid (Metamucil) are examples of bulk-forming laxatives. Patients with hypercalcemia should avoid calcium polycarbophil because of the calcium in the drug. Metamucil is a nondigestible and nonabsorbent substance that, when mixed with water, becomes a viscous solution. Protein binding and half-life for this drug are unknown. It is excreted in the feces. There are no systemic effects. Nausea can occur with excessive use. The dry form can cause abdominal cramps.

Emollients

Emollients (surfactants) are stool softeners (surface-acting drugs) and lubricants used to prevent constipation and decrease straining during defecation by lowering surface tension and promoting water accumulation in the intestine and stool.

Emollients are frequently prescribed for patients after a myocardial infarction (heart attack) or surgery and are also given prior to administration of other laxatives in treating fecal impaction. Docusate calcium (Surfak), docusate potassium (Dialose), docusate sodium (Colace), and docusate sodium with casanthranol (Peri-Colace) are examples of stool softeners.

Lubricants such as mineral oil increase water retention in the stool. Mineral oil absorbs essential fat-soluble vitamins A, D, E, and K. Some of the minerals can be absorbed into the lymphatic system. Side effects include nausea, vomiting, diarrhea, and abdominal cramping. They are not indicated for children, the elderly, or patients with debilitating conditions because these patients can aspirate the mineral oil, resulting in lipid pneumonia.

Emollients are contraindicated in patients with inflammatory disorders of the GI tract, such as appendicitis, ulcerative colitis, undiagnosed severe pain that could be due to an inflammation of the intestines (diverticulitis, appendicitis), pregnancy, spastic colon, or bowel obstruction.

A list of stimulant drugs is provided in the Appendix. Detailed tables show doses, recommendations, expectations, side effects, contraindications, and more and are available on the book's website (see URL in Appendix).

Peptic Ulcer

A *peptic ulcer* is a sore or hole in the lining of the stomach or duodenum; this term is used to describe a lesion in the esophagus, stomach, or duodenum. More specific names are used to describe an ulcer located at a specific site. Duodenal ulcers (the first part of the small intestine) are more common than other types of peptic ulcers. Peptic ulcers are caused by hypersecretion of hydrochloric acid and pepsin that erode the GI mucosal lining.

Anyone can get an ulcer. Most ulcers are caused by an infection with the bacterium *Helicobacter pylori*—not spicy food, acid, or stress—and can be cured with antibiotics in about 2 weeks. The most common ulcer symptom is burning pain in the stomach: 0.5–1.5 hours after eating with gastric ulcers; 2–3 hours for a duodenal ulcer.

Gastric secretions in the stomach maintain a pH between 2 and 5. Pepsin, a digestive enzyme, activates at pH 2, and the acid-pepsin complex of gastric secretions causes mucosal damage. If gastric secretions increase to pH 5, pepsin declines. The *gastric mucosal barrier* (GMB) is a thick, viscous, mucous lining and serves as defense against corrosive substances. The two sphincter muscles—cardiac and pyloric—act as barriers to prevent reflux of acid into the esophagus and the duodenum. Esophageal ulcers result from reflux of acidic gastric secretion into the esophagus as a result of a defective or incompetent cardiac sphincter.

Gastric ulcers frequently occur because of a breakdown of the GMB.

Duodenal ulcers are caused by hypersecretion of acid from the stomach that passes to the duodenum because of the following conditions:

- Insufficient buffers to neutralize the gastric acid in the stomach
- A defective or incompetent pyloric sphincter
- Hypermotility of the stomach

Treatment of peptic ulcers is given in two-drug, three-drug, and four-drug regimens, or a combination medication consisting of multiple drugs combined into one package.

However, the American College of Gastroenterology no longer recommends two-drug regimens since they are not as effective as other treatment regimens. The different classes of medication that may be combined are described in the following paragraphs.

Gastroesophageal Reflux Disease

Gastroesophageal reflux disease (GERD) is an inflammation of the esophageal mucosa caused by reflux of stomach contents into the esophagus. It is caused by a malfunction of the esophageal sphincter brought about by smoking and obesity.

Gastrointestinal reflux disease is treated by administering common antiulcer drugs that neutralize the gastric contents and reduce gastric acid secretion. Once the content is neutralized, the esophageal mucosa has time to heal—freeing the patient of symptoms of GERD.

There are eight groups of anti-ulcer drugs used to treat GERD.

Tranquilizers

Tranquilizers have minimal effect preventing and treating ulcers. However, they reduce vagal stimulation and decrease anxiety. Librax (benzodiazepine) is a commonly prescribed tranquilizer to treat GERD. Librax is a combination of the anxiolytic chlordiazepoxide (Librium) and the anticholinergic clidinium (Quarzan) and is used in the treatment of ulcers.

Anticholinergics

Anticholinergics (antimuscarinics, parasympatholytics) relieve pain by decreasing GI motility and secretion and by inhibiting acetylcholine and blocking histamine and hydrochloric acid. Anticholinergics delay gastric emptying time and are used frequently to treat duodenal ulcers.

Anticholinergics should be taken before meals to decrease the acid secretion that occurs with eating. They should not be taken with antacids because antacids can slow the absorption of anticholinergic administration. Side effects include dry mouth, decreased secretions, tachycardia, urinary retention, and constipation. However, because gastric emptying time is delayed, gastric secretions can be stimulated and actually aggravate the ulceration.

Antacids

Antacids promote ulcer healing by neutralizing hydrochloric acid and reducing pepsin activity. Antacids don't coat the ulcer. There are two types of antacids: those that have a systemic effect and those that do not. A systemic effect occurs when the antacid is absorbed.

Sodium bicarbonate is a systemic antacid that has many side effects, including sodium excess, which causes hypernatremia and water retention. Sodium bicarbonate also causes metabolic alkalosis related to the excess bicarbonate. Therefore, sodium bicarbonate is seldom used to treat peptic ulcers.

Calcium carbonate is most effective in neutralizing acid; however, one-third to one-half of the drug can be systemically absorbed, resulting in acid rebound. Hypercalcemia and "milk-alkali syndrome" can result from excessive use of calcium carbonate. Calcium carbonate is intensified if taken with milk products.

Nonsystemic antacids consist of alkaline salts such as aluminum (aluminum hydroxide, aluminum carbonate) and magnesium (magnesium hydroxide, magnesium carbonate, magnesium trisilicate, and magnesium phosphate). A small degree of systemic absorption occurs with these drugs—mainly with aluminum.

Magnesium hydroxide has greater neutralizing power than aluminum hydroxide; however, magnesium compounds can be constipating in long-term use. A combination of magnesium and aluminum salts neutralizes gastric acid without causing constipation or severe diarrhea. Simethicone (an antigas agent) is found in many antacids.

Histamine2 (H2 Blockers)

Histamine2 blockers prevent acid reflux in the esophagus by blocking the H2 receptors of the parietal cells in the stomach. This results in a reduction of gastric acid secretion and concentration. Histamine2 blockers also cause headaches, dizziness, constipation, pruritus, skin rash, gynecomastia, decreased libido, and impotence. Examples include cimetidine (Tagamet), famotidine (Pepcid), and ranitidine (Zantac).

Proton Pump Inhibitors

Proton pump inhibitors (gastric acid secretion inhibitors, gastric acid pump inhibitors) inhibit gastric acid secretion 90% greater than the H2 blockers because they block the final step of acid production. Both omeprazole (Prilosec) and lansoprazole (Prevacid) are proton pump inhibitors used for the treatment of peptic ulcers and GERD. Those with hepatic impairment should take these drugs with caution and have liver enzymes monitored regularly.

Pepsin Inhibitor

Pepsin inhibitors such as sucralfate (Carafate) are mucosal protective drugs that are nonabsorbable and combine with protein to form a viscous substance that covers the ulcer. This protects it from acid and pepsin. Pepsin inhibitors do not neutralize acid or decrease acid secretions.

Prostaglandin E1 Analog

Prostaglandin analog antiulcer drugs, such as misoprostol (Cytotec), prevent and treat peptic ulcers by suppressing gastric acid secretion and increasing cytoprotective mucus in the GI tract. Prostaglandin analog also moderately decreases pepsin secretion. Prostaglandin analog is an ideal alternative for patients who have gastric distress from taking NSAIDs such as aspirin or indomethacin. Prostaglandin analog should not be taken during pregnancy and by any women of childbearing age.

Gastrointestinal Stimulants

Gastrointestinal stimulants are used to treat nocturnal heartburn caused by GERD and primarily prescribed for patients who do not respond to other drugs or nondrug therapy. Gastrointestinal stimulants increase gastric emptying time, preventing acid reflux into the esophagus. Gastrointestinal stimulants also enhance the release of acetylcholine at the mesenteric plexus. Cisapride (Propulsid) is an example of a gastrointestinal stimulant (ie, gastroprokinetic agent).

Gastrointestinal stimulants should not be used for patients who have cardiac dysrhythmias, especially ventricular tachycardia, ventricular flutter, or fibrillation. Nor should it be used for patients with ischemic heart disease, congestive heart failure, uncorrected electrolyte disorders (hypokalemia, hypomagnesemia), and renal or respiratory failure. An EKG should be done before and during therapy.

See the list of inhibitor drugs in the Appendix. Detailed tables show doses, recommendations, expectations, side effects, contraindications, and more and are available on the book's website (see URL in Appendix).

Summary

The gastrointestinal (GI) system consists of the alimentary canal, and the digestive tract that begins with the oral cavity and extends to the anus. When the GI system malfunctions or is invaded by a microorganism, the patient might experience vomiting, diarrhea, constipation, peptic ulcers, and gastroesophageal reflux disease.

Vomiting (emesis) is the expulsion of gastric contents of the stomach through the esophagus and out the oral cavity. It is caused by motion sickness, viral and bacterial infections, food intolerance, surgery, pregnancy, pain, shock, and the effects of selected drugs, radiation, and disturbances of the middle ear affecting equilibrium. Antiemetic medication is administered to prevent or stop vomiting.

Vomiting can be induced by stimulating the patient to regurgitate ingested toxins by administering an emetic; however, the use of emetics is no longer recommended. Activated charcoal is the drug of choice if the patient ingested an overdose of medications of any type, including caustic materials.

Diarrhea is a frequent liquid stool that can be caused by foods, fecal impaction, bacteria, a virus, or a number of other conditions. Diarrhea can be stopped by administering antidiarrhea medication and treating the underlying cause. Caution should be exercised when using antidiarrhea medication if the patient has experienced only 1–2 diarrhea stools.

Constipation is the accumulation of hard fecal material in the large intestine. Constipation can be relieved by administering laxatives to promote a soft stool and cathartics to promote a soft-to-watery stool with some cramping.

A *peptic ulcer* is a sore or hole in the lining of the stomach or duodenum or a lesion in the esophagus, stomach, or duodenum. Most ulcers are caused by a bacterial infection. Treatment of peptic ulcers is to give a two-drug, three-drug, and four-drug regimen, or combination medication consisting of multiple drugs combined into one package.

Gastroesophageal reflux disease (GERD) is an inflammation of the esophageal mucosa caused by reflux of stomach content into the esophagus. One of eight groups of antiulcer drugs is used to treat GERD.

QUIZ

1. **What cells produce hydrochloric acid in the stomach?**
    (a) Gastrin-producing cells
    (b) Parietal cells
    (c) Mucus-producing cells
    (d) None of the above

2. **Vomiting is caused by**
    (a) viral and bacterial infections.
    (b) motion sickness.
    (c) surgery.
    (d) all of the above.

3. **Ipecac should not be taken with**
    (a) ≥8 oz of water.
    (b) ≥8 oz of juice.
    (c) milk.
    (d) none of the above.

4. **Laxatives should be avoided if there is any question that the patient has an intestinal obstruction or severe abdominal pain.**
    (a) True
    (b) False

5. **Stimulant laxatives increase peristalsis by irritating sensory nerve endings in the intestinal mucosa.**

    (a) True

    (b) False

6. **GERD is caused by**

    (a) a malfunctioning of the stomach mucosa.

    (b) a malfunctioning of the pepsin pump.

    (c) a malfunctioning of the esophageal sphincter.

    (d) none of the above.

7. **Dopamine antagonists suppress emesis by blocking dopamine receptors in the CTZ.**

    (a) True

    (b) False

8. **Serotonin antagonists suppress nausea and vomiting by**

    (a) blocking the glucocorticoids.

    (b) blocking the serotonin receptors in the CTZ and the afferent vagal nerve terminals in the upper GI tract.

    (c) blocking the dexamethasone.

    (d) blocking the dopamine receptors.

9. **An emetic is administered to a patient who ingests toilet cleaner.**

    (a) True

    (b) False

10. **Emollients are frequently prescribed for patients after a myocardial infarction.**

    (a) True

    (b) False

19

Cardiac Circulatory Medications

The cardiovascular system is the highway within the body that distributes oxygen, nutrients, and hormones and transports waste products, such as carbon dioxide, so that they can be removed from the body.

When this highway falters, the flow of traffic slows down, sometimes coming to a complete stop, backing up other systems of the body, and ultimately causing death to tissues and organs.

Fortunately, there are medications available that can treat and prevent cardiovascular disorders. In this chapter, you'll learn about drugs that affect the heart and drugs that keep the vascular system humming.

1. A Brief Look at the Cardiovascular System

The *cardiovascular system* includes the heart, blood vessels (arteries and veins), and blood. Blood rich in oxygen, nutrients, and hormones moves through vessels called *arteries* that narrow to arterioles. Capillaries transport oxygenated blood to cells and absorb waste products such as CO_2, urea, creatinine, and ammonia. The deoxygenated blood is returned to the circulation by the venules and veins for elimination of waste products by the lungs and kidneys. The pumping action of the heart circulates blood through the blood vessels.

333

The heart is divided into four chambers:

1. **Right Atrium:** The right atrium receives deoxygenated blood from the circulation.

2. **Right Ventricle:** The right ventricle pumps unoxygenated blood to the pulmonary artery to the lungs for gas exchange (CO_2 for O_2).

3. **Left Atrium:** The left atrium receives oxygenated blood via the pulmonary vein.

4. **Left Ventricle:** The left ventricle pumps the blood into the aorta for systemic circulation.

The Heart

The heart muscle, called the *myocardium*, has a fibrous covering called the *pericardium*. The endocardium is a three-layered membrane that lines the interior of the heart chambers.

The heart has four valves—two atrioventricular (tricuspid and mitral) and two semilunar (pulmonic and aortic). Atrioventricular valves control blood flow between the atria and the ventricles. Semilunar valves control the blood flow between the ventricles and the pulmonary artery and the aorta.

There are three major coronary arteries: right, left, and circumflex. Each provides nutrients to the myocardium. Blockage in one or more of these arteries can result in a *myocardial infarction* (commonly known as a "heart attack").

The myocardium is capable of generating and conducting its own electrical impulses. The impulse begins in the sinoatrial (SA) node and moves to the atrioventricular (AV) node. The heart beats about 60–80 beats per minute. The ventricle can beat independently at a rate of about 30–40 bpm.

Drugs can affect cardiac contraction by stimulating or inhibiting the heart. Contractions are also influenced by the autonomic nervous system (ANS). The sympathetic nervous system increases heart rate, and the parasympathetic nervous system decreases heart rate (see Chapter 15).

Blood Pressure and Cardiac Performance

Resistance develops as the blood travels through the circulatory system. This resistance is known as *blood pressure*. The average systemic arterial pressure (blood pressure) is 120/80 mmHg. The higher the resistance, the higher the blood pressure.

The total volume of blood expelled by the heart in a minute is referred to as *cardiac output*. The average cardiac output is 4–8 L/min. The amount of blood ejected from the left ventricle during each heartbeat is called the *stroke volume*. The average stroke volume is 70 mL/beat.

As blood flows into the ventricles, the ventricles fill and stretch. The force with which blood flows into the ventricle is called *preload*. The force used to contract the ventricle is called the heart's *contractility*. The resistance to blood ejected by the ventricle is called the *afterload*. Afterload is the opposing pressure in the aorta and systemic circulation to the contraction of the ventricle. These relationships can be expressed in equation format:

[Cardiac output (amount of blood that the heart beats each minute)] = [stroke volume (amount pumped per beat)] × [heart rate (number of beats per minute)]

A change in stroke volume can affect the cardiac output, and a change in the heart rate affects cardiac output. Later in this chapter we will discuss medications that can affect this equation.

Drugs can be used to ease the workload of the heart by increasing or decreasing the preload and afterload, resulting in adjusting the stroke volume and cardiac output. Vasodilators decrease the preload and afterload, thereby decreasing the arterial pressure and cardiac output. Vasopressors increase the preload and afterload, thus increasing the arterial pressure and cardiac output.

Circulation

There are two types of circulation:

1. **Pulmonary Circulation:** In *pulmonary circulation*, the heart pumps deoxygenated blood that contains CO_2 from the right ventricle through the pulmonary artery to the lungs. Oxygenated blood returns to the left atrium by the pulmonary vein.

2. **Systemic (Peripheral) Circulation:** In *systemic circulation*, the heart pumps blood from the left ventricle to the aorta into the general circulation. Blood is carried by the arteries to the arterioles down to the capillary beds, where nutrients in the blood are exchanged with waste products at the cellular level. Blood then returns through the venules to the veins back to the heart.

Blood

Blood is composed of plasma, red blood cells (erythrocytes), white blood cells (WBCs; leukocytes), and platelets. *Plasma* is the fluid component of blood that consists of 90% water and 10% solutes, and constitutes 55% of the total blood volume.

Plasma contains glucose, protein, lipids, amino acids, electrolytes, minerals, lactic and pyruvic acids, hormones, enzymes, oxygen, and carbon dioxide.

Blood provides nutrients, including oxygen, to body cells. Oxygen is carried in the hemoglobin of red blood cells (RBCs). The WBCs are the major defense mechanism of the body and act by engulfing microorganisms. Platelets are present in the blood. They gather at the site of a wound and aggregate (stitch together) to form a clot to stop the bleeding.

Cardiac Drugs

Cardiac drugs regulate heart contraction, heart rate, and heart rhythm. Cardiac drugs also regulate blood flow to the heart muscle. There are three groups of cardiac drugs: glycosides, antianginals, and antidysrhythmics.

Glycosides, known also as *digitalis glycosides*, inhibit the sodium-potassium pump and increase intracellular calcium. This causes the cardiac muscle fibers to contract better. Glycosides have three effects on the heart:

1. A positive inotropic action that increases cardiac muscle contraction.
2. A negative chronotropic action that decreases the heart rate.
3. A negative dromotropic action that decreases conduction of the electrical stimulus.

The effects of glycosides improve heart, peripheral, and kidney function because

- Cardiac output is increased.
- Preload is decreased, improving blood flow to the periphery and kidneys.
- Edema decreases.
- Fluid excretion increases.
- Fluid retention in the lung and extremities is decreased.

Glycoside preparations are also used to correct atrial fibrillation and atrial flutter (cardiac dysrhythmia).

Glycosides include digoxin (Lanoxin), inamrinone lactate (Inocor) and milrinone lactate (Primacor), and positive inotropic bipyridines. The antidote for glycoside toxicity is digoxin immune Fab (Ovine, Digibind).

A list of drugs utilized in the treatment of the heart is provided in the Appendix. Detailed tables show doses, recommendations, expectations, side effects, contraindications, and more; they are available on the book's website (see URL in Appendix).

Heart Failure Medication

Heart failure is treated by using vasodilators to decrease venous blood return to the heart. This results in a decrease in cardiac filling, decreased ventricular stretching, and decreased oxygen demand on the heart.

Vasodilators work in three ways:

- They reduce cardiac afterload, which increases cardiac output.
- They dilate the arterioles of the kidneys to improve renal perfusion and increase fluid loss.
- They improve circulation to the skeletal muscles.

Examples of vasodilators include hydralazine (Apresoline) and minoxidil (Loniten).

Heart failure is also treated with angiotensin-converting enzyme (ACE) inhibitors. These ACE inhibitors dilate venules and arterioles to improve renal blood flow and decrease blood fluid volume; they also moderately decrease the release of aldosterone; sodium retention is reduced, as is fluid retention.

Diuretics are also prescribed to treat heart failure. Diuretics, which will be discussed in detail later in this chapter, are the first line of treatment for reducing fluid volume and are frequently prescribed with digoxin. Spironolactone (Aldactone) is a potassium-sparing diuretic and is effective in treating moderate to severe heart failure. It is more effective than ACE inhibitors. Use of β blockers has been contraindicated for patients in heart failure.

Antianginal Drugs Antianginal drugs (see Table 19–1) are used to treat angina pectoris by increasing blood flow by either increasing oxygen supply to or decreasing oxygen demand of the heart. *Angina pectoris* is acute cardiac pain caused by inadequate blood flow as a result of plaque occlusion in the coronary arteries of the myocardium or spasms of the coronary arteries. The decreased blood flow causes a decrease in oxygen to the myocardium, which is the cause of the pain. Anginal attacks may last for a few minutes and can lead to myocardial infarction (heart attack).

There are three types of angina:

1. **Classic (Stable):** Classic angina occurs with stress and exertion and is caused by the narrowing or partial occlusion of coronary arteries.

2. **Unstable (Preinfarction):** Unstable angina occurs over the course of a day with progressive severity and is caused by the narrowing or partial occlusion of coronary arteries. This often indicates an impending heart attack—a medical emergency.

3. **Variant (Prinzmetal, Vasospastic):** Variant angina occurs at rest and is due to a vessel spasm (vasospasm).

TABLE 19–1 Effects of Antianginal Drugs on Angina		
Drug Group	**Variant (Vasospastic) Angina**	**Classic (Stable) Angina**
Nitrates	Relaxation of coronary arteries, which decreases vasospasms and increases oxygen supply	Dilation of veins, which decreases preload and decreases oxygen demands
β blockers	Not effective	Decreases heart rate and contractility, which decreases oxygen demand
Calcium channel blockers	Relaxation of coronary arteries, which decreases vasospasms and increases oxygen supply	Dilation of arterioles, which decreases afterload and decreases oxygen demand. Verapamil and diltiazem decrease heart rate and contractility

Stress tests, cardiac profile laboratory tests, and cardiac catheterization may be needed to determine the degree of blockage in the coronary arteries. A combination of pharmacologic and nonpharmacologic measures (avoiding heavy meals, smoking, extremes in weather changes, strenuous exercise, and emotional stress) is necessary to control and prevent anginal attacks. Proper nutrition, moderate exercise, adequate rest, and relaxation techniques are also recommended as preventive measures.

Antianginals

Nitrates Nitrates reduce venous tone, resulting in decreased workload of the heart and increased vasodilation. They are used to treat variant angina pectoris. The most commonly prescribed nitrate is nitroglycerin, which can be administered sublingually, intravenously, or topically with patches. There are various types of organic nitrates. Isosorbide dinitrate (Isordil, Sorbitrate) can be administered sublingually (SL) by tablets and orally by chewable tablets, immediate-release tablets, sustained-release tablets, and capsules. Isosorbide mononitrate (Monoket, Imdur) can be given orally by immediate-release or sustained-release tablets.

β Blockers The heart's workload and oxygen demand are decreased by β blockers (see Chapter 15). Examples of β blockers include atenolol (Tenormin), metoprolol tartrate (Lopressor), nadolol (Corgard), and propranolol HCl (Inderal).

Calcium Channel Blockers Calcium channel blockers also decrease the heart's workload and oxygen demands and are used to treat variant angina pectoris. Calcium channel blockers include amlodipine (Norvasc), bepridil HCl (Vascor), and diltiazem HCl (Cardizem), Felodipine (Plendil), and verapamil HCl (Calan, Isoptin).

See "Nitrates" and "Calcium Channel Blocker" entries in the Appendix. Detailed tables show doses, recommendations, expectations, side effects, contraindications, and more and are available on the book's website (see URL in Appendix).

Antidysrhythmics

Antidysrhythmics are drugs that restore normal cardiac rhythm and are used to treat cardiac dysrhythmias. A *cardiac dysrhythmia* is a disturbed heart rhythm. It is also known as *arrhythmia*—absence of heart rhythm. A disturbed heart rhythm is any deviation from the normal heart rate or heart pattern, including slow rates (bradycardia) and fast rates (tachycardia). The electrocardiogram (EKG) is used to identify the type of dysrhythmia.

Table 19–2 lists the actions of antidysrhythmics, and Table 19–3 describes classes of antidysrhythmic drugs.

Cardiac dysrhythmias frequently follow a myocardial infarction (heart attack) or result from hypoxia (lack of oxygen to body tissues), hypercapnia (increased carbon dioxide in the blood), excess catecholamines, or electrolyte imbalance.

TABLE 19–2 Antidysrhythmic Actions
Mechanisms of Action
Block adrenergic stimulation of the heart
Depress myocardial excitability and contractility
Decrease conduction velocity in cardiac tissue
Increase recovery time (repolarization) of the myocardium
Suppress automaticity (spontaneous depolarization to initiate beats)

Antidysrhythmics are grouped into four classes:

1. **Fast (Sodium) Channel Blockers:** Fast channel blockers are 1A (I) (quinidine and procainamide), 1B (II) (lidocaine), and 1C (III) (encainide, flecainide).

2. **β Blockers:** β blockers were discussed previously in this chapter and also in Chapter 15. They include propranolol (Inderal).

3. **Prolonged Repolarization:** *Prolonged repolarization* is the time when the electrical impulse returns to normal and is ready to fire again. The drug of choice for this dysrhythmia is amiodarone (Cordarone).

4. **Slow (Calcium) Channel Blockers:** Slow channel blockers were discussed previously in this chapter and include verapamil (Calan, Isoptin) and diltiazem (Cardizem).

Antihypertensive Drugs

Antihypertensive drugs are used to treat hypertension. Hypertension is classified as follows:

1. **Essential Hypertension:** Essential hypertension affects 90% of patients who are hypertensive and is caused by conditions other than those related to renal and endocrine disorders.

2. **Secondary Hypertension:** Secondary hypertension affects 10% of patients who are hypertensive and is caused by secondary disorders of the renal and endocrine systems.

The exact cause of essential hypertension is unknown. However, there are nine factors that contribute to hypertension:

- Family history of hypertension
- Hyperlipidemia
- African-American ethnicity
- Diabetes
- Obesity

TABLE 19–3 Classes and Actions of Antidysrhythmic Drugs

Classes	Actions	Examples/Side Effects
Class I Sodium channel blockers IA IB IC	 Slows conduction; prolongs repolarization Slows conduction and shortens repolarization Prolongs conduction with little to no effect on repolarization	Procainamide (Pronestyl, Procan) (*less cardiac depression than quinidine, abdominal pain/cramping, nausea, diarrhea, vomiting, flushing, rash, pruritus, lupus-like syndrome with rash*) Quinidine sulfate, polygalactorate, gluconate (Quinidex, Cadioquin) (*nausea, vomiting, diarrhea, confusion, and hypotension*) Lidocaine (Xylocaine) (*cardiovascular depression, bradycardia, and hypotension; dizziness, lightheadedness, and confusion*) Flecainide (Tambocor) (*nausea, vomiting, diarrhea, confusion*)
Class II β blockers	Reduces calcium entry; decreases conduction velocity, automaticity, and recovery time (refractory period)	Esmolol (Brevibloc) (*Generally well tolerated, with transient and mild side effects*) Propranolol HCl (Inderal) (*Decreased sexual ability, drowsiness, difficulty sleeping, unusual tiredness/weakness*)
Class III Prolong repolarization	Prolongs repolarization during ventricular dysrhythmias. Prolongs action potential duration	Adenosine (Adenocard) (*Facial flushing, shortness of breath/dyspnea*) Amiodarone HCl (Cordarone) (*Corneal microdeposits are noted in almost all patients treated for >6 months [can lead to blurred vision], hypotension, nausea, fever, bradycardia, constipation, headache, decreased appetite, nausea, vomiting, numbness of fingers/toes, photosensitivity, muscular incoordination*) Bretylium tosylate (Bretylol) (*Transitory hypertension followed by postural and supine hypotension in 50% of patients observed as dizziness, lightheadedness, faintness, vertigo*)
Class IV Calcium channel blockers	Blocks calcium influx; slows conduction velocity, decreases myocardial contractility (negative inotropic), and increases refraction in the AV node	Verapamil HCl (Calan) (*Constipation, dizziness, lightheadedness, headache, asthenia [loss of strength, energy]*) Diltiazem (Cardizem) (*Peripheral edema, dizziness, lightheadedness, headache, bradycardia, asthenia [loss of strength, weakness], nausea, constipation, flushing, altered EKG*)

- Aging

- Stress

- Diet

- Excessive smoking and alcohol ingestion

There are three stages of hypertension. Along with normal blood pressure (systolic and diastolic), these are as follows:

1. Normal: between <120 and <80

2. Prehypertension: 120–129/80–89 mmHg

3. Stage 1 hypertension: 140–159/90–99 mmHg

4. Stage 2 hypertension: ≥160–179/100–109 mm Hg

Kidneys and Blood Pressure

The kidneys use the renin-angiotensin system needed to maintain blood pressure. The renin-angiotensin system increases blood pressure by retaining sodium and water. Once baroreceptors in the aorta and carotid sinus detect adequate blood pressure, the baroreceptors signal the vasomotor center in the medulla to signal the renin-angiotensin system to excrete sodium and water, thereby lowering the blood pressure.

Hypertension is treated using a stepped-care approach. Each step uses a different group of antihypertensive drugs to control hypertension. There are four steps:

Step 1: Diuretic, β blocker, calcium blocker, angiotensin-converting enzyme (ACE)
Step 2: Diuretic with β blocker, sympatholytics
Step 3: Direct-acting vasodilator; sympatholytic with diuretic
Step 4: Adrenergic neuron blocker; combinations from steps 1, 2, and 3

Combining Antihypertensive Drugs

An antihypertensive drug can be used alone or in combination with one or more drugs that fall into one of five categories.

Diuretics

Diuretics promote sodium depletion, which decreases extracellular fluid volume. It is the first-line drug for treating mild hypertension. Hydrochlorothiazide (HydroDIURIL), a thiazide, is the most frequently prescribed diuretic to control mild hypertension.

Thiazides are not used in patients who have renal insufficiency. Loop diuretics, such as furosemide (Lasix), are usually recommended for these patients because they do not depress renal flow.

Diuretics are not used if hypertension is the result of renal-angiotensin-aldosterone involvement because these drugs tend to elevate the serum renin level. Hydrochlorothiazides are combined with β blockers and ACE inhibitors. ACE inhibitors tend to increase serum potassium (K) levels. When they are combined with the thiazide diuretic, serum potassium loss is minimized.

Sympathetic Depressants (Sympatholytics)

Sympatholytics (see Chapter 15) are divided into five groups:

- β-Adrenergic blockers: acebutolol HCl (Sectral), atenolol (Tenormin), metoprolol (Lopressor), Nadolol (Corgard), propranolol (Inderal)
- Centrally acting sympatholytics (adrenergic blockers): clonidine HCl (Catapres), methyldopa (Aldomet)
- α-Adrenergic blockers: phentolamine (Regitine), doxazosin mesylate (Cardura), terazosin HCl (Hytrin)
- Adrenergic neuron blockers (peripherally acting sympatholytics): guanethidine monosulfate (Ismelin), reserpine (Serpasil)
- α- and β-adrenergic blockers: carteolol HCl (Cartrol, Ocupress)

Direct-Acting Arteriolar Vasodilators

Direct-acting arteriolar vasodilators are step 3 drugs that act by relaxing the smooth muscles of the blood vessels—mainly the arteries—causing vasodilation. Direct-acting arteriolar vasodilators promote an increase in blood flow to the brain and kidneys. Diuretics can be given with direct-acting vasodilators to decrease edema. Reflex tachycardia is caused by vasodilation and the decrease in blood pressure. β blockers are frequently prescribed with arteriolar vasodilators to decrease the heart rate, counteracting the effect of reflex tachycardia. Nitroprusside and diazoxide are prescribed for acute hypertensive emergencies.

A list of drugs utilized in the treatment of hypertension is provided in the Appendix. Detailed tables show doses, recommendations, expectations, side effects, contraindications, and more and are available on the book's website (see URL in Appendix).

Angiotensin Antagonists

Drugs in this group inhibit ACE, which, in turn, inhibits the formation of angiotensin II (vasoconstrictor) and blocks the release of aldosterone. When aldosterone is blocked, peripheral resistance is lowered.

Calcium Channel Blockers

These drugs dilate coronary arteries and arterioles and decrease total peripheral vascular resistance by vasodilation.

Stepped-Care Treatment

The prescribed method of treating hypertension begins with a nonpharmacological approach such as lifestyle changes: losing weight, reducing sodium intake, limiting alcohol intake, smoking cessation, and increasing physical activity.

If blood pressure remains elevated, then treatment moves to the next step. The patient is administered diuretics or β blockers.

If blood pressure still remains high, then the dose of diuretics or β blockers is increased or a calcium channel blocker, ACE inhibitor, angiotensin II blocker, or combination drug replaces or is added to the treatment plan.

If blood pressure does not decrease, the patient is given a diuretic with a β blocker or a second drug is added such as a calcium channel blocker, ACE inhibitor, α blocker, or centrally acting sympatholytic.

If blood pressure still does not decrease, two or three additional drugs are administered to the patient. These include α blockers, direct-acting vasodilators, or adrenergic neuron blockers.

A list of drugs utilized in the treatment of high blood pressure is provided in the Appendix. Detailed tables show doses, recommendations, expectations, side effects, contraindications, and more and are available on the book's website (see URL in Appendix).

Angiotensin Antagonists, ACE Inhibitors, and Angiotensin II Blockers

Angiotensin antagonists (angiotensin-converting enzyme inhibitors) and ACE inhibitors inhibit the formation of angiotensin II (vasoconstrictor) and block the release of aldosterone. Aldosterone promotes sodium retention and potassium excretion. When aldosterone is blocked, sodium is excreted along with water and potassium is retained. These drugs cause little change in cardiac output or heart rate and lower peripheral resistance. They can be used in patients with elevated serum renin levels.

They are used primarily to treat hypertension; some of the agents are also effective in treating heart failure. Examples of these drugs include benazepril (Lotensin), captopril (Capoten), enalapril maleate (Vasotec), enalaprilat (Vasotec IV), lisinopril (Prinivil, Zestril), and ramipril (Altace).

Losartan (Cozaar), valsartan (Diovan), and irbesartan (Avapro) are angiotensin II blockers that block angiotensin II at the receptor site. ACE inhibitors and angiotensin II receptor antagonists are less effective for treating hypertension in African-American persons. They both may cause angioedema. Angioedema is very similar to urticaria, with which it often coexists and overlaps. The swelling occurs especially in the lips and other parts of the mouth and throat, the eyelids, the genitals, and the hands and feet. Angioedema is life-threatening if swelling in the mouth or throat makes it difficult to breathe. Less often the sheer amount of swelling means that so much fluid has moved out of the blood circulation that blood pressure drops dangerously.

Calcium Channel Blockers

As discussed previously in this chapter, calcium channel blockers decrease calcium levels and promote vasodilation. Calcium channel blockers include verapamil (Calan), diltiazem (Cardizem), nifedipine (Procardia), amlodipine (Norvasc), felodipine (Plendil), nicardipine HCl (Cardene), and nisoldipine (Sular).

Calcium channel blockers can be combined with ACE inhibitors. Such combinations include benazepril with amlodipine (Lotrel), enalapril with diltiazem (Teczem), enalapril with felodipine (Lexxel), and trandolapril with verapamil (Tarka).

A list of ACE inhibitor drugs is included in the Appendix. Detailed tables show doses, recommendations, expectations, side effects, contraindications, and more and are available on the book's website (see URL in Appendix).

Diuretics

Diuretics lower blood pressure and decrease peripheral and pulmonary edema in congestive heart failure and renal or liver disorders by inhibiting sodium and water reabsorption from the kidney tubules, resulting in increased urine flow (diuresis).

Most sodium and water reabsorption occurs throughout the renal tubular segments. Diuretics affect one or more of these segments. Every 1.5 hours, the kidneys (glomeruli) clean the body's extracellular fluid (ECF).

Small particles—such as electrolytes, drugs, glucose, and waste products from protein metabolism—are filtered in the glomeruli during this process. Sodium and water are the largest filtrate substances. Larger products—such as protein and blood—are not filtered with normal renal function. Instead, they remain in the circulation.

Nearly all filtered sodium is reabsorbed. Half occurs in the proximal tubules, approximately 40% in the loop of Henle, about 7% in the distal tubules, and the remaining in the collecting tubules.

Diuretics, such as mannitol, that act on the tubules closest to the glomeruli, have the greatest effect in causing sodium loss in the urine (natriuresis).

Diuretics have an antihypertensive effect by promoting sodium and water loss. They block sodium and chloride reabsorption, causing a decrease in fluid volume, a lowering of blood pressure, and a decrease of edema. If sodium is retained, water is also retained in the body and blood pressure increases.

Many diuretics cause loss of other electrolytes, including potassium, magnesium, chloride, and bicarbonate. The diuretics that promote potassium excretion are classified as *potassium-wasting* diuretics. *Potassium-sparing* diuretics promote the reabsorption of potassium. Combination diuretics have been marketed that have both actions.

There are five categories of diuretics that remove water and sodium.

Thiazide and Thiazide-Like Diuretics

Thiazide diuretics include chlorothiazide (Diuril), hydrochlorothiazide (HydroDIURIL, HCTZ), bendroflumethiazide (Naturetin), benzthiazide (Aquatag, Dihydrex), hydroflumethiazide (Saluron, Diucardin); methyclothiazide (Aquatensen, Enduron), polythiazide (Renese-R), trichlormethiazide (Metahydrin, Naqua); thiazide-like diuretics: chlorthalidone (Hygroton), indapamide (Lozol), metolazone (Zaroxolyn), and quinethazone (Hydromox).

Loop or High-Ceiling Diuretics

Loop or high-ceiling diuretics include bumetanide (Bumex), ethacrynic acid (Edecrin), furosemide (Lasix), and torsemide (Demadox).

Osmotic Diuretics

Osmotic diuretics include mannitol and urea (Ureaphil).

Carbonic Anhydrase Inhibitors

Carbonic anhydrase inhibitors include acetazolamide (Diamox), dichlorphenamide (Daranide, Oratrol), and methazolamide (Neptazane).

Potassium-Sparing Diuretics

Potassium-sparing diuretics include amiloride HCl (Midamor), spironolactone (Aldactone), and triamterene (Dyrenium). Combination diuretics include: amiloride HCl and hydrochlorothiazide (Moduretic); spironolactone and hydrochlorothiazide (Aldactazide); and triamterene and hydrochlorothiazide (Dyazide, Maxzide).

Thiazide Diuretics

Thiazides influence the distal convoluted renal tubule beyond the loop of Henle to promote sodium, chloride, and water excretion. Thiazides are used in the treatment of hypertension and peripheral edema, but are not effective for immediate diuresis and should be used mainly with patients with normal kidney function.

Thiazides cause a loss of sodium, potassium, and magnesium and promote calcium reabsorption. They affect glucose tolerance and should be used with caution in clients with diabetes mellitus. Laboratory tests for electrolytes and glucose should be monitored.

Side effects and adverse reactions of thiazides are electrolyte imbalances, hyperglycemia, hyperuricemia (elevated serum uric acid level), and hyperlipidemia (elevated blood lipid levels). They affect the metabolism of carbohydrates.

Other side effects include dizziness, headaches, nausea, vomiting, constipation, and rarely urticaria (hives) and blood dyscrasias.

A list of thiazide diuretic drugs is provided in the Appendix. Detailed tables show doses, recommendations, expectations, side effects, contraindications, and more and are available on the book's website (see URL in Appendix).

Loop or High-Ceiling Diuretics

Loop or high-ceiling diuretics act on the ascending loop of Henle by inhibiting chloride transport of sodium into the circulation. Sodium, potassium, calcium, and magnesium are lost. Loop or high-ceiling diuretics have little effect on blood sugar, but increase the uric acid level.

Loop or high-ceiling diuretics are potent and cause marked depletion of water and electrolytes. They are more potent than thiazides and 2–3 times more effective when inhibiting reabsorption of sodium. However, loop or high-ceiling diuretics are less effective as antihypertensive agents.

Loop or high-ceiling diuretics can increase renal blood flow by ≤40%. This drug is commonly the choice for patients who have decreased kidney function or end-stage renal disease.

Loop or high-ceiling diuretics cause excretion of calcium and have a great saluretic (sodium-losing) effect that causes rapid diuresis, decreases vascular fluid volume, and decreases cardiac output and blood pressure.

Loop or high-ceiling diuretics cause a vasodilatory effect and increase renal blood flow before diuresis. The most common side effects are fluid and electrolyte imbalances such as hypokalemia, hyponatremia, hypocalcemia, hypomagnesemia, and hypochloremia. Hypochloremic metabolic alkalosis may result. Orthostatic hypotension can also occur. Thrombocytopenia, skin disturbances, and transient deafness are seen rarely. Prolonged use can cause thiamine deficiency.

A list of loop diuretic drugs is provided in the Appendix. Detailed tables show doses, recommendations, expectations, side effects, contraindications, and more and are available on the book's website (see URL in Appendix).

Osmotic Diuretics

Osmotic diuretics increase the concentration (osmolality) of the plasma and fluid in the renal tubules. Sodium, chloride, potassium (to a lesser degree), and water are excreted. Osmotic diuretics are used to prevent kidney failure, decrease intracranial pressure (ICP) (cerebral edema), and decrease intraocular pressure (IOP), as is the case with glaucoma.

Mannitol is a potent potassium-wasting osmotic diuretic used in emergencies to treat intraocular pressure. Mannitol is also used with cisplatin and carboplatin in cancer chemotherapy to induce a frank diuresis for decreased side effects of treatment.

Mannitol is the most frequently prescribed osmotic diuretic. The side effects and adverse reactions include fluid and electrolyte imbalance, pulmonary edema from rapid shift of fluids, nausea, vomiting, tachycardia from rapid fluid loss, and acidosis.

Carbonic Anhydrase Inhibitors

The carbonic anhydrase inhibitors block the action of the enzyme carbonic anhydrase, which is needed to maintain acid-base balance (hydrogen and bicarbonate ion balance). Inhibition of this enzyme causes increased sodium, potassium, and bicarbonate excretion. Prolonged use can result in metabolic acidosis.

Carbonic anhydrase inhibitors include acetazolamide dichlorphenamide (Diamox) and methazolamide (Daranide).

Carbonic anhydrase inhibitors are used to decrease intraocular pressure in patients with open-angle (chronic) glaucoma and are not used in narrow-angle or acute glaucoma. Other uses include inducing diuresis, management of epilepsy, and treatment of high-altitude or acute mountain sickness.

Carbonic anhydrase inhibitors can cause fluid and electrolyte imbalance, metabolic acidosis, nausea, vomiting, anorexia, confusion, orthostatic hypotension, and crystalluria. Hemolytic anemia and renal calculi can also occur. Carbonic anhydrase inhibitors are contraindicated in the first trimester of pregnancy.

A list of drugs for carbonic anhydrase inhibitors is provided in the Appendix. Detailed tables show doses, recommendations, expectations, side effects, contraindications, and more and are available on the book's website (see URL in Appendix).

Potassium-Sparing Diuretics

Potassium-sparing diuretics act primarily in the collection of distal duct renal tubules to promote sodium and water excretion and potassium retention. The drugs interfere with the sodium-potassium pump that is controlled by mineralocorticoid hormone aldosterone (sodium retained and potassium excreted). Potassium is reabsorbed and sodium is excreted.

Potassium-sparing diuretics are weaker than thiazides and loops and are used as mild diuretics or in combination with antihypertensive drugs. Continuous use of potassium-wasting diuretics requires a daily oral potassium supplement because potassium, sodium, and body fluid are excreted through the kidneys. However, potassium supplements are not used when the patient takes potassium-sparing diuretics.

When potassium-sparing diuretics are used alone, they are less effective in reducing body fluid and sodium than when used in combination. They are usually combined with a potassium-wasting diuretic, such as a thiazide or loop. The combination intensifies the diuretic effect and prevents potassium loss. The main side effect of these drugs is hyperkalemia.

Caution should be exercised with patients who have poor kidney function. Urine output should be at least 600 mL per day. Patients should not use potassium supplements while taking this group of diuretics. If potassium supplements are given with an ACE inhibitor, hyperkalemia could become severe or life-threatening because both drugs retain potassium. Gastrointestinal disturbances (anorexia, nausea, vomiting, diarrhea) can occur.

A list of potassium-sparing diuretic drugs is provided in the Appendix. Detailed tables show doses, recommendations, expectations, side effects, contraindications, and more and are available on the book's website (see URL in Appendix).

2. Circulatory Disorders

Circulatory disorders impair the flow of blood throughout the body. Circulatory drugs are used to restore and maintain circulation. There are four groups of circulatory drugs:

1. **Anticoagulants and Antiplatelets (Antithrombotics):** Anticoagulants and antiplatelets prevent platelets from clumping together and lower the risk that a patient will develop blood clots.

2. **Thrombolytics:** Thrombolytics are sometimes called "clot busters" because they attack and dissolve blood clots that have already formed.

3. **Antilipemics:** Antilipemics decrease blood lipid concentrations.

4. **Peripheral Vasodilators:** Peripheral vasodilators dilate vessels that have been narrowed by vasospasm.

Anticoagulants and Antiplatelets

A *clot* is a thrombus that has formed in an arterial or venous vessel and is caused by decreased circulation (blood stasis). Anticoagulants such as warfarin and heparin inhibit clot formation but do not dissolve clots that have already formed.

Anticoagulants are given to patients who are at risk for deep venous thrombosis and pulmonary embolism. These patients may have had a myocardial infarction

(MI, heart attack), a cerebrovascular accident (CVA or stroke), or have an artificial heart valve.

Antiplatelet drugs such as aspirin, dipyridamole (Persantine), and sulfinpyrazone (Anturane) are prescribed for the prevention and formation of blood clots (platelet aggregation).

Patients who have chronic or acute atrial fibrillation are also given anticoagulants to prevent the formation of mural thrombi (blood clots in the heart).

Anticoagulants can be administered orally (Coumadin) or parenterally (heparin) to combine with antithrombin III, thus inactivating thrombin and other clotting factors. This prevents the formation of a fibrin clot.

Anticoagulants are poorly absorbed through the GI mucosa and are destroyed by liver enzymes, so they are administered subcutaneously or intravenously. Anticoagulants can be given as an IV bolus or infusion. Clotting time is prolonged, and partial thromboplastin time (PTT) and activated partial thromboplastin time (aPTT) are monitored during therapy.

Anticoagulants decrease platelet count, thereby causing thrombocytopenia. The antidote for heparin is protamine sulfate, which is given intravenously.

When IV therapy is to be discontinued, oral warfarin (Coumadin) and dicumarol are administered simultaneously. However, you must monitor lab values as heparin is gradually stopped and Coumadin is added. The dose of Coumadin is adjusted according to PT values.

The International Normalized Ratio (INR) is the laboratory test used to monitor patients on anticoagulant therapy. Normal INR is 1.3–2.0, and patients on warfarin therapy are maintained at an INR of 2.0–3.0. Monitoring the lab values at regular intervals is required for the duration of drug therapy.

Patients should also be observed for petechiae and ecchymosis, tarry stools, and hematemesis, which all could be indicative of occult (hidden) bleeding. The antidote for the oral anticoagulants is vitamin K (phytonadione) (AquaMEPHYTON).

Low-molecular-weight heparins (LMWHs) are derivatives of standard heparin and include enoxaparin sodium (Lovenox) and dalteparin sodium (Fragmin). They are used for prevention of deep venous thrombosis (DVT).

Low-molecular-weight heparins can be administered at home because PTT monitoring is not necessary. They are given subcutaneously in the abdomen twice a day. The average treatment is for 7–14 days. The half-life of LMWH is 2–4 times longer than that of heparin. Patients should not take antiplatelet drugs such as aspirin while on LMWH medication. Bleeding is less likely to occur, and overdose is rare. However, protamine sulfate is the antidote if necessary, and the dose is 1 mg of protamine for every 1 mg of LMWH given.

A list of anticoagulant low-molecular-weight drugs is provided in the Appendix. Detailed tables show doses, recommendations, expectations, side effects, contraindications, and more and are available on the book's website (see URL in Appendix).

Thrombin Inhibitors

Thrombin inhibitors are anticoagulants that bind to and inhibit the activity of thrombin, thereby preventing clot formation. They are used to prevent arterial and venous thrombosis, prevent and treat DVT, or prevent thromboembolism in atrial fibrillation. Dabigatran (Pradaxa) is an example of a thrombin inhibitor. A list of thrombin inhibitors is provided in the Appendix. Detailed tables show doses, recommendations, expectations, side effects, contraindications, and more and are available on the book's website.

Factor Xa Inhibitors

Factor Xa inhibitors are anticoagulants that block the activity of clotting factor Xa and prevent blood clots from developing or getting worse. They are generally used as prophylaxis in patients having hip or knee replacement. Rivaroxaban (Xarelto) is an example of a factor Xa inhibitor.

A list of thrombin inhibitors is provided in the Appendix. Detailed tables show doses, recommendations, expectations, side effects, contraindications, and more and are available on the book's website (see URL in Appendix).

Thrombolytics

When a blood clot is mobilized, it is called a *thrombus* or *embolus*. It moves through blood vessels, eventually causing a blockage, called a *thromboembolism*, resulting in decreased blood flow (ischemia) that causes death (necrosis) of tissues in the affected area. Thromboembolisms disintegrate naturally in about 2 weeks through the fibrinolytic mechanism, which breaks down fibrin.

Thrombolytics are drugs that promote the fibrinolytic mechanism if administered within 4 hours following an acute myocardial infarction (AMI). An AMI (heart attack) can be caused by a thromboembolism blocking a coronary artery. This results in decreased circulation to that part of the heart. The ischemic (oxygen-devoid) tissue becomes necrotic (dies) if left without an oxygen supply. Thrombolytics prevent or minimize necrosis that results from the blocked artery and therefore decreases hospitalization time. After thrombolytic treatment, the patient is evaluated for cardiac bypass or coronary angioplasty procedures.

Thrombolytics are also used for pulmonary embolism, DVT, and noncoronary arterial occlusion from an acute thromboembolism.

Commonly used thrombolytics are streptokinase, urokinase, tissue plasminogen activator (t-PA, Alteplase), anisoylated plasminogen streptokinase activator complex (APSAC, Anistreplase), and reteplase (Retavase).

All of these drugs induce fibrin breakdown (fibrinolysis).

Allergic reactions can complicate thrombolytic therapy. Anaphylaxis (vascular collapse) occurs more frequently with streptokinase than with the other thrombolytics.

Reperfusion dysrhythmia or hemorrhagic infarction can result if thrombolytics break up the clot after an MI. The major complication using thrombolytics is hemorrhage. The hemorrhage is stopped by using amino(caproic acid) (Amicar) to inhibit plasminogen activation. The use of heparin with thrombolytic medications is commonly done and can prevent formation of new clots but requires intensive care and close monitoring of the patient.

A list of thrombolytic drugs is provided in the Appendix. Detailed tables show doses, recommendations, expectations, side effects, contraindications, and more and are available on the book's website (see URL in Appendix).

Antilipemics

Antilipemics are drugs that lower abnormal blood lipid levels (see Table 19–4). Lipids, composed of cholesterol, triglycerides, and phospholipids, are bound to lipoproteins (see Table 19–5) and are transported in the body. These lipoproteins are classified as follows:

- Chylomicrons
- Very-low-density lipoproteins (VLDLs)
- High-density lipoproteins (HDL)

The HDL ("friendly" or "good" lipoproteins) has a higher percentage of protein and fewer lipids. HDL removes cholesterol from the bloodstream and delivers cholesterol to the liver. The other three lipoproteins are composed of cholesterol and triglycerides and contribute to atherosclerotic plaque in the blood vessels ("bad" lipoproteins).

TABLE 19–4 Serum Lipid Values				
Lipids	Normal Value (mg/dL)	Low Risk (mg/dL)	Level of Risk for CAD Moderate Risk	Level of Risk for CAD High Risk (mg/dL)
Cholesterol	150–240	<200	200–240	>240
Triglycerides	40–190	Values vary with age		>190
Lipoproteins LDL	60–160	<130	130–159	>160
Lipoproteins HDL	29–77	>60	35–50	<35

TABLE 19–5	Hyperlipidemia: Association of Lipoprotein Types II and IV With Coronary Artery Disease
Type	**Major Lipids**
I	Increased chylomicrons and increased triglycerides. Uncommon.
IIA	Increased low-density lipoprotein (LDL) and increased cholesterol.
IIB	Increased very low-density lipoprotein (VLDL), increased LDL, increased cholesterol and triglycerides. Very common.
III	Moderately increased cholesterol and triglycerides. Uncommon.
IV	Increased VLDL and markedly increased triglycerides. Very common.
V	Increased chylomicrons, VLDL, and triglycerides. Uncommon.

When cholesterol, triglycerides, and LDL are elevated, the patient is at increased risk for coronary artery disease.

Before antilipemics are administered, patients are treated with nonpharmacological methods to reduce cholesterol and saturated fats in their diets. Total fat intake should be 30%. They are also encouraged to exercise. Hereditary factors significantly influence cholesterol levels and are considered nonmodifiable risk factors.

Antilipemics include cholestyramine (Questran), colestipol (Colestid), clofibrate (Atromid-S), gemfibrozil (Lopid), nicotinic acid, and niacin (vitamin B$_2$).

Clofibrate is not used for long-term treatment because of its many side effects such as cardiac dysrhythmias, angina, thromboembolism, and gallstones.

Nicotinic acid is effective in lowering cholesterol levels, but it, too, has numerous side effects, including GI disturbances, flushing of the skin, abnormal liver function (elevated serum liver enzymes), hyperglycemia, and hyperuricemia. Required large doses make it intolerable for most patients.

Probucol is poorly absorbed and is not as effective as the other antilipemic drugs. Probucol also causes diarrhea and is contraindicated in patients with cardiac dysrhythmias.

Cholestyramine lowers cholesterol levels, but causes constipation and peptic ulcer.

Statin drugs inhibit the enzyme HMG CoA reductase in cholesterol biosynthesis. They inhibit cholesterol synthesis in the liver, decrease the concentration of cholesterol, decrease the LDL, and slightly increase the HDL cholesterol.

Reduction of LDL is seen in as early as 2 weeks.

Statins include atorvastatin calcium (Lipitor), cerivastatin (Baycol), fluvastatin (Lescol), lovastatin (Mevacor), pravastatin sodium (Pravachol), and simvastatin (Zocor).

A list of antihyperlipidemic HMG-CoA reductase inhibitor drugs is provided in the Appendix. Detailed tables show doses, recommendations, expectations, side effects, contraindications, and more and are available on the book's website (see URL in Appendix).

Peripheral Vascular Disease

A common problem in the elderly is peripheral vascular disease. It is characterized by numbness and coolness of the extremities, intermittent claudication (pain and weakness of limbs when walking and absence of symptoms when the patient is at rest), and possible leg ulcers. The primary cause is hyperlipidemia, resulting in atherosclerosis and arteriosclerosis. The arteries become occluded.

Peripheral vasodilators increase blood flow to the extremities and are used for venous and arterial disorders. They are more effective for disorders resulting from vasospasm (Raynaud's disease) than from vessel occlusion or arteriosclerosis [arteriosclerosis obliterans, thromboangiitis obliterans (Buerger's disease)]. Some of the drugs that promote vasodilation include tolazoline (Priscoline), an α-adrenergic blocker (Chapter 15); isoxsuprine (Vasodilan) and nylidrin (Arlidin); β-adrenergic agonists (Chapter 15); and cyclandelate (Cyclan), nicotinyl alcohol, and papaverine (Cerespan, Genabid), direct-acting peripheral vasodilators. The α blocker prazosin (Minipress) and the calcium channel blocker nifedipine (Procardia) have also been used.

A list of vasodilator drugs is provided in the Appendix. Detailed tables show doses, recommendations, expectations, side effects, contraindications, and more and are available on the book's website (see URL in Appendix).

Summary

The cardiovascular system consists of the heart, blood vessels, and blood that are used to distribute oxygen, nutrients, and hormones and to transport waste products so that they can be removed from the body.

Cardiac drugs regulate heart contraction, heart rate, and heart rhythm and regulate blood flow to the heart muscle. There are three groups of cardiac drugs: glycosides, antianginals, and antidysrhythmics.

Glycosides are known as *digitalis glycosides*. They inhibit the sodium-potassium pump and increase intracellular calcium. As a result, there is an increase in cardiac muscle contraction, a decrease in heart rate, and a decrease in conduction of electrical stimulus to the heart.

Antianginal drugs are used to treat angina pectoris by increasing blood flow by either increasing oxygen supply or decreasing oxygen demand of the heart. *Antidysrhythmics* are drugs that restore normal cardiac rhythm and are used to treat cardiac dysrhythmias.

Antihypertensive drugs are used to treat hypertension by employing a stepped-care approach where groups of antihypertensive drugs are used in succession if blood pressure is not decreased. Angiotensin antagonists are used primarily to treat hypertension, and some are also effective in treating heart failure.

Diuretics lower blood pressure and decrease peripheral and pulmonary edema in congestive heart failure. In patients with renal or liver disorders, diuretics inhibit sodium and water reabsorption from the kidney tubules, resulting in an increase in urine flow.

Circulatory disorders impair the flow of blood throughout the body. Circulatory drugs are used to restore and maintain circulation. There are four groups of circulatory drugs: *anticoagulants* and *antiplatelets*, which prevent blood clots from forming; *thrombolytics*, which dissolve blood clots; *antilipemics*, which decrease blood lipids; and *peripheral vasodilators*, which dilate vessels narrowed by vasospasm.

QUIZ

1. **Vasodilators work by**
   (a) reducing cardiac afterload.
   (b) dilating the arterioles of the kidneys.
   (c) improving circulation to the skeletal muscles.
   (d) all of the above.

2. **What type of angina occurs over the course of a day?**
   (a) Stable
   (b) Preinfarction
   (c) Class angina
   (d) Distal angina

3. **β blockers**
   (a) decrease the workload of the heart and decrease the heart's oxygen demands.
   (b) increase the workload of the heart and decrease the heart's oxygen demands.
   (c) decrease the workload of the heart and increase the heart's oxygen demands.
   (d) do none of the above.

4. **Repolarization is the time when the electrical impulses return to normal.**
   (a) True
   (b) False

5. **Thiazides are not used with patients who have renal insufficiency.**
   (a) True
   (b) False

6. **Many diuretics cause a loss of**

    (a) potassium.

    (b) magnesium.

    (c) bicarbonate.

    (d) all of the above.

7. **Loop diuretics increase renal blood flow before diuresis.**

    (a) True

    (b) False

8. **Carbonic anhydrase inhibitors**

    (a) decrease intraocular pressure in patients with open-angle glaucoma.

    (b) decrease intraocular pressure in patients with narrow-angle glaucoma.

    (c) decrease intraocular pressure in patients with acute glaucoma.

    (d) increase intraocular pressure in patients with open-angle glaucoma.

9. **Potassium-sparing diuretics act primarily in the collection of distal duct renal tubules to promote sodium and water excretion and potassium retention.**

    (a) True

    (b) False

10. **Osmotic diuretics increase the concentration of the plasma and fluid in the renal tubules.**

    (a) True

    (b) False

chapter 20

Skin Disorders

The least appreciated organ in the body is your skin. Yet your skin is the largest organ of the integumentary system and first line of defense against infection. Injury to the skin can have far more resounding repercussions than leaving an unflattering blemish. When the integrity of the skin is disrupted, it leaves an open door to infection and fluid loss, which can be life-threatening.

There are many disorders that can affect your skin, including acne; dry skin; a rash; and injuries such as cuts, scrapes, puncture wounds, and burns. Some disorders are annoying, while others endanger your existence.

You'll learn about common disorders in this chapter and about the medications used to help treat those disorders.

1. A Brief Look at the Skin

Skin is the largest organ of the body. It is composed of two major layers: the *epidermis*, which is the outer layer; and the *dermis*, which is beneath the epidermis. The skin protects the body from the environment, aids in controlling the body's temperature, and prevents the body's fluid loss.

The epidermis has four layers: the *basal layer* (stratum germinativum), which is the deepest layer covering the dermis; the *spinous layer* (stratus spinosum); the *outer layer*; and the *cornified layer* (stratum corneum).

Epidermal cells migrate from the basal layer to the surface of the skin, where cells die. Their cytoplasm is converted to *keratin*, which is the hard, rough texture that forms keratinocytes. Eventually keratinocytes slough off and new layers of epidermal cells migrate upward.

The dermis has two layers: the *papillary layer*, which is next to the epidermis; and the *reticular layer*, which is the deeper layer of the dermis. Dermal layers are composed of fibroblasts, collagen fibers, and elastic fibers. Collagen and elastic fibers give the skin strength and elasticity. The dermal layer contains sweat glands, hair follicles, sebaceous glands, blood vessels, and sensory nerve terminals.

Subcutaneous tissue lies under the dermis and supports and protects the dermis. Subcutaneous tissue consists of fatty tissue, blood and lymphatic vessels, nerve fibers, and elastic fibers.

2. Skin Disorders

The skin is the site of several common disorders that include acne vulgaris, psoriasis, eczema dermatitis, contact dermatitis, drug-induced dermatitis, and burns. Some disorders result from viral infections such as herpes simplex and herpes zoster. Some result from fungal infections such as tinea pedis (athlete's foot) and tinea capitis (ringworm).

Lesions may also appear on the skin as macules (flat with varying colors), papules (raised, palpable, and <1 cm in diameter), vesicles (raised, filled with fluid, and <1 cm in diameter), or plaques (hard, rough raised, and flat on top).

Nearly all the disorders can be treated using mild or aggressive drug therapy in the form of topical creams, ointments, pastes, lotions, and solutions—some of which are available over the counter.

Acne Vulgaris

Acne vulgaris, commonly called "acne," is inflammation of the pilosebaceous glands. These are the glands that produce oil for the hair. Acne is more likely to occur in adolescent males. Genetics appear to be the cause of 80% of acne cases. Diet and smoking do not have any clear association with acne, nor do cleanliness and exposure to sun.

Inflammation of the pilosebaceous glands form papules, nodules, and cysts on the face, neck, shoulders, and back as a result of keratin plugs at the base of the pilosebaceous oil glands near the hair follicles.

The increase in androgen production that occurs during adolescence increases the production of sebum, an oily skin lubricant. Sebum combines with keratin to form a keratin plug. An individual has little control over acne breakouts. Acne is significantly influenced by age, heredity, stress, hormonal changes, and onset of puberty. All of these factors are beyond the patient's control.

TABLE 20-1 Medication for Systemic Therapy	
Nonhormonal Treatment	Hormonal Treatment
Antibiotics, oral	Corticosteroids
Tetracycline	Anti-inflammatory actions: high dose
Erythromycin	Androgen suppressant action: low dose
Minocycline	Sex hormones (for women only)
Trimethoprim-sulfamethoxazole	Estrogen (oral contraceptive medication)
Isotretinoin, oral	Antiandrogens

Acne is treated by gently applying a cleansing agent several times a day to the skin. Vigorous scrubbing should be avoided. In addition, the patient can administer topical antiacne medication such as keratolytics. These include benzoyl peroxide, resorcinol, and salicylic acid that dissolves keratin, the outer layer of the epidermis.

A patient who has a severe case of acne vulgaris that results in scarring has persistent hyperpigmentation, or whose acne persists despite topical treatment should undergo systemic treatment (see Table 20–1).

A list of drugs utilized in the treatment of skin disorders is provided in the Appendix. Detailed tables show doses, recommendations, expectations, side effects, contraindications, and more and are available on the book's website (see URL in Appendix).

Psoriasis

Psoriasis is a chronic skin disorder characterized by erythematous papules and plaques covered with silvery scales appearing on the scalp, elbows, palms of the hands, knees, and soles of the feet. It is caused by an accelerated growth of epidermal cells—more than 5 times its normal rate. Less than 3% of the population of the United States is affected by psoriasis. More Caucasians are affected than African-Americans, and onset occurs between 10 and 30 years of age.

Patients who have psoriasis are treated with antipsoriatic medications that loosen erythematous papules and plaques. However, patients usually experience periods of exacerbation and remission.

- **Vitamin D Analogs:** These synthetic forms of vitamin D slow down the growth of skin cells. Calcipotriene (Dovonex) is a prescription cream or solution containing a vitamin D analog that may be used alone to treat mild to moderate psoriasis or in combination with other topical medications or phototherapy. This treatment can irritate the skin. Calcitriol (Rocaltrol) is expensive but may be equally effective and possibly less irritating than calcipotriene.

- **Anthralin:** This medication is believed to normalize DNA activity in skin cells. Anthralin (Dritho-Scalp) also can remove scale, making the skin smoother. However, anthralin can irritate skin, and it stains virtually anything it touches, including skin, clothing, countertops, and bedding. For that reason, physicians often recommend short-contact treatment, allowing the cream to stay on the skin for a brief time before washing it off.

- **Topical Retinoids:** These are commonly used to treat acne and sun-damaged skin, but tazarotene (Tazorac, Avage) was developed specifically for the treatment of psoriasis. Like other vitamin A derivatives, it normalizes DNA activity in skin cells and may decrease inflammation. The most common side effect is skin irritation. It may also increase sensitivity to sunlight, so sunscreen should be applied while using the medication. Although the risk of birth defects is far lower for topical retinoids than for oral retinoids, tazarotene is not recommended for someone who is or intends to become pregnant or is breastfeeding.

- **Calcineurin Inhibitors:** Currently, calcineurin inhibitors—tacrolimus (Prograf) and pimecrolimus (Elidel)—are approved only for the treatment of atopic dermatitis, but studies have shown them to be effective at times in the treatment of psoriasis. Calcineurin inhibitors are thought to disrupt the activation of T cells, which, in turn, reduces inflammation and plaque buildup.

Calcineurin inhibitors are not recommended for long-term or continuous use because of a potential increased risk for skin cancer and lymphoma. They may be especially helpful in areas of thin skin, such as around the eyes, where steroid creams or retinoids may be too irritating or cause harmful effects.

- **Salicylic Acid:** Available over the counter (OTC; nonprescription) and by prescription, salicylic acid promotes sloughing of dead skin cells and reduces scaling. Sometimes it is combined with other medications, such as topical corticosteroids or coal tar, to increase its effectiveness. Salicylic acid is available in medicated shampoos and scalp solutions to treat scalp psoriasis.

- **Coal Tar:** A thick, black by-product of the manufacture of petroleum products and coal, coal tar is probably the oldest treatment for psoriasis. It reduces scaling, itching, and inflammation. Exactly how it works is unknown. Coal tar has few known side effects, but it is messy, stains clothing and bedding, and has a strong odor. Coal tar is available in OTC shampoos, creams, and oils. It is also available in higher concentrations by prescription. This treatment is not recommended for women who are pregnant or breastfeeding.

- **Moisturizers:** By themselves, moisturizing creams will not heal psoriasis, but they can reduce itching and scaling and can help combat the dryness that results from other therapies. Moisturizers in an ointment base are usually more effective than are lighter creams and lotions.

See "Antipsoriatic" in the Appendix. Detailed tables show doses, recommendations, expectations, side effects, contraindications, and more and are available on the book's website (see URL in Appendix).

Warts

A *wart* is a benign lesion characterized as a hard, horny nodule that may appear anywhere on the body, but particularly on the hands and feet. Warts are removed by freezing, electrodesiccation, or surgical excision.

Salicylic acid, podophyllum resin, and cantharidin are three medications commonly used to remove warts. Salicylic acid promotes desquamation. However, salicylic acid is also absorbed through the skin, and this can result in salicylism (toxicity).

Podophyllum resin is used to remove venereal warts, but it is not as effective against the common wart. Podophyllum also can be absorbed through the skin, resulting in toxic symptoms such as peripheral neuropathy, blood dyscrasias, and kidney impairment. Podophyllum can cause teratogenic effects and should not be used during pregnancy.

Cantharidin (Cantharone, Verr-Canth) is used to remove the common wart, but it can be harmful to the normal skin. Cantharidin is applied topically, allowed to dry, and covered with a nonporous tape for 24 hours. This treatment is repeated in a week or two.

Dermatitis

Dermatitis is a skin eruption that is caused by medications (drug-induced dermatitis) or by a chemical agent coming in contact with the skin (contact dermatitis).

Drug-induced dermatitis is characterized by skin lesions that can be a rash, urticaria, papules, vesicles or life-threatening skin eruptions such as erythema multiforme (red blisters over a large portion of the body), or Stevens-Johnson syndrome (large blisters in the oral and anogenital mucosa, pharynx, eyes, and viscera). As a result of having a hypersensitive reaction to a drug, the patient may form sensitizing lymphocytes.

If the patient received multiple drug therapy, the last drug administered to the patient may have caused hypersensitivity and skin eruptions. Drug-induced dermatitis may take a few minutes, several hours, or a day for urticaria (hives) to appear. Certain drugs such as penicillin are known to cause hypersensitivity.

Other types of drug-induced dermatitis include discoid lupus erythematosus (DLE) and exfoliative dermatitis. Hydralazine hydrochloride (Apresoline), isoniazid (INH), phenothiazines, anticonvulsants, and antidysrhythmics such as procainamide (Pronestyl) may cause lupus-like symptoms. If lupus-like symptoms occur, the drug should be discontinued.

Certain antibacterials and anticonvulsants may cause exfoliative dermatitis, resulting in erythema of the skin, itching, scaling, and loss of body hair.

Contact dermatitis, also called *exogenous dermatitis*, is caused by chemical or plant irritation and is characterized by a skin rash with itching, swelling, blistering, oozing, or scaling at the affected skin sites. The chemical contact may include cosmetics, cleansing products (soaps and detergents), perfume, clothing, dyes, and topical drugs. Plant contacts include poison ivy, poison oak, and poison sumac.

Nonpharmacological treatment of contact dermatitis includes avoiding direct contact with the causative irritant. The patient should use protective gloves and clothing if the chemical agent is associated with his/her employment.

At the first sign of contact dermatitis, clean the skin area immediately. Patch testing may be needed to determine the causative factor. Apply wet dressings containing Burow's solution (aluminum acetate), lotions such as calamine that contain zinc oxide, calcium hydroxide solution, and glycerin. Calamine lotion may contain the antihistamine diphenhydramine and is used primarily for plant irritations. If itching persists, antipruritics [topical or systemic diphenhydramine (Benadryl)] may be used. Topical antipruritics should not be applied to open wounds or near the eyes or genital area.

Other medications used as antipruritics are as follows:

- Systemic drugs such as cyproheptadine hydrochloride (Periactin) and trimeprazine tartrate (Temaril)

- Antipruritic baths of oatmeal such as Alpha-Keri

- Solutions of potassium permanganate, aluminum subacetate, or normal saline

- Glucocorticoid ointments, creams, or gels

Topical glucocorticoids can aid in alleviating dermatitis (see Table 20–2). These include dexamethasone (Decadron) cream, hydrocortisone ointment or cream, methylprednisolone acetate (Medrol) ointment, triamcinolone acetonide (Aristocort), and flurandrenolide (Cordran).

Topical glucocorticoids are systemically absorbed into the circulation depending on whether it is a cream or a lotion, drug concentration, drug composition, and skin area to which the glucocorticoid is applied.

Absorption is greater at the face, scalp, eyelids, neck, axilla, and genitalia with prolonged use of the topical drug and if the drug is continuously covered with a dressing. Prolonged use of topical glucocorticoids can cause thinning of the skin with atrophy of the epidermis and dermis, and purpura from small-vessel eruptions.

TABLE 20–2 Topical Glucocorticoids		
Potency	**Drug Name**	**Drug Form**
High	Amcinonide 0.1% (Cyclocort)	Cream, ointment
	Betamethasone dipropionate 0.05% (Diprosone)	Cream, ointment, lotion
	Desoximetasone 0.25% (Topicort)	Cream, ointment
	Desoximetasone 0.05%	Gel
	Diflorasone diacetate 0.05% (Florone)	Cream, ointment
	Halcinonide 0.1% (Halog)	Cream, ointment
	Triamcinolone acetonide 0.5% (Aristcort A, Kenalog)	Cream, ointment
Moderate	Betamethasone benzoate 0.025% (Benisone)	Cream, ointment
	Betamethasone valerate 0.1% (Valisone)	Cream, ointment, lotion
	Desoximetasone 0.05% (Topicort LP)	Cream, gel
	Fluocinolone acetonide 0.025% (Fluonid)	Cream, ointment
	Flurandrenolide 0.025% (Cordran, Cordran SP)	Cream, ointment, lotion
	Halcinonide 0.025% (Halog)	Cream, ointment
	Hydrocortisone valerate 0.2% (Westcort)	Cream, ointment
	Mometasone furoate 0.1% (Elocon)	Cream, ointment, lotion
	Triamcinolone acetonide (0.025–0.1%) (Aristocort A, Kenalog)	Cream, ointment, lotion
Low	Dexamethasone 0.1% (Decadron)	Cream
	Desonide 0.05% (Tridesilon)	Cream
	Fluocinolone acetonide 0.02% (Fluonid)	Solution
	Hydrocortisone 0.25%, 0.5%, 1.0%, 2.5% (Cortef, Hytone)	Cream, ointment
	Methylprednisolone acetate 0.25%, 1.0% (Medrol)	Ointment

Eczema

The term *eczema* is used in two different ways. It can be used widely to describe any rash-like skin conditions. Or it can be used to describe atopic dermatitis, a chronic skin condition that commonly starts during infancy and continues into childhood. The specific cause of eczema remains unknown, but it is believed to develop because of a combination of hereditary (genetic) and environmental factors. Children are more likely to develop eczema if a parent has had it or another atopic disease. If both parents have an atopic disease, the chances increase further. Environmental factors are also known to bring out the symptoms of eczema, including the following:

- *Irritants*—soaps, detergents, shampoos, disinfectants, juices from fresh fruits, meats, or vegetables can irritate the skin.
- *Allergens*—infestation or contact with dust mites, pets, pollens, mold, and dandruff can lead to eczema.

- *Microbes*—bacteria such as *Staphylococcus aureus*, viruses, and certain fungi can infect the skin.
- *Hot and cold temperatures*—hot weather, high and low humidity, and perspiration from exercise are also predisposing factors.
- *Foods*—dairy products, eggs, nuts and seeds, soy products, and wheat can produce allergic reactions that lead to eczema.
- *Stress*—this is not a cause of eczema but can exacerbate the symptoms.
- *Hormones*—women can experience worsening of eczema symptoms at times when their hormone levels are changing, such as during pregnancy and at certain points in the menstrual cycle.

There is no cure for eczema. Treatment can include home therapies and medications:

- Taking regular warm baths
- Applying moisturizer within 3 minutes of bathing to "lock in" moisture
- Moisturizing the skin every day
- Wearing cotton and soft fabrics and avoiding rough, scratchy fibers, and tight-fitting clothing
- Using mild soap or a nonsoap cleanser when washing
- Air drying or gently patting skin dry with a towel, rather than rubbing skin dry after bathing
- Avoiding rapid changes of temperature and activities that induce perspiration (where possible)
- Learning individual eczema triggers and avoiding them
- Using a humidifier in dry or cold weather
- Keeping fingernails short to prevent scratching from breaking skin

There are several medications that can be prescribed by physicians to treat the symptoms of eczema:

- Topical corticosteroid creams and ointments can be applied. These agents are a type of anti-inflammatory medication and should relieve the main symptoms of eczema, such as skin inflammation and itchiness.
- If these medications are ineffective, systemic corticosteroids can be prescribed. These are either injected or taken by mouth; they are used only for short periods of time.
- Antibiotics can be administered if there is an overlying bacterial skin infection.
- Medications can be applied to treat fungal and viral infections.

- Antihistamines that cause drowsiness are often recommended as these drugs can help to reduce the risk of nighttime scratching.

- Topical calcineurin inhibitors, a type of drug that suppresses the activities of the immune system, which decreases inflammation and helps prevent flare-ups, can be administered.

- Barrier repair moisturizers, which reduce water loss and work to repair the skin, can be applied.

- Phototherapy can be prescribed to treat mild to moderate dermatitis. It involves exposure to ultraviolet A or B waves, alone or combined. The skin should be monitored carefully.

Alopecia (Male Pattern Baldness)

Alopecia occurs when the hair shaft is lost and the hair follicle cannot regenerate. This results in permanent hair loss. Alopecia is associated with a familial history and the aging process. Some patients experience alopecia earlier than others.

Some medications can cause temporary alopecia. These include anticancer (antineoplastic) agents, gold salts, sulfonamides, anticonvulsants, aminoglycosides, and nonsteroidal anti-inflammatory drugs (NSAIDs) such as indomethacin.

Severe febrile illnesses, pregnancy, myxedema (a condition resulting from hypothyroidism), and cancer therapies are conditions contributing to temporary hair loss.

A 2% minoxidil (Rogaine) solution has been approved by the FDA for treating alopecia. Minoxidil causes vasodilation. This increases cutaneous blood flow and stimulates hair follicle growth. However, alopecia returns within 3–4 months after the patient stops using minoxidil. Systemic absorption of minoxidil is minimal, and adverse reactions seldom occur.

Burns

A burn causes lesions that break down skin, exposing the body to infection. There are three causes of burns: heat (thermal), electricity (electrical), and chemicals. All cause the same kind of skin lesion.

Burns are classified by degree, which is based on the tissue depth of the burn. There are three burn classifications: first-degree, second-degree, and third-degree. Burns are assessed by the percentage of body area that has been burned. This is commonly referred to as the "rule of nines" (see Table 20–3). For example, if a patient's left leg is burned, then 18% of the patient's body is burned.

First-Degree (Superficial) Burns

First-degree burns affect only the epidermis (outer layer) of skin. The burn site is red, painful, dry, and devoid of blisters such as those seen in a mild sunburn. Rarely is there

TABLE 20–3 Rule of Nines	
Body Area	Percentage Assessed
Head	9%
Front torso	18%
Back torso	18%
Right arm	9%
Left arm	9%
Right leg	18%
Left leg	18%
Groin	1%

any long-term tissue damage, and it usually results in an increase or decrease in the skin color.

Treatment involves placing a cold, wet compress on the burned area in order to constrict blood vessels and reduce swelling and pain. Less tissue damage occurs if the burned area is cooled quickly. Remove clothing immediately and flush the burned area with water if a chemical agent caused the burn.

Do not apply greasy ointments, butter, or a dressing to the burned area. This inhibits heat loss and increases tissue damage. Bacitracin with polymyxin B (Polysporin) and similar OTC antibiotics should be used.

Second-Degree (Partial-Thickness) Burns

Second-degree burns expose the epidermis and part of the dermis layer of skin. The burn site appears red and blistered and may be swollen and painful.

These burns can be quite painful and can become infected easily. They should be cleaned with a nonabrasive solution, treated with antibiotic ointment such as silver sulfadiazine (Silvadine) and protected with a nonstick dressing, and the patient should be given an analgesic according to the amount of area burned and the pain experienced.

Third-Degree (Full-Thickness) Burns

Third-degree burns destroy the epidermis and dermis and may also damage underlying nerves, bones, muscles, and tendons. The burn site appears white or charred, and the patient has no sensation in the area since the nerve endings are destroyed.

Third-degree burns can be very painful because they are generally mixed (that is, second and third-degree). Analgesics are used to manage the pain (see Chapter 16). Burn patients are susceptible to infection. With the skin gone, the patient is exposed to infection.

Third-degree burns are treated by first removing the charred skin (eschar), which is called *debridement*. This is a painful procedure. The patient is then given multiple antibiotics to prevent infections. The patient is also at risk for fluid and electrolyte imbalances (see Chapter 10) and at high risk for stress ulcers (see Chapter 18). Burn patients must be assessed for possible smoke inhalation. If it exists, the patient is treated with respiratory medications (see Chapter 14).

Burned areas must be cleansed with sterile saline solutions and an antiseptic such as povidone-iodine (Betadine). Broad-spectrum topical antibiotics should then be applied to burn areas. These include antibacterials such as mafenide acetate (Sulfamylon), silver sulfadiazine (Silvadene), silver nitrate 0.5% solution, and nitrofurazone (Furacin).

Third-degree burns are best managed in a designated burn center by a burn specialist or surgeon.

A list of drugs utilized in the treatment of burns is provided in the Appendix. Detailed tables show doses, recommendations, expectations, side effects, contraindications, and more and are available on the book's website (see URL in Appendix).

Abrasions and Lacerations

The most common skin injuries are abrasions and lacerations that are the result of accidents such as "road rash." This is caused by the body scraping along the roadway such as in a motorcycle accident. Patients who receive an abrasion or laceration are exposed to the same risk as a burn patient.

The site of the abrasion and laceration must be cleansed very carefully and treated with topical and sometimes systemic antibiotics and analgesics. Incomplete cleansing can result in tattoo-type scars.

Lacerations, commonly referred to as "cuts," are interruptions in the integrity of the skin and should be monitored for signs of infection after they are cleansed and treated with antibiotics. Infection will cause the wound to appear red and swollen, and to undergo purulent drainage (pus) and produce persistent pain.

Most minor cuts and abrasions are treated by cleansing the area with hydrogen peroxide or betadine and applying a topical antibiotic such as Neosporin (bacitracin, etc).

Some lacerations need to be sutured to close the open areas of the skin or topical skin adhesives are used to bring the edges together. Before suturing, the area must be flushed with copious amounts of normal saline. Sutures remain in place for about 7–10 days before they dissolve or are removed.

Puncture wounds do not cause a large area of visible injury to the skin but can carry a risk of damage to underlying tissues and infection. Puncture wounds should be cleansed carefully and monitored for signs of infection. The need for a tetanus toxoid booster immunization should be assessed whenever the skin is "broken" such as in a burn or puncture wound.

Summary

Skin is the largest organ of the body composed of two major layers—the epidermis and dermis. Skin controls body temperature, provides protection against infection, the environment, and prevents the loss of bodily fluids.

There are many skin disorders. The more common are acne vulgaris, psoriasis, warts, dermatitis, alopecia, burns, abrasions, and lacerations.

Acne vulgaris is an inflammation of the pilosebaceous glands and is treated by using a cleansing agent and applying topical antiacne medication.

Psoriasis is a chronic skin disorder characterized by erythematous papules and plaques covered with silvery scales appearing on the scalp, elbows, palms of the hands, knees, and soles of the feet. Psoriasis is treated by using antipsoriatic medication to loosen the psoriasis scales.

A *wart* is a benign lesion characterized as a hard, horny nodule on the hand or foot. Warts are removed by freezing, electrodesiccation, or surgical excision using topical treatments with salicylic acid, podophyllum resin, and cantharidin.

Dermatitis is a skin eruption that is caused by medications (drug-induced dermatitis) or by a chemical agent coming in contact with the skin (contact dermatitis). Dermatitis can be treated by using topical glucocorticoids.

The term *eczema* is used in two different ways: (1) to describe any rash-like skin conditions or (2) to describe *atopic dermatitis*, a chronic skin condition that commonly starts during infancy and continues through childhood. The specific cause of eczema remains unknown, but it is believed to develop as the result of a combination of hereditary (genetic) and environmental factors.

Alopecia is male pattern baldness and occurs when the hair shaft is lost and the hair follicle cannot regenerate. Minoxidil (Rogaine) returns hair growth, but alopecia returns within 3–4 months after the patient stops using the drug.

A burn causes lesions that break down skin and expose the body to infection. Burns are classified by degree, which is based on the tissue depth of the burn. There are three burn classifications: first-degree (superficial), second-degree (partial-thickness), and third-degree (full-thickness) burns. Burns are treated by cleansing the burn site, removing charred skin, and then administering anti-infectives to prevent infection.

An *abrasion* is a scrape and a *laceration* is a cut. Both are cleansed and treated with topical antibiotics.

QUIZ

1. **Acne vulgaris is associated with**

    (a) foods containing trans–fatty acids (TFA).

    (b) testosterone level.

    (c) genetics.

    (d) smoking.

2. **Keratolytics**

    (a) loosen psoriasis scales.

    (b) are used to treat burn patients.

    (c) remove warts.

    (d) protect lesions from becoming infected.

3. **Contact dermatitis is caused by**

    (a) pollen.

    (b) sunlight.

    (c) plants.

    (d) none of the above.

4. **First-degree burns affect only the epidermis of skin.**

    (a) True

    (b) False

5. **Podophyllum resin is used to remove venereal warts.**

    (a) True

    (b) False

6. **Absorption of topical glucocorticoids is greater at the**

    (a) axilla.

    (b) feet.

    (c) eyelids.

    (d) all of the above.

7. **A patient who has burns over 36% of her/his body may have a burned right leg and right arm.**

    (a) True

    (b) False

8. A wound that appears red and swollen and has purulent drainage (pus) and produces persistent pain is said to be

    (a) infected.

    (b) healed.

    (c) starting to heal.

    (d) nearly healed.

9. The patient has little control over acne vulgaris.

    (a) True

    (b) False

10. There is no cure for eczema.

    (a) True

    (b) False

Endocrine Medications

When the hormones kick in and the adrenals begin pumping, practically nothing can stand in your way. However, you can quickly feel out of sorts and behave strangely if your body either doesn't produce enough hormones or produces too many.

Hormones are messengers that influence how tissues, organs, and other parts of the human body function. An overproduction of hormones causes an overreaction such as growing too tall. An underproduction of hormones causes an underreaction such as producing insufficient insulin to metabolize glucose.

In this chapter, you'll learn about disorders caused by hormone imbalance, as well as the drugs used to correct the imbalance.

1. A Brief Look at the Endocrine System

Glands of the endocrine system produce hormones that are distributed throughout the body in circulating blood. Hormones, synthesized from amino acids and cholesterol, affect cellular activity of tissues and organs.

There are two types of hormones: proteins (which are also known as *small peptides*) and steroids. Steroids are secreted from the adrenal glands and the gonads.

Endocrine glands are ductless glands that include the pituitary (hypophysis), thyroid, parathyroid, adrenals, gonads, and pancreas. Table 21–1 lists the endocrine glands, and also their location and the hormone(s) secreted by the gland.

TABLE 21−1 Endocrine Glands and Their Secretions

Gland	Location	Secretes
Pituitary (hypophysis)	Base of the brain	Thyroid-stimulating hormone (TSH) Adrenocorticotropic hormone (ACTH)
Anterior (adenophypophysis)		Gonadotropins [follicle-stimulating hormone (FSH) and luteinizing hormone (LH)]. Growth hormone (GH), prolactin, melanocyte-stimulating hormone (MSH)
Posterior (neurohypophysis)		Antidiuretic hormone (ADH), vasopressin, oxytocin
Thyroid gland	Anterior to the trachea (2 lobes)	Thyroxine (T4) and triodothyroinine (T3)
Parathyroid gland	Lie on the dorsal surface of the thyroid gland (4 glands—2 pairs)	Parathormone (PTH)
Adrenal glands	Top of each kidney (2 sections—medulla is inner and 2 cortex surrounds medulla)	Cortex secretes corticosteroids (glucosteroids and mineralcorticoids); small amounts of androgen, estrogen, and progestin
Pancreas	Left of and behind the stomach (exocrine and endocrine gland)	Exocrine secretes digestive enzymes into the duodenum; endocrine has cell clusters called islets of Langerhans; α islet cells produce glucagons; β cells secrete insulin

2. Drugs and Hormones

Think of hormones as messengers that can increase or decrease tissue, organ, and cellular activities by the number of hormones that are carried by the blood. Sometimes, through aging or disease, an inappropriate number of hormones are produced, causing the patient to experience adverse reactions.

Hormonal drug therapy is used to return the patient to hormonal balance by either replacing the missing hormone or inhibiting the secretion of the hormone. Hormonal drug therapy is used for hormones produced by the pituitary, thyroid, parathyroid, and adrenal glands.

Drugs and the Pituitary Gland

Growth hormone (GH) is secreted by the pituitary gland to influence growth. Gigantism (during childhood) and acromegaly (after puberty) can occur with GH hypersecretion. They are frequently caused by a pituitary tumor. If the tumor cannot be destroyed by radiation, or bromocriptine, a prolactin-releasing inhibitor can inhibit the release of GH from the pituitary. Octreotide (Sandostatin) is a potent synthetic somatostatin used to suppress growth hormone release. It is very expensive, and gastrointestinal side effects are common.

If the pituitary gland produces too little GH, the patient will not reach a normal height. This is referred to as *GH deficiency*. Patients with this deficiency undergo GH replacement by taking somatrem (Protropin) and somatropin (Humatrope) to replenish the missing GH and enable normal growth to occur.

The posterior pituitary gland secretes antidiuretic hormone (ADH) and oxytocin. ADH is a vasopressin. Oxytocin is released to start labor contractions. ADH promotes water reabsorption from the renal tubules to maintain water balance in the body's fluids. A deficiency of ADH, called *diabetes insipidus* (DI), causes the kidneys to excrete large amounts of water. This leads to severe fluid volume deficit and electrolyte imbalances.

Diabetes insipidus can also be caused by head injury and brain tumors, resulting in trauma to the hypothalamus and pituitary gland. You must monitor fluid and electrolyte balance in patients who have diabetes insipidus. ADH replacement may be needed.

Some of the drugs used for pituitary disorders include desmopressin acetate (DDAV), desmopressin (Stimate), lypressin (Diapid), vasopressin (aqueous) (pitressin), and vasopressin tannate/oil (pitressin tannate).

A list of anterior pituitary hormone and posterior pituitary hormone drugs is provided in the Appendix. Detailed tables show doses, recommendations, expectations, side effects, contraindications, and more and are available on the book's website (see URL in Appendix).

Drugs and the Adrenal Gland

There are two adrenal glands, located near the top of each kidney. The adrenal gland is composed of two parts: the adrenal medulla and the adrenal cortex.

The *adrenal cortex* produces glucocorticoids (cortisol) and mineralocorticoids (aldosterone). Corticosteroids promote sodium retention and potassium excretion. Corticotropin (Acthar) is an adrenocorticotropic hormone (ACTH) drug that is used to diagnosis adrenal gland disorders.

Corticotropin (Acthar) is also used to treat adrenal gland insufficiency and as an anti-inflammatory drug in the treatment of allergic reactions such as anaphylaxis shock.

ACTH given intravenously increases the serum cortisol levels in 30–60 minutes if the adrenal gland is functioning properly. ACTH will eventually stimulate cortisol production if pituitary insufficiency causes steroid deficiency.

TABLE 21–2 Effects of Adrenal Hyposecretion and Hypersecretion		
Body System	Hyposecretion	Hypersecretion
Metabolism Glucose Protein Fat	Hypoglycemia muscle weakness	Hyperglycemia Muscle wasting; thinning of the skin; fat accumulation in face, neck, and trunk (protruding abdomen, buffalo hump); hyperlipidemia; high cholesterol
Central nervous system	Apathy, depression, fatigue	Increased neural activity; mood elevation; irritability; seizures
Gastrointestinal	Nausea, vomiting, abdominal pain	Peptic ulcers
Cardiovascular	Tachycardia, hypotension, cardiovascular collapse	Hypertension; edema; heart failure
Eyes	None	Cataract formation
Fluids and Electrolytes	Hypovolumia; hyponatremia; hyperkalemia	Hypervolemia; hypernatremia; hypokalemia
Blood cells	Anemia	Increased red blood cell count and neutrophils; impaired clotting

Table 21–2 shows the effects of an adrenal gland that produces too much (hypersecretion) or too little (hyposecretion) hormone. Adrenal hyposecretion is called *Addison's disease*, and hypersecretion is called *Cushing's syndrome*.

The ACTH hormone is released by the anterior pituitary gland that influences the glucocorticoids that are secreted by the adrenal gland. Glucocorticoids affect carbohydrate, protein, and fat metabolism in addition to muscle and blood cell activity.

Glucocorticoids can cause sodium absorption from the kidney that result in water retention, potassium loss, and increased blood pressure. Cortisol, the primary glucocorticoid, has anti-inflammatory, antiallergic, and antistress effects.

Glucocorticoid therapy is used in trauma, surgery, infections, emotional upsets, and anxiety. Most glucocorticoid drugs are produced synthetically and are administered orally, IM, IV, topically (see Chapter 20), intranasally (see Chapter 14), and as aerosol inhalers (see Chapter 14).

Glucocorticoid drugs include beclomethasone dipropionate (Vanceril), betamethasone (Celestone), cortisone acetate (Cortone Acetate), dexamethasone (Decadron), fludrocortisone acetate (Florinef Acetate), hydrocortisone (Hydrocortone), methylprednisolone (Medrol, Solu-Medrol, Depo-Medrol), prednisolone, and prednisone. The adrenal medulla synthesizes, stores, and releases epinephrine and norepinephrine. Hypersecretion causes prolonged or continual sympathetic nervous system responses. A lack of secretion from the adrenal medulla has no significant effects.

Drugs and the Thyroid Gland

The thyroid gland secretes two hormones that regulate protein synthesis and enzymatic activity and stimulate mitochondrial oxidation. These are thyroxine (T4) and triiodothyronine (T3). The thyroid gland secretes 20% of the circulating T3. The remaining 80% comes from degradation of T4 hormone. Approximately 40% of T4 is degraded and becomes T3.

Both T3 and T4 are carried in the blood by thyroxine-binding globulin (TBG) and albumin, which protects the hormones from being degraded. T3 is more potent than T4. Only unbound free T3 and T4 are active and produce a hormonal response.

A decreased amount of T3 and T4 is produced in a condition called *hypothyroidism*. This is caused by a disorder of the thyroid gland or a secondary lack of TSH secretion. *Hyperthyroidism* is an increase in circulatory T4 and T3 caused by an overactive thyroid gland or an excessive output of thyroid hormones.

Hypothyroidism

Primary hypothyroidism is characterized by a decrease in T4 and an increase in TSH levels. Primary hypothyroidism is caused by acute or chronic inflammation of the thyroid gland, radioiodine therapy, excess intake of antithyroid drugs, and surgery.

Myxedema is a severe form of hypothyroidism characterized by lethargy, apathy, memory impairment, emotional changes, slow speech, deep coarse voice, edema of the eyelids and face, thick dry skin, cold intolerance, slow pulse, constipation, weight gain, and abnormal menses.

In children, hypothyroidism can have a congenital (cretinism) or prepubertal (juvenile hypothyroidism) onset.

Hypothyroidism is treated by administering levothyroxine sodium (Levothroid, Synthroid), which increases levels of T3 and T4. Levothyroxine sodium (Levothroid, Synthroid) is also used to treat simple goiter and chronic lymphocytic (Hashimoto's) thyroiditis.

Liothyronine sodium (Cytomel) is a synthetic T3 that is used for short-term treatment of hypothyroidism. It is not used for maintenance therapy because liothyronine has a short half-life and duration.

Liotrix (Euthroid, Thyrolar) is a mixture of levothyroxine sodium and liothyronine sodium with no significant advantage over levothyroxine sodium. Thyroid and thyroglobulin (Proloid) are seldom used.

A list of drugs utilized in the treatment of hypothyroidism is provided in the Appendix. Detailed tables show doses, recommendations, expectations, side effects, contraindications, and more and are available on the book's website (see URL in Appendix).

Hyperthyroidism

Hyperthyroidism is an increase in circulating T4 and T3 levels, resulting from an overactive thyroid gland or excessive output of thyroid hormones. Hyperthyroidism may be mild with few symptoms or severe, leading to vascular collapse and death.

Graves' disease or thyrotoxicosis is the most common type of hyperthyroidism and is caused by a hyperfunctioning thyroid gland. Graves' disease is characterized by a rapid pulse (tachycardia), palpitations, excessive perspiration, heat intolerance, nervousness, irritability, exophthalmos (bulging eyes), and weight loss. Treatment involves surgical removal of a portion of the thyroid gland (subtotal thyroidectomy), radioactive iodine therapy, or antithyroid drugs that inhibit either the synthesis or the release of thyroid hormones.

Antithyroid drugs reduce the excessive secretion of T4 and T3 by inhibiting thyroid secretion. Thiourea derivatives (thioamides) are the drugs of choice used to decrease thyroid production.

Propylthiouracil (PTU) and methylthiouracil (Tapazole) are effective thioamide antithyroid drugs used for treating thyrotoxic crises and in preparation for subtotal thyroidectomy. Methimazole does not inhibit peripheral conversion of T4 to T3 as does PTU, but it is 10 times more potent and has a longer half-life than PTU. Prolonged use of thioamides may cause development of goiter because of the increased thyroid-stimulating hormone (TSH) secretion that inhibits T4 and T3 syntheses. Minimal doses should be given when indicated to avoid goiter formation.

Strong iodide preparations such as Lugol's solution are used to suppress thyroid function in patients with a history of subtotal thyroidectomy for Graves' disease. Sodium iodide administered intravenously is useful for the management of thyrotoxic crises.

A list of drugs utilized in the treatment of hyperthyroidism is provided in the Appendix. Detailed tables show doses, recommendations, expectations, side effects, contraindications, and more and are available on the book's website (see URL in Appendix).

Drugs and the Parathyroid Glands

The parathyroid glands secrete parathyroid hormone (PTH), which regulates calcium levels in the blood. A decrease in serum calcium stimulates the release of PTH. A decrease of PTH is called *hypoparathyroidism*; an increase in PTH is termed *hyperparathyroidism*.

Hypoparathyroidism is treated with PTH drugs, and hyperparathyroidism is treated with calcitonin. Calcitonin decreases serum calcium levels by promoting renal excretion of calcium.

Deficiency of PTH can cause *hypocalcemia*, which is a deficit of serum calcium. Hypocalcemia can also be caused by vitamin D deficiency, renal impairment, or diuretic therapy.

Hypocalcemia is treated with PTH replacement that corrects the calcium deficit by promoting calcium absorption from the GI tract, promotes calcium reabsorption from the renal tubules, and activates vitamin D. Calcitriol is a vitamin D analog that promotes calcium absorption from the GI tract and secretion of calcium of bone to the bloodstream.

Hyperparathyroidism is caused by malignancies of the parathyroid glands or ectopic PTH hormone secretion from lung cancer, hyperthyroidism, or prolonged immobility during which calcium is lost from bone.

Drugs and the Pancreas

The pancreas secretes insulin that is used to metabolize glucose. The patient contracts diabetes mellitus if insufficient insulin is produced. Diabetes mellitus is a chronic disease resulting from deficient glucose metabolism caused by insufficient insulin secretion from the β cells of the pancreas. Table 21–3 illustrates hypoglycemic and hyperglycemic reactions caused by a deficient glucose metabolism.

There are two types of diabetes mellitus: types 1 and 2.

Type 1 Diabetes Mellitus

Type 1 diabetes mellitus is referred to as *insulin-dependent diabetes mellitus* (IDDM) or *juvenile-onset diabetes* because the initial onset usually occurs in childhood or adolescence. In type 1 diabetes mellitus, the pancreas produces little or no insulin.

TABLE 21–3 Hypoglycemic Reactions and Diabetic Ketoacidosis	
Reaction	**Signs and Symptoms**
Hypoglycemic reaction (insulin shock)	Headache, lightheadedness, nervousness, apprehension, tremor, excess perspiration; cold, clammy skin, tachycardia, slurred speech, memory lapse, confusion, seizures Blood sugar <60 mg/dL
Diabetic ketoacidosis (hyperglycemic reaction)	Extreme thirst, polyuria, fruity breath odor, Kussmaul breathing (deep, rapid, labored, distressing, dyspnea), rapid, thready pulse, dry mucous membranes, poor skin turgor Blood sugar level >250 mg/dL

Type 1 diabetes mellitus is characterized by a sudden onset that occurs more frequently in populations descended from northern European countries (Finland, Scotland, Norway, and Sweden) than in those from southern European countries, the Middle East, or Asia.

Approximately 3 in 1000 people in the United States develop type 1 diabetes and are dependent on regular insulin injections.

Type 2 Diabetes Mellitus

Type 2 diabetes mellitus, sometimes called *age-onset* or *adult-onset diabetes*, is the most common form of diabetes mellitus that effects approximately 5% of Americans under the age of 50 and 15% of those 50 and older. More than 90% of the diabetics in the United States have type 2 diabetes mellitus.

Patients with type 2 diabetes mellitus are often overweight and do not exercise sufficiently. They can produce insulin but are unable to utilize it effectively. Type 2 diabetes mellitus is more common in people of Aboriginal, Hispanic, and African-American descent. People who have emigrated to the West from India, Japan, and Australia are more likely to develop type 2 diabetes mellitus than those who remain in their original countries.

Type 2 diabetes mellitus is considered a milder form of diabetes mellitus because of its slow onset (sometimes developing over the course of several years) and because it can usually be controlled with diet and oral medication. Type 2 diabetes mellitus is also called *non-insulin-dependent diabetes mellitus* (NIDDM), a term that is somewhat misleading. Many people with type 2 diabetes mellitus can control the condition with diet and oral medications. However, insulin injections are sometimes necessary if treatment with diet and oral medication is not adequate.

Uncontrolled and untreated type 2 diabetes mellitus is as serious as type 1 diabetes mellitus.

Gestational Diabetes Mellitus

Gestational diabetes mellitus develops during pregnancy and resolves after delivery. Gestational diabetes mellitus develops during the second or third trimester of pregnancy in about 2% of pregnancies and is treated by diet. However, insulin injections may be required. Women who have gestational diabetes mellitus are at higher risk for developing type 2 diabetes mellitus within 5–10 years.

Signs and Symptoms of Diabetes Mellitus

The signs and symptoms of diabetes are polyuria (increased urine output), polydipsia (increased thirst), and polyphagia (increased hunger). Certain drugs increase blood sugar and can cause hyperglycemia in prediabetic persons. These include glucocorticoids (cortisone, prednisone), thiazide diuretics [hydrochlorothiazide (HydroDIURIL)], and epinephrine. Usually the blood sugar returns to normal after the drug is discontinued.

Insulin

Insulin is a protein that cannot be administered orally because GI secretions destroy the insulin structure. Insulin is therefore administered subcutaneously in a special insulin syringe (see Chapter 6). The site and depth of the injection affect the absorption and are greater in the deltoid and abdominal areas than in the thighs and buttocks. Heat and massage can increase subcutaneous absorption. Cooling the area can decrease absorption.

Insulin can also be delivered via insulin pump. An insulin pump is surgically implanted in the abdomen and delivers an insulin infusion and bolus doses with meals either intraperitoneally or intravenously.

Insulin can also be administered intranasally to provide a rapid-onset effect for a short duration, although this method is expensive and rarely used.

Insulin injectors deliver insulin under high pressure through the skin into fatty tissue without a needle. Insulin injectors can cause bruising, pain, and burning and are not indicated for children or the elderly. They are also expensive.

Insulin Types

There are three standard types of insulin:

- **Rapid-Acting:** The drug of choice is regular or lispro (HumaLOG) insulin, onset 0.5–1 hour, peak 2–4 hours, with a duration of 6–8 hours.

- **Intermediate-Acting:** The drug of choice is NPH, Humulin N, Lente, and Humulin L insulin, onset 1–2 hours, peak 6–12 hours, duration 18–24 hours.

- **Long-Acting:** The drug of choice is Ultralente insulin, onset 5–8 hours, peak 14–20 hours, duration 30–36 hours.

There are also combinations that include Humulin 70/30 (NPH 70%, regular 30%) and Humulin 50/50 (NPH 50%, regular 50%).

Unopened insulin vials are refrigerated until needed. Once an insulin vial has been opened, it may be kept at room temperature for 1 month or in the refrigerator for 3 months. An open insulin vial should not be placed in the freezer, in direct sunlight, or in a high-temperature area.

A list of drugs utilized in the treatment of diabetes is provided in the Appendix. Detailed tables show doses, recommendations, expectations, side effects, contraindications, and more and are available on the book's website (see URL in Appendix).

Oral Antidiabetics

Oral antidiabetic drugs such as sulfonylureas are administered to patients who have type 2 diabetes mellitus to stimulate β cells to secrete insulin. This results in an increase in insulin cell receptors, enabling cells to bind to insulin during glucose metabolism. Sulfonylureas are chemically related to sulfonamides but lack antibacterial activity.

Sulfonylureas are classified as first- and second-generation drugs, and each generation is divided into short-acting, intermediate-acting, and long-acting antidiabetics.

The following drugs are first-generation sulfonylureas:

- Tolbutamide (Orinase)
- Acetohexamide (Dymelor)
- Tolazamide (Tolinase)
- Chlorpropamide (Diabinese)

Second-generation sulfonylureas include the following:

- Glipizide (Glucotrol)
- Glyburide nonmicronized (DiaBeta, Micronase)
- Glimepiride (Amryl)

Second-generation sulfonylureas increase tissue response to insulin and decrease glucose production by the liver. This results in greater hypoglycemic potency at smaller doses. Second-generation sulfonylureas have a longer duration of action and cause few side effects, but should not be used if the patient has liver or kidney dysfunction.

Nonsulfonylureas are new drugs that affect the hepatic and GI production of glucose. For example, metformin (Glucophage) is a nonsulfonylurea biguanide compound that acts by decreasing hepatic production of glucose from stored glycogen. The result is a reduced increase in serum glucose following a meal and limits the degree of postprandial (postmeal) hyperglycemia.

Metformin (Glucophage) also decreases the absorption of glucose from the small intestine and may increase insulin receptor sensitivity as well as peripheral glucose uptake at the cellular level. Metformin does not produce hypoglycemia or hyperglycemia and can cause GI disturbances. Metformin can be used alone and is considered the first line of drugs for those with type 2 diabetes.

α-Glucosidase inhibitors [acarbose (Precose)] inhibit α-glucosidase, the digestive enzyme in the small intestine that is responsible for the release of glucose from the complex carbohydrates in the diet. With inhibition of α-glucosidase, carbohydrates cannot be absorbed and instead, pass into the large intestine. Acarbose has no systemic effects, is not absorbed into the body in significant amounts, and does not cause a hypoglycemic reaction.

Thiazolidinediones, such as pioglitazone (Actos), decrease insulin resistance and help muscle cells respond to insulin and utilize glucose more effectively. Thiazolidinediones may be used in addition to sulfonylurea, metformin, or insulin for insulin-resistant patients. Pioglitazone (Actos) has no significant side effects or adverse effects.

Repaglinide (Prandin) is used alone or in combination with metformin as a short-acting drug similar to sulfonylureas; however, Repaglinide does not cause a hypoglycemic reaction.

Glucagon

Glucagon is a hyperglycemic hormone secreted by the α cells of the islets of Langerhans in the pancreas and increases blood sugar by stimulating glycogenolysis (glycogen breakdown) in the liver.

Glucagon protects the body cells, especially those in the brain and retina, by providing the nutrients and energy needed to maintain body function. Glucagon, available for parenteral use, treats insulin-induced hypoglycemia when other methods of providing glucose are not available. Glucagon can increase blood glucose levels in patients who are semiconscious or unconscious and unable to ingest carbohydrates.

Oral diazoxide (Proglycem) increases blood sugar by inhibiting insulin release from the β cells and stimulating release of epinephrine (Adrenalin) from the adrenal medulla. Oral diazoxide (Proglycem) is used to treat chronic hypoglycemia caused by hyperinsulinism due to islet cell cancer or hyperplasia, but not for hypoglycemic reactions. Patients do not experience hypotension when taking oral diazoxide (Proglycem).

A list of antidiabetic second-generation drugs is provided in the Appendix. Detailed tables show doses, recommendations, expectations, side effects, contraindications, and more and are available on the book's website (see URL in Appendix).

Summary

Glands of the endocrine system produce hormones that are distributed throughout the body by blood vessels. Hormones are messengers that influence how tissues, organs, and other parts of the body function. Glands can overproduce or underproduce hormones, causing parts of the body to behave inappropriately.

Hormonal drug therapy is used to return the patient to hormonal balance by either replacing the missing hormone or inhibiting the secretion of the hormone. Hormonal drug therapy is used for hormones produced by the pituitary, thyroid, parathyroid, and adrenal glands.

The pituitary gland secretes the growth hormone. Octreotide (Sandostatin) is used to suppress growth hormone release. Somatrem (protropin) and somatropin (Humatrope) are used to replenish missing growth hormone.

The adrenal glands produce a number of hormones. Cortiocotropin (Acthar) is used to treat adrenal gland insufficiency.

The thyroid gland secretes two hormones that regulate protein synthesis and enzymatic activity and stimulate mitochondrial oxidation: thyroxine (T4) and triiodothyronine (T3). Levothyroxine sodium (Levothroid, Synthroid) is used to increase the production of T3 and T4. Thiourea derivatives (thioamides) inhibit T3 and T4.

The parathyroid glands secrete parathyroid hormone (PTH), which regulates calcium levels in the blood. Calcitonin increases the level of PTH.

The pancreas secretes insulin that is used to metabolize glucose. Insulin is used to treat a decreased output of insulin by the pancreas.

QUIZ

1. **An overproduction of GH results in**
   - (a) acromegaly.
   - (b) gigantism.
   - (c) abnormal growth.
   - (d) all of the above.

2. **ADH replacement is needed for trauma to the**
   - (a) hypothalamus and pituitary gland.
   - (b) pancreas.
   - (c) liver.
   - (d) adrenal gland.

3. **Addison's disease is caused by**
   - (a) underproduction of the adrenal gland.
   - (b) overproduction of the adrenal gland.
   - (c) overproduction of the pancreas.
   - (d) underproduction of the pancreas.

4. **Glucocorticoids therapy is used for trauma, surgery, infections, emotional upset, and anxiety.**
   - (a) True
   - (b) False

5. Liothyronine (Cytomel) is a synthetic T3 that is used for short-term treatment of hypothyroidism.

   (a) True

   (b) False

6. Graves' disease is caused by

   (a) overproduction of the thyroid gland.

   (b) underproduction of the thyroid gland.

   (c) overproduction of the parathyroid gland.

   (d) underproduction of the parathyroid gland.

7. In type 1 diabetes mellitus, the pancreas produces little or no insulin.

   (a) True

   (b) False

8. Type 2 is considered a milder form of diabetes mellitus because

   (a) the pancreas secretes a normal amount of insulin after the patient gives birth.

   (b) it affects only children.

   (c) it has a slow onset and is usually controlled by diet and oral medication.

   (d) none of the above.

9. Diabetes insipidus (DI) is a deficiency of ADH.

   (a) True

   (b) False

10. Hormonal drug therapy inhibits the secretion of a hormone.

    (a) True

    (b) False

22

Disorders of the Eye and the Ear

Most of us become anxious whenever anything happens to our vision or hearing and tend to avoid reporting the condition to our healthcare professional, fearing devastating news—we're going blind or deaf.

The truth is that common eye and ear disorders rarely result in loss of sight or hearing once the disorder is diagnosed and treated with the proper medication. Some conditions heal without intervention, while others are eliminated after a few weeks of treatment.

This chapter takes a look at common disorders that affect the eyes and the ears and discusses drugs that are used to treat them.

1. Eye Disorders

The eye has three layers. The first layer contains the cornea and sclera. The second layer contains the choroid, the iris, and the ancillary body. The third layer contains the retina, which connects to the brain through the optic nerve.

There are three common disorders of the eye: glaucoma, conjunctivitis, and corneal abrasion.

Glaucoma

The eye is under constant intraocular pressure (IOP) that increases in patients who have glaucoma. This increased pressure damages the optic nerve, resulting in decreased peripheral vision and eventually blindness.

Approximately 3 million Americans have glaucoma, and 120,000 have lost their eyesight. Glaucoma is the leading cause of blindness. There are two types of glaucoma: chronic (primary) open-angle glaucoma (POAG) and acute closed-angle glaucoma.

Chronic Open-Angle Glaucoma

Chronic open-angle glaucoma is the most common form of glaucoma. The "open" drainage angle of the eye can become blocked, leading to a gradual increase in eye pressure. If this increased pressure results in optic nerve damage, it is known as *chronic open-angle glaucoma*. The optic nerve damage and vision loss usually occurs so gradually and painlessly that the patient is unaware of any problem until the optic nerve is already badly damaged.

Angle-Closure Glaucoma

Angle-closure glaucoma results when the drainage angle of the eye narrows and becomes completely blocked. In the eye, the iris may close off the drainage angle and cause a dangerously high eye pressure. When the drainage angle of the eye suddenly becomes completely blocked, pressure builds up rapidly, and this condition is called *acute angle-closure glaucoma*. The symptoms include severe eye pain, blurred vision, headache, rainbow halos around lights, nausea, and vomiting. Unless an ophthalmologist treats the acute angle-closure glaucoma immediately, blindness can result. When the drainage angle of the eye gradually becomes completely blocked, pressure builds up gradually; this condition is called *chronic angle-closure glaucoma*. This form of glaucoma occurs more frequently in people of African and Asian ancestry, and in certain eye conditions.

Acute angle-closure glaucoma is a medical emergency. If IOP is not reduced within hours of onset, the patient's vision can be permanently damaged.

Conjunctivitis

Conjunctivitis, commonly known as "pink eye," is an inflammation of the thin, clear membrane that covers the white part of the eye and the eyelids (the conjunctiva). This inflammation causes the white of the eye and the undersides of the eyelids to become pink or red. The patient's eyes may be itchy or painful.

There are four types of conjunctivitis:

1. **Viral Conjunctivitis:** Viral conjunctivitis affects only one eye, causing excessive eye watering and a light discharge from the eye.

2. **Bacterial Conjunctivitis:** Bacterial conjunctivitis affects both eyes, causing a heavy greenish discharge.

3. **Allergic Conjunctivitis:** Allergic conjunctivitis also affects both eyes, causing itching and redness and excessive tearing. The patient may also experience an itchy and red nose.

4. **Giant Papillary Conjunctivitis:** Giant papillary conjunctivitis (GPC) affects both eyes, causing contact lens intolerance, itching, heavy discharge, tearing, and red bumps on the underside of the eyelids.

Corneal Abrasion

A *corneal abrasion* is a cut or scratch on the cornea, which is the clear, protective membrane covering the colored part of the eye (iris). Corneal abrasion can be caused by sand, dust, dirt, and shavings from materials such as metal. Fingernails, tree branches, rubbing the eyes, and even contact lenses can also scratch the cornea. Some patients have a weak outer layer of the cornea that can sustain an abrasion for no apparent reason.

Most corneal abrasions heal properly with the proper treatment. However, if the treatment is not successful, the abrasion can reappear months after the original injury.

Corneal abrasions are painful because of the sensitivity of the cornea. Patients may feel as if there is sand in their eyes. Their eyes become teary and red. Their vision is blurred, and light causes pain in their eyes (photophobia). Corneal abrasions have been known to cause headaches.

Fluorescein sodium and Fluress (fluorescein sodium and benoxinate HCl) are used to diagnose corneal abrasions and to locate lesions or foreign objects in the eye.

Fluorescein is a dye used to demonstrate defects in corneal epithelium and is excreted in nasal secretions if the lacrimal (tear) duct is patent.

When fluorescence strips are used to examine the eye, the following phenomena may occur:

- Corneal scratches turn bright red.
- Foreign bodies are surrounded by a green ring.
- Loss of conjunctiva appears orange-yellow.

Fluress is a dye and a local anesthetic and is used for short corneal and conjunctival procedures such as removing foreign bodies from the eye.

Eye Medication

Eye disorders are treated by using one of various medications (Table 22–1).

TABLE 22–1 Ophthalmic Medications

Antibacterials	Antifungals	Antivirals	Anti-inflammatories
Chloramphenicol (Chlormycetin Ophthalmic) Ciprofloxacin (Cipro) Erythromycin Gentamicin sulfate (Garamycin Ophthalmic) Norfloxacin (Chibroxin) Tobramycin (Nebcin, Tobrex) Silver nitrate 1% (used in neonates to prevent ophthalmia neoatorum) Tetracycline HCl (Achromycin Ophthalmic)	Natamycin (Natacyn Ophthalmic)	Idoxuridine (IDU) Trifluridine (Viroptic) Vidarabine monohydrate (Vira-A)	Dexamethasone Diclofenac Na (Voltaren) Suprofen (Profenal) Ketorolac tromethamine (Acular) Olopatadine HCl Ophthalmic solution Medrysone (HMS Liquifilm) Prednisolone acetate Prednisolone Na phosphate Combination: TobraDex (tobramycin 0.3% and dexamethasone 0.1%)
Miotics: Cholinergics and β-adrenergic blockers	Indirect-acting cholinesterase inhibitors: Short-acting	β-adrenergic blockers	Carbonic anhydrase inhibitors
Acetylcholine HCl (Miochol) Carbachol intraocular (Miostat) Pilocarpine HCl (Isopto Carpine) Pilocarpine nitrate (Ocusert Pilo-20) Echothiophate iodide (Phospholine Iodide)	Physostigmine salicylate (Osopto Eserine)	Betaxolol HCl (Betoptic) Levobunolol HCl Timolol maleate (Timoptic)	Acetazolamide (Diamox) Brinzolamideophthalmic suspension 1% Dichlorphenamide (Daranide) Dorzolamide (Trusopt) Methazolamide (Neptazane)
Osmotics	Mydriatics and Cycloplegics		
Glycerin Isosorbide (Ismotic) Mannitol (Osmitrol) Urea (Ureaphil)	Atropine sulfate Cyclopentolate HCl Dipivefrin HCl Epinephrine HCl Epinephrine borate Homatropine hydrobromide (Isopto Homatropine) Scopolamine hydrobromide Tropicamide (Mydriacyl Ophthalmic)		

Topical Anesthetics   *Topical anesthetics* are used to anesthetize the eye for comprehensive eye examinations and for removal of foreign bodies from the eye. Onset occurs in about 1 minute and lasts for 15 minutes. During this time, the blink reflex is temporarily lost and the corneal epithelium is temporarily dried. The patient is required to wear a protective eye patch until the effects of the drug wear off.

Anti-infectives and Antimicrobials   *Anti-infectives* and *antimicrobials* are administered for eye infections such as conjunctivitis. These drugs can cause local skin and eye irritation. You learned about anti-infective and antimicrobial medication in Chapters 12 and 13.

Lubricants   *Lubricants* are used to reduce the discomfort that is associated with dry eyes and to moisten contact lenses and artificial eyes. Lubricants are also used to maintain the integrity of the epithelial surface and to moisten the eye during anesthesia and unconsciousness.

Miotics   *Miotics* lower intraocular pressure in open-angle glaucoma, allowing increased blood flow to the retina. This results in less retinal damage and prevents the loss of vision. There are two types of miotics: direct-acting cholinergics and cholinesterase inhibitors. *Direct-acting cholinergics* constrict the pupils, whereas cholinesterase inhibitors dilate the pupils. Patients who take miotics might experience headache, eye pain, decreased vision, brow pain, and less frequently hyperemia of the conjunctiva (red eye). Miotics can be absorbed systemically, resulting in the patient experiencing nausea, vomiting, diarrhea, frequent urination, precipitation of asthma attacks, increased salivation, diaphoresis, muscle weakness, and respiratory difficulty.

Carbonic Anhydrase Inhibitors   *Carbonic anhydrase inhibitors* are used for long-term treatment of open-angle glaucoma by decreasing intraocular pressure (IOP). The IOP is reduced by interference with the production of aqueous humor. Patients who take carbonic anhydrase inhibitors can experience lethargy, anorexia, drowsiness, paresthesia, depression, polyuria, nausea, vomiting, hypokalemia, and renal calculi. It is because of these adverse side effects that patients frequently discontinue taking carbonic anhydrase inhibitors. Carbonic anhydrase inhibitors are contraindicated in the first trimester of pregnancy and for patients who are allergic to sulfonamides.

Osmotics   *Osmotics* are preoperative and postoperative medications used to reduce intraocular pressure by decreasing vitreous humor volume. They are also used in the emergency treatment of closed-angle glaucoma. Patients who are administered osmotics can experience headache, nausea, vomiting, and diarrhea. Elderly patients can become disoriented.

Anticholinergic Mydriatics and Cycloplegics   Anticholinergic mydriatics and cycloplegics are used in diagnostic procedures and ophthalmic surgery. *Anticholinergic mydriatics* dilate the pupils. *Cycloplegics* paralyze eye muscles. Patients who are treated with these medications experience tachycardia, photophobia, dryness of the mouth, edema, conjunctivitis, and dermatitis. You learned about anticholinergics in Chapter 15.

A list of eye disorder drugs is provided in the Appendix. Detailed tables show doses, recommendations, expectations, side effects, contraindications, and more and are available on the book's website (see URL in Appendix).

2. Patient Education for Eye Medication

It is important that patients understand the effects of their eye disorders and the effects of the medications that they are taking to treat them. Patients may be anxious about their eye disorders, fearing a possible loss of vision.

The healthcare provider should demonstrate the proper technique for administering eyedrops and ointment and ensure that the patient knows how to maintain a sterile technique so the eyedropper does not become contaminated.

Patients should be informed about expected side effects such as blurred vision and that administering the medication at bedtime could avoid problems that could arise from temporary loss of vision.

Patient should also be asked to keep a record of the times when they administer the medication. This is especially important for patients who are confused or forgetful and could accidentally receive an overdose of the medication. The patient should not stop taking the medication without consulting the healthcare provider.

Patients should be instructed to wear MedicAlert bracelets if they are taking glaucoma medications or if they are allergic to any medication.

3. Ear Disorders

The ear consists of three parts: the external, middle, and inner ear. The *external ear* consists of the pinna and the external auditory canal that transmits sound to the middle ear. The *middle ear* has an air-filled cavity that contains auditory ossicles, which are the malleus, incus, and stapes bones. The auditory ossicles forward the sound to the *inner ear*, where the eardrum is located. Pressure on both sides of the eardrum is equalized by the *eustachian tube*, which connects to the nasopharynx. The eardrum could rupture if pressure becomes unequal. The inner ear also contains a series of canals called *labyrinths*, which are made up of the vestibule, the cochlea, and the semicircular canals. The vestibule maintains equilibrium and balance, and the cochlea is the principal hearing organ.

Common ear disorders are cerumen (ear wax) impaction, otitis external, otitis media (infections of the external and middle ear), and vestibular disorders of the inner ear.

Cerumen Impaction

Cerumen (ear wax) is produced by glands in the outer portion of the ear canal. Cerumen moves down the canal to the external os (opening), where the cerumen is washed away. When this process fails, cerumen becomes impacted and must be loosened by administering ceruminolytics such as a hydrogen peroxide solution (3% diluted to 50% strength with water). The ear canal is irrigated with *ceruminolytics*, which flush the cerumen deposits out of the ear canal. Patients who have chronic cerumen impaction are treated with drops of olive oil or mineral oil or by Cerumenex and Debrox. Cerumenex is available by prescription, and Debrox is an OTC medication.

Otitis Externa and Otitis Media

Otitis externa and *otitis media* are infections of the external and middle ear, respectively. These disorders are treated with analgesics and antibiotics. Antibiotics are discussed in Chapter 13. Analgesics are discussed in Chapter 16. Table 22–2 lists commonly used antibiotics for ear infections. Most ear infections are caused by a virus and should not be treated with antibiotics.

Vestibular Disorders

The most frequently reported symptoms of vestibular disorders are dizziness, unsteadiness or imbalance when walking, vertigo, and nausea. These symptoms may be quite mild, lasting only minutes, or quite severe, resulting in total disability.

Because the vestibular system interacts with many other parts of the nervous system, symptoms may also be experienced as problems with vision, muscles, thinking, and memory. In addition, people with vestibular disorders may suffer headaches and

TABLE 22–2 Common Medications Used to Treat Ear Infections	
External Ear	**Internal Ear**
Acetic acid and aluminum acetate (Otic Deomboro)	Amoxicillin (Amoxil, Augmentin)
Boric acid (Ear-Dry), Carbamide peroxide (Debrox)	Ampicillin trihydrate (Polycillin)
	Cefaclor (Ceclor)
Chloramphenical (Chloromycetin Otic)	Erythromycin (E-Mycin)
Polymyxin B	Penicillin (Pentids, Pen-V)
Tetracycline (Achromycin)	Sulfonamides (Azulfidine, Bactrim)
	Clarithromycin (Biaxin)
Trolamine polypeptide oleate-condensate (Cerumenex)	Amoxicillin and potassium clavulanate (Augmentin)
	Loracarbef (Lorabid)

muscular aches in the neck and back, increased tendency to suffer from motion sickness, and increased sensitivity to noise and bright lights. Patients with vestibular disorders often report fatigue and loss of stamina and an inability to concentrate. Difficulty with reading and speech may occur during times of fatigue. When these symptoms are constant and disabling, they may be accompanied by irritability, loss of self-esteem, and/or depression. Ménière's disease, labyrinthitis, and inner-ear infections usually cause vestibular disorders.

Ear Pain

Ear pain usually resolves itself between 48 and 72 hours from the onset of the pain. However, analgesics such as acetaminophen or ibuprofen should be administered to relieve the pain in the interim.

Ear Congestion

Ear congestion can be caused by the improper drainage of the eustachian tube. This can be relieved by administering antihistamine-decongestant medications such as Actifed, Allerest, Dimetapp, Drixoral, Novafed, Ornade, and Triaminic, all of which are available OTC.

4. Patient Education for Ear Medication

Patients should understand that no foreign objects should be placed inside the ear canal, including Q-Tips. Ceruminolytics should be used to remove cerumen. Patients who are prone to swimmer's ear (otitis externa) should keep the ear canal dry by placing 2 drops of alcohol in the ear canal.

Many medications used to treat ear disorders increase sensitivity to light. Therefore, they should be kept in a light-resistant container.

All antibiotics must be taken for the prescribed length of time (10–14 days). The patient should not stop taking antibiotics once the pain has subsided.

The patient should report any change in hearing. Some patients may not report the loss to their healthcare professionals because they might consider the hearing loss as a normal part of aging or due to exposure to environmental noise.

Summary

There are three common eye disorders: glaucoma, conjunctivitis, and corneal abrasion. *Glaucoma* is characterized by an increase in intraocular pressure that, if left untreated, can damage the optic nerve and lead to blindness.

Conjunctivitis is inflammation of the thin, clear membrane that covers the white part of the eye and the eyelids. There are four types of conjunctivitis: viral conjunctivitis, bacterial conjunctivitis, allergic conjunctivitis, and giant papillary conjunctivitis. A *corneal abrasion* is a cut or scratch on the cornea caused by debris, fingernails, contact lenses, or rubbing the eye. Most corneal abrasions heal with the proper treatment.

Eye disorders are treated using a topical anesthetic, anti-infectives, antimicrobials, lubricants, miotics, carbonic anhydrase inhibitors, osmotics, anticholinergic mydriatics, or cycloplegics.

There are four common ear disorders: cerumen impaction, otitis external, otitis media, and vestibular disorders. *Cerumen impaction* is the overproduction of earwax. *Otitis externa* and *otitis media* are infections of the external ear and middle ear, respectfully. Vestibular disorders include Ménière's disease, labyrinthitis, and inner-ear infections.

Cerumen impaction is treated by administering ceruminolytics to flush the cerumen from the canal. Otitis externa and otitis media are treated with analgesics. If a bacterial infection is suspected, antibiotics may be ordered.

QUIZ

1. **What type of conjunctivitis causes a heavy greenish discharge?**
   (a) Viral conjunctivitis
   (b) Bacterial conjunctivitis
   (c) Allergic conjunctivitis
   (d) None of the above

2. **What type of conjunctivitis causes itching and redness and excessive tearing?**
   (a) Viral conjunctivitis
   (b) Bacterial conjunctivitis
   (c) Allergic conjunctivitis
   (d) None of the above

3. **What medication lowers intraocular pressure?**
   (a) Cholinesterase inhibitors
   (b) Direct-acting cholinergics
   (c) Miotics
   (d) All of the above

4. Blurred vision is an expected side effect of some eye medications.

   (a) True

   (b) False

5. Topical anesthetics are used to anesthetize the eye for a comprehensive eye examination.

   (a) True

   (b) False

6. Which medication is used to treat cerumen impaction?

   (a) Hydrogen peroxide solution

   (b) Olive oil

   (c) Debrox

   (d) All of the above

7. Administration of 2 drops of alcohol in the ear canal helps to prevent swimmer's ear.

   (a) True

   (b) False

8. Which medication relieves ear congestion?

   (a) Allerest

   (b) Phenergan

   (c) Novafed

   (d) All of the above

9. Ear pain usually resolves itself within 48–72 hours from the onset of the pain.

   (a) True

   (b) False

10. A virus causes nearly all ear infections.

   (a) True

   (b) False

chapter 23

Geriatric Considerations

When you visit your grandparents you probably don't realize that they are part of the most rapidly growing segment of our society. More and more people are living to an advanced age and they are healthier and more active than ever before despite their increased susceptibility to multiple chronic conditions. Advances in healthcare allow the >65-year-old population to live longer, but they consume more resources, especially medications.

The term polypharmacy means the result of taking an increased or excessive number of medications simultaneously, including medications that are not really necessary. The elderly are at increased risk of negative health consequences due to polypharmacy. In this chapter you will learn about the most commonly prescribed medications in the elderly population as well as their physiological response to multiple medications.

1. Normal Aging Versus Pathology

Aging changes are caused by multiple factors. Genetics, or inherited factors, play a major role. If your grandmother lived to be 100, there's a good chance that you will have a long life. Just plain wear and tear on the body is also an issue. It is important to stay in good shape by maintaining a normal weight and keeping physically active.

Even the environment plays a role in keeping individuals healthy and active for many years. Sun exposure can have a negative effect on individuals and speed up the aging process. Other factors that hasten the process, and thus shorten lifespan, include smoking, alcohol consumption, and stress. Finally, metabolism affects the aging process and is definitely involved in an individual's ability to manage multiple medications.

We can start with the skin and the common disorders that affect the elderly as well as the medications used to treat these conditions. *Rosacea* is a common condition found in fair-skinned people. It involves reddened areas on the cheek, forehead, and chin. It can also involve the eye. It is commonly treated with oral antibiotics (Chapter 13) such as tetracyclines and erythromycin or topical agents such as clindamycin and metronidazole. Medications such as oral niacin, which is used to treat dyslipidemia, can also cause this condition. This is an example of polypharmacy in reverse. The medications used to treat a chronic condition can now cause another chronic condition and require the use of more medications. Table 23–1 includes more examples of skin disorders that affect the elderly who are already taking multiple medications for other chronic diseases.

TABLE 23–1 Common Dermatologic Diseases and Disorders in the Elderly and Drugs Used to Treat Them		
Disease/Disorder	Treatment	Causes
Seborrheic dermatitis	Selenium sulfide, ketoconazole, and various tar shampoos	
Xerosis (dry skin)	Mild topical corticosteroids	Too frequent washing and other environmental factors
Bullous pemphigoid	Topical corticosteroids	Diuretics, analgesics, antibiotics, and ACE inhibitors can cause this disorder
Herpes zoster	Valacyclovir or famciclovir are prodrugs of acyclovir used to treat this condition; narcotics, NSAIDs, epidural injection of local anesthetics, glucocorticoids, low-dose tricyclic antidepressants, capsaicin, and acupuncture are some of the therapies used to treat herpes zoster	Zostavax (live zoster vaccine) immunization is used to prevent this debilitating condition

Abbreviations: ACE—angiotensin-converting enzyme; NSAID—nonsteroidal anti-inflammatory drug.

Teeth age, along with the rest of the body, and untreated dental disease can have a serious effect on an elderly person. The mouth is the site where food intake occurs, speech is produced, and the salivary glands affect the alimentary tract and upper airway. Older patients are susceptible to candidiasis due to denture use, hypofunction of the salivary glands, diabetes mellitus, and the use of antibiotics for pulmonary and urologic diseases. Patients who use inhaled corticosteroids for chronic pulmonary diseases are at high risk. Treatment for candidiasis involves administration of topical or system antifungal agents. Side effects of antifungal agents can include abdominal pain and diarrhea, headaches, a rash, and indigestion, all of which can make an already compromised patient less able to function.

2. Pulmonary Disorders

Age-related pulmonary changes include a decrease in *forced vital capacity,* which is the forced expiratory volume of air in 1 second. Approximately 5–10% of those over 65 meet the criteria for asthma. The size of the airways is reduced because of a decrease in connective tissue, and the alveolar sacs become shallow. The ability of the chest wall to expand is reduced for several reasons, including arthritic changes. The intercostal muscles atrophy (shrink), thus reducing the strength of the diaphragm by 25%. The PaO_2 (oxygen in the blood) also decreases with age. These changes lead to an increased occurrence of respiratory (pulmonary) disorders in the elderly.

Following are a few terms related to pulmonary disorders commonly found in the elderly:

- **Dyspnea:** Difficulty in breathing, which becomes prominent in end-stage lung diseases such as chronic obstructive pulmonary disease (COPD) and pulmonary fibrosis.
- **Chronic Cough:** Common causes are postnasal drip, asthma, and gastroesophageal reflux. Angiotensin-converting enzyme (ACE) inhibitors (medication for high blood pressure) and heart failure can also cause a chronic cough in the elderly.
- **Wheezing:** This is a high-pitched whistling sound made while breathing. This is common in all age groups who are asthmatic, but it is more common in the elderly because of postnasal drip and heart failure.

Medications administered to treat these pulmonary disorders are generally β-adrenergic agonists, which are medications that relax muscles of the airways, widen the airway, and make it easier to breathe. They are administered with metered-dose inhalers. Examples of these drugs are albuterol (Proventil, Ventolin), levalbuterol (Xopenex), and salmeterol (Serevent). The side effects include anxiety, hypertension, increased heart rate, and insomnia. These effects can be very serious for an elderly patient who is already taking medication for high blood pressure and a rapid heart rate. Insomnia (inability to fall asleep or stay asleep) is also a common problem for the elderly population. This is another example of polypharmacy, namely, where one medication leads to problems and interactions with other medications.

Corticosteroids are also used for pulmonary disorders. Examples are beclomethasone (Beclovent), budesonide (Pulmicort), and triamcinolone (Azmacort). The side effects of inhaled corticosteroids are a major problem for the elderly patient. Long-term use can result in cataracts (clouding of the lens in one or both eyes); high blood sugar, which can trigger or worsen diabetes and increase the risk of infections; and osteoporosis (thinning bones) and fractures. All of these side effects are problems that the elderly patient may already be experiencing. Oral corticosteroids can cause glaucoma (elevated pressure in the eyes); fluid retention in the lower legs; high blood pressure; problems with mood, memory, behavior, thin skin, and bruising and delayed wound healing; and weight gain. The risks of using these medications in the elderly must be balanced with the benefits. Is it worth it to give them a medication that may increase their chronic problems? They may already be taking medications to lower their blood pressure.

3. Infectious Diseases

Finally, the elderly are at an increased risk for infectious diseases as the immune function (structures and processes to protect against disease and infection) is reduced. Infection is the major cause of death in 40% of those over 65 years of age. It is also a major cause of morbidity (disease) in older adults. Infections make underlying illness worse and often lead to hospitalization. Older adults may not have the same signs and symptoms of infection. Fever may be absent in 30–50% of older patients. Drug distribution, metabolism, excretion, and interactions may be changed with age. Decreased renal function (kidneys) in the aged may require a reduction in antibiotic dose (see Chapter 2). Also, drug interactions occur with many medications commonly prescribed for elderly patients, such as digoxin, warfarin, oral hypoglycemic (antidiabetic) agents, theophylline, antacids, lipid-lowering agents, antihypertensive medications (high blood pressure), and H2-receptor antagonists (which block histamine in the stomach) such as cimetidine, ranitidine, or famotidine. Treating an elderly patient with antibiotics can be a very risky process. A nurse needs to be very aware of these interactions and should check on the interactions of any medications that the patient is taking before giving them.

Summary

Managing medications for elderly patients is complicated and requires careful attention to the changes that occur in the body with aging. Older patients need to be educated about all medications that they are taking and advised not to add OTC drugs without talking to a healthcare provider about the risks and benefits. They must also be educated about the side effects of all medications. Written instructions in clear and understandable language should be offered. It is important to use a feedback method when teaching patients about their medications. Ask them to list the medications that they are currently taking and understand why they are taking them. Help them update the list regularly, and remove the medications that have been discontinued. Nurses need to be vigilant advocates for the elderly and understand the effects of aging.

QUIZ

1. **Polypharmacy is common among elderly patients.**

   (a) True

   (b) False

2. **Heredity can be a factor in living a long life.**

   (a) True

   (b) False

3. **Xerosis is a life-threatening disorder of the elderly.**

   (a) True

   (b) False

4. **Zostavax is an immunization used for herpes zoster.**

   (a) True

   (b) False

5. **Decreased renal function can be a major concern in elderly patients who are taking many medications.**

   (a) True

   (b) False

Final Exam

1. A patient who requires a higher dose to achieve the same therapeutic effect is said to
   (a) be cured.
   (b) be addicted to the drug.
   (c) have developed a tolerance to the drug.
   (d) be none of the above.

2. A patient who is allergic to shellfish is not likely to be allergic to some medications.
   (a) True
   (b) False

3. What type of injection is used to prevent medication from leaking back onto the tissue?
   (a) IM
   (b) Z-track
   (c) SC
   (d) None of the above

4. Order: 1000 mL of IV fluid q12h. Available: 1000 mL of IV fluid and microdrip tubing. At a rate of how many drops (gtt) per minute will the nurse regulate the IV?

   (a) 83 gtt/min

   (b) 83.3 gtt/min

   (c) 8.33 gtt/min

   (d) 0.833 gtt/min

5. Peppermint may relieve migraine headaches when rubbed on the forehead.

   (a) True

   (b) False

6. Water-soluble vitamins are excreted in urine shortly after they are absorbed.

   (a) True

   (b) False

7. Blenderized enteral feedings are

   (a) lactose-free liquid.

   (b) powdered mixed with milk.

   (c) liquids that are individually prepared according to the nutritional needs of the patient.

   (d) powered mixed with water.

8. When administered enteral feedings, the patient may become dizzy if

   (a) large amounts of solution are administered rapidly.

   (b) the solution is too concentrated.

   (c) the patient is supine (lying flat on her/his back).

   (d) none of the above.

9. Which of the following medications prevents the formation of blood clots?

   (a) Analgesic

   (b) Antipyretic

   (c) Anticoagulant

   (d) All of the above

10. An infant does not receive a full dose of the drug given to its mother when it is breastfeeding.

   (a) True

   (b) False

11. The desired action of a medication is called its

    (a) medication reaction.

    (b) safety action.

    (c) addictive action.

    (d) therapeutic effect.

12. What may be given to a patient prior to administering bad-tasting medication?

    (a) Nothing

    (b) Water

    (c) Ice chips

    (d) None of the above

13. When installing drops in a 7-year-old child, the nurse should pull the child's earlobe

    (a) downward and back.

    (b) upward and back.

    (c) upward and forward.

    (d) downward and forward.

14. A patient reports taking herbal medications and complains of having palpitations. The nurse suspects that the patient may be taking which herb?

    (a) Ma huang

    (b) Comfrey

    (c) Chamomile

    (d) Ginkgo biloba

15. Vitamin K is the antidote for Coumadin.

    (a) True

    (b) False

16. Which of the following is not a sign of inflammation?

    (a) Redness

    (b) Warmth

    (c) Headache

    (d) Swelling

17. All antibiotics kill all bacteria.

    (a) True

    (b) False

18. A runny nose is not caused by nasal congestion.

    (a) True
    (b) False

19. A correct dose of medication for a pediatric patient is determined by the patient's

    (a) weight.
    (b) height.
    (c) age.
    (d) sex.

20. An undesired outcome of a medication is called

    (a) an emergency.
    (b) a risk factor.
    (c) an adverse reaction to a medication.
    (d) a side effect to a medication.

21. Order: 1000 mL D$_5$W q8h. Using tubing that delivers 15 gtt/mL, the nurse will regulate the IV to _____ gtt/min?

    (a) 31 gtt/min
    (b) 31.25 gtt/min
    (c) 310 gtt/min
    (d) 10 gtt/min

22. What vitamin is acquired through sunlight?

    (a) Vitamin A
    (b) Vitamin E
    (c) Vitamin D
    (d) Vitamin C

23. A serum potassium level higher than normal is called

    (a) hyperkalemia.
    (b) hypokalemia.
    (c) hypernatremia.
    (d) none of the above.

24. Potassium is not necessary for conduction of nerve impulses.

    (a) True
    (b) False

25. **Blood in the pleural cavity is called**

    (a) pneumothorax.

    (b) hemothorax.

    (c) hydrothorax.

    (d) all of the above.

26. **A healthy, well-nourished person has a nutritional level to last 4 days before beginning to show signs of malnutrition.**

    (a) True

    (b) False

27. **Antibiotics may fight bacteria by**

    (a) inhibiting the ability to make protein, called protein synthesis.

    (b) inhibiting the growth of a cell wall.

    (c) disrupting or altering the permeability of the membrane.

    (d) all the above.

28. **What triggers respiration in a patient who has emphysema?**

    (a) A decrease in CO_2

    (b) A decrease in O_2

    (c) An increase in O_2

    (d) An increase in CO_2

29. **Naloxone (Narcan) is the antidote to an overdose of opioid narcotics.**

    (a) True

    (b) False

30. **When administering a vaccination, which of the following should you have on hand?**

    (a) Immune globulin

    (b) Whole blood

    (c) Plasma

    (d) Epinephrine

31. **A malfunctioning of the esophageal sphincter causes**

    (a) dizziness.

    (b) GERD.

    (c) rickets.

    (d) none of the above.

32. How many doses of nitroglycerin should a patient take for an angina attack?

   (a) 3

   (b) 5

   (c) 1

   (d) None

33. Thiazides should not be used with patients who have renal insufficiency.

   (a) True

   (b) False

34. The nurse should not massage the site after giving a heparin injection.

   (a) True

   (b) False

35. Order: Duricef 0.4g. On hand: Duricef 200-mg capsules. How many capsules should the nurse give?

   (a) 1 capsule

   (b) 2 capsules

   (c) 5 capsules

   (d) 20 capsules

36. Comfrey causes swelling associated with abrasions and sprains.

   (a) True

   (b) False

37. Electrolytes are found in

   (a) intracellular fluid.

   (b) interstitial fluid.

   (c) intravascular fluid.

   (d) all of the above.

38. A pain diary may be helpful for

   (a) HIV patients.

   (b) patients whose pain has been relieved.

   (c) patients who expect to be in pain.

   (d) patients who are in chronic pain.

39. A newborn whose mother is HIV-positive should be treated for HIV unless the newborn shows signs and symptoms of HIV.

   (a) True

   (b) False

40. **A patient's condition after medication is administered is compared to**
    (a) baseline patient data.
    (b) drug manufacturer's statistics.
    (c) the conditions of other patients who have received the same medication.
    (d) statistics provided by the hospital.

41. **The nurse should pinch the patient's skin when giving an insulin injection.**
    (a) True
    (b) False

42. **Herbal therapies**
    (a) do not require FDA approval.
    (b) are safe to self-medicate as long as the patient is undergoing conventional therapy.
    (c) require a prescription from a specially certified physician.
    (d) are none of the above.

43. **The ingredient in a drug that gives it shape is called**
    (a) filler.
    (b) excipient.
    (c) D-active.
    (d) particle.

44. **All drugs are not absorbed immediately when they are administered.**
    (a) True
    (b) False

45. **A patient demonstrates the ability to self-medicate by**
    (a) explaining the film on self-medication.
    (b) explaining to the patient's family how to medicate.
    (c) knowing the name of the medication.
    (d) showing the nurse how to self-medicate.

46. **Using a prescribed pain management routine**
    (a) helps prevent a patient from becoming dependent on a drug.
    (b) helps the patient afford the medication.
    (c) increases the risk of becoming drug-dependent.
    (d) is most likely to give the patient pain relief.

47. **What can inadvertently cause a patient to receive an insufficient dose of a medication?**
    (a) Genetic substitution of a brand medication
    (b) Allergies
    (c) Obesity
    (d) Underweight

48. **Ordered: 1 L of normal saline (NS) q7h. Available: 1 L of NS and IV tubing with a drip factor of 10. You would regulate the IV at 24 gtt/min.**
    (a) True
    (b) False

49. **Potassium levels are higher intracellularly than extracellularly.**
    (a) True
    (b) False

50. **NNRTs arrest the progression of rheumatoid arthritis.**
    (a) True
    (b) False

51. **Superinfection is**
    (a) an infection that spreads to more than one organ.
    (b) infection caused by a bacterium that has become resistant to antibiotics.
    (c) a hospital-acquired infection.
    (d) none of the above.

52. **Rhinitis is**
    (a) nose surgery.
    (b) insertion of an nasogastric (NG) tube.
    (c) a sinus infection.
    (d) a common cold.

53. **Patients with emphysema lack the**
    (a) trypsin protein.
    (b) β_1-antitrypsin protein
    (c) α_1-antitrypsin protein
    (d) trypsin-7 protein

54. **Smooth muscles are stimulated by**
    (a) muscarinic receptors.
    (b) antimuscarinic receptors.
    (c) barrel receptors.
    (d) all of the above.

55. Nonpharmacological pain relief treatments are based on the

   (a) pain oppression theory.
   (b) pain suppression theory.
   (c) brain suppression theory.
   (d) gate control theory.

56. Cell-mediated immunity uses T leukocytes referred to as *natural-killer cells.*

   (a) True
   (b) False

57. Parietal cells produce

   (a) hydrochloric acid in the gallbladder.
   (b) hydrochloric acid in the liver.
   (c) hydrochloric acid in the stomach.
   (d) none of the above.

58. Many diuretics cause loss of

   (a) potassium.
   (b) magnesium.
   (c) bicarbonate.
   (d) all of the above.

59. IM glucocorticoids resin is used to remove venereal warts.

   (a) True
   (b) False

60. Graves' disease is caused by an

   (a) overactive thyroid gland.
   (b) underactive thyroid gland.
   (c) overactive parathyroid gland.
   (d) underactive parathyroid gland.

61. HIV is transmitted via

   (a) injection of infected blood or blood products.
   (b) sexual contact.
   (c) maternal-fetal transmission.
   (d) all of the above.

62. Music cannot help relieve pain.

   (a) True
   (b) False

63. Pain occurring from skeletal muscles, fascia, ligaments, vessels, and joints is called

    (a) neuropathic pain.

    (b) visceral pain.

    (c) chronic pain.

    (d) none of the above.

64. Antibiotics fight off viruses.

    (a) True

    (b) False

65. Calcium is not necessary for conduction of nerve impulses.

    (a) True

    (b) False

66. Ordered: Ceclor (cefaclor) 2 mg/kg for a child who weighs 20 lb. Available: Ceclor 20 mg/2 mL. You would administer 1.8 mL.

    (a) True

    (b) False

67. A piggyback infusion is connected to

    (a) the IV tubing.

    (b) the patient's arm.

    (c) the patient's leg.

    (d) none of the above.

68. A nurse may administer medication to a patient who is prepared by another licensed practitioner.

    (a) True

    (b) False

69. St. John's wort has action similar to that of

    (a) sage.

    (b) Prozac.

    (c) psyllium.

    (d) kava kava.

70. What vitamin is given to help alleviate symptoms of neuritis caused by isoniazid therapy for TB?

    (a) Vitamin A

    (b) Vitamin E

    (c) Vitamin D

    (d) None of the above

71. **Vitamin A may be used to treat acne.**
    (a) True
    (b) False

72. **Insulin and glucose administered parenterally**
    (a) force potassium out of the cell.
    (b) force potassium into the cell.
    (c) correct the acidosis balance.
    (d) do none of the above.

73. **It is dangerous to suddenly interrupt parenteral nutrition therapy.**
    (a) True
    (b) False

74. **Which of the following symptoms are possible side effects of an antibiotic?**
    (a) Rash
    (b) Fever
    (c) Hives and itching
    (d) All of the above

75. **The saddle block is never used during childbirth.**
    (a) True
    (b) False

76. **The HIV virus enters the cell through the CD4 molecule on the cell surface.**
    (a) True
    (b) False

77. **Prolonged exposure to a drug decreases the excretion of the drug from the body.**
    (a) True
    (b) False

78. **If a medication order is unclear, the nurse should**
    (a) ask a colleague to explain it.
    (b) review it with the patient.
    (c) ask the prescriber to clarify the order.
    (d) try to figure it out.

79. A pregnant patient tells the nurse that she is taking gingko to keep her mind sharp. The nurse's best response would be

    (a) "That's fine. It should help."
    (b) "Take it in small doses."
    (c) "You should not take any herbal therapies while you are pregnant."
    (d) "Check the label carefully before you take it."

80. Monomeric is a very expensive enteral solution.

    (a) True
    (b) False

81. During what phase of the inflammation response do the red blood cells infiltrate the injured tissue?

    (a) Anti-inflammatory phase
    (b) Vascular phase
    (c) Delayed phase
    (d) None of the above

82. Ringing in the ear can be a side effect of salicylates.

    (a) True
    (b) False

83. What chemical mediators bring about the inflammatory response by causing vasodilatation, smooth-muscle relaxation, capillary permeability, and sensitized nerve cells within the affected area to pain?

    (a) PCN
    (b) Sulfonamides
    (c) Prostaglandin inhibitors
    (d) Prostaglandins

84. Compliance is

    (a) the ability of the lungs to be contracted.
    (b) the ability of the lungs to be distended.
    (c) the ability of the lungs to exchange gases.
    (d) all of the above.

85. β-adrenergic blockers

    (a) decrease blood pressure.
    (b) decrease heart rate.
    (c) cause bronchoconstriction.
    (d) do all of the above.

86. Chamomile can be taken by a patient who is allergic to ragweed.

    (a) True
    (b) False

87. Valerian has a therapeutic effect similar to that of

    (a) ginseng.
    (b) zingiber.
    (c) Benadryl.
    (d) none of the above.

88. The concentration of a hypotonic intravenous solution does not have the same concentration as intracellular fluid.

    (a) True
    (b) False

89. The nurse should instruct the patient to monitor for adverse side effects of herbal therapies.

    (a) True
    (b) False

90. If the patient cannot absorb oral medication ordered by the provider, the nurse should

    (a) use a rectal suppository.
    (b) postpone administering medication.
    (c) insert a GI tube.
    (d) call the physician.

91. What can be used to relieve swelling associated with abrasions and sprains?

    (a) Ginseng
    (b) Comfrey
    (c) Zingiber
    (d) Valerian

92. A good source of dietary potassium is

    (a) bread.
    (b) milk.
    (c) eggs.
    (d) bananas.

93. Spinach is a source of iron.

    (a) True
    (b) False

94. A drug that causes a nonspecific physiological response is called

    (a) an agonist.

    (b) a metabolite.

    (c) a protein.

    (d) a molecule.

95. A medical diagnosis

    (a) is the same as a nursing diagnosis.

    (b) identifies the patient's disease or medical condition.

    (c) is a problem statement that identifies the potential or actual health problem.

    (d) none of the above.

96. A patient undergoing withdrawal from hashish can be treated by

    (a) administering a lower dose of hashish.

    (b) administering a sedative.

    (c) doing nothing.

    (d) prescribing exercise.

97. Healthcare providers never use drugs for recreational purposes.

    (a) True

    (b) False

98. If the dose of a transdermal patch is more than the prescriber's medication order,

    (a) cut the patch to an appropriate length.

    (b) contact the prescriber.

    (c) do nothing.

    (d) apply the patch anyway.

99. The nursing process is a circular process.

    (a) True

    (b) False

100. Commonly used medications for relieving headaches are aspirin, acetaminophen, and ibuprofen.

    (a) True

    (b) False

Answers to Quiz and Final Exam Questions

Chapter 1

1. b	2. b	3. d	4. b	5. b
6. d	7. b	8. c	9. b	10. a

Chapter 2

1. b	2. c	3. c	4. b	5. a
6. d	7. b	8. a	9. b	10. a

Chapter 3

1. b	2. b	3. d	4. b	5. b
6. a	7. a	8. d	9. a	10. b

Chapter 4

1. c	2. d	3. c	4. b	5. a
6. a	7. a	8. a	9. a	10. a

Chapter 5

1. c	2. c	3. a	4. b	5. a
6. c	7. b	8. b	9. a	10. b

Chapter 6

1. c	2. b	3. a	4. a	5. a
6. a	7. b	8. a	9. b	10. a

Chapter 7

1. b	2. d	3. a	4. a	5. a
6. c	7. a	8. b	9. b	10. a

Chapter 8

1. d	2. b	3. d	4. a	5. b
6. c	7. b	8. c	9. a	10. a

Chapter 9

1. b	2. c	3. b	4. a	5. a
6. a	7. b	8. d	9. b	10. a

Chapter 10

1. b	2. b	3. d	4. a	5. b
6. c	7. a	8. b	9. a	10. a

Chapter 11

1. b	2. b	3. a	4. b	5. a
6. d	7. a	8. d	9. a	10. a

Chapter 12

1. c	2. c	3. a	4. a	5. a
6. b	7. a	8. d	9. b	10. a

Chapter 13

1. b	2. a	3. d	4. b	5. a
6. d	7. b	8. d	9. a	10. a

Chapter 14

1. b   2. b   3. c   4. a   5. a
6. c   7. a   8. c   9. a   10. a

Chapter 15

1. b   2. a   3. a   4. a   5. a
6. d   7. a   8. b   9. a   10. a

Chapter 16

1. a   2. d   3. d   4. a   5. a
6. d   7. a   8. b   9. a   10. a

Chapter 17

1. c   2. a   3. d   4. a   5. a
6. c   7. b   8. d   9. b   10. a

Chapter 18

1. b   2. d   3. c   4. a   5. a
6. c   7. a   8. b   9. b   10. a

Chapter 19

1. d   2. b   3. a   4. a   5. a
6. d   7. a   8. a   9. a   10. a

Chapter 20

1. d   2. a   3. c   4. a   5. a
6. c   7. b   8. a   9. a   10. b

Chapter 21

1. d   2. a   3. a   4. a   5. a
6. a   7. a   8. c   9. a   10. b

Chapter 22

1. b   2. c   3. d   4. a   5. a
6. d   7. a   8. d   9. a   10. a

Chapter 23

1. a   2. a   3. b   4. a   5. a

FINAL EXAM

1. c	2. b	3. b	4. a	5. b
6. a	7. c	8. a	9. c	10. a
11. d	12. c	13. b	14. a	15. a
16. c	17. b	18. b	19. a	20. c
21. a	22. c	23. a	24. b	25. b
26. b	27. d	28. a	29. a	30. d
31. b	32. a	33. a	34. a	35. b
36. b	37. d	38. d	39. a	40. a
41. a	42. a	43. a	44. a	45. d
46. d	47. c	48. a	49. a	50. a
51. b	52. d	53. c	54. a	55. d
56. a	57. c	58. d	59. b	60. a
61. d	62. b	63. d	64. b	65. b
66. a	67. a	68. b	69. b	70. d
71. a	72. b	73. a	74. d	75. b
76. a	77. b	78. c	79. c	80. a
81. d	82. a	83. d	84. b	85. d
86. b	87. c	88. a	89. a	90. d
91. b	92. b	93. a	94. a	95. b
96. d	97. b	98. b	99. a	100. a

Appendix

Drug-Specific Tables

Chapter 16: Narcotic Agonists

Non-Narcotic Analgesic
Narcotic Agonist-Opiate Analgesic
Opioid Agonist
Narcotic Agonist-Antagonists

Chapter 17: Immunologic Agents

Integrase Inhibitors (INSTIs)
Chemokine Receptor Antagonists (CCR5 Antagonists)
Pharmacokinetic Enhancers
Combination HIV Medicines

Chapter 18: Gastrointestinal System

Anticholinergic
Serotonin Antagonist
Antihistamine
Antidiarrheals
GI Stimulant-Laxative
GI Osmotic: Laxative/Antacid, Anticonvulsant, Electrolyte
Proton Pump Inhibitor (PPIs)
Antiulcers: Histamine$_2$ Blocker

Chapter 19: Cardiac Circulatory Medications

Cardiac Glycoside
Nitrates
Calcium Channel Blocker
Fast (Sodium) Channel Blocker I
Direct-Acting Arteriolar Vasodilators
ACE Inhibitors
Thiazide Diuretic
Loop Diuretic
Carbonic Anhydrase Inhibitors
Potassium-Sparing Diuretic
Anticoagulant Low Molecular Weight
Thrombolytic
Antihyperlipemic HMG-CoA Reductase Inhibitor
Vasodilator

Chapter 20:   Skin Disorders

Acne Vulgaris (Systemic Preparation)
Antipsoriatic
Antiinfective

Chapter 21:   Endocrine Medications

Anterior Pituitary Hormone
Posterior Pituitary Hormone
Hypothyroidism
Hyperthyroidism
Antidiabetic Drugs
Antidiabetic: Second Generation Sulfonylurea

Chapter 22:   Disorders of the Eye and Ear

Direct-Acting Miotic (Cholinergics)
Osmotic (Osmotic Diuretic, Antiglaucoma, Antihemolytic)

Chapter 23:   Geriatric Considerations

Normal Aging Versus Pathology
Pulmonary Disorders
Infectious Diseases

Index

Page numbers followed by *f* denote figures; those followed by *t* denote tables.

CPSIA information can be obtained
at www.ICGtesting.com
Printed in the USA
LVHW061930080119
603173LV00006B/42/P

9 781259 862595